A WEALTH OF HEALTH

SELF-HEALING, UNIVERSAL THERAPIES FOR PAIN, STRESS AND INSOMNIA

USE CHINESE MEDICINE FOR A HEALTHY & HAPPY LIFE

BY FRIEDA MAH,

L.Ac., NGH C.I., Dream Builder Coach, Life Mastery Consultant, Energy Healer

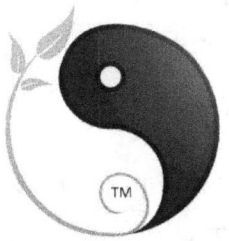

Universal Acupuncture and TCM Corp
Cerritos, CA 90703, USA

A WEALTH OF HEALTH

SELF-HEALING, UNIVERSAL THERAPIES FOR PAIN, STRESS AND INSOMNIA

Author: Frieda Mah

© 2015 Universal Acupuncture and TCM Corp,
Cerritos, CA 90703, USA

Printed by
Best Seller Publishing
1346 Walnut St. #205
Pasadena, CA 91106

Phone: (626) 765-9750
Fax: (561) 828-8180

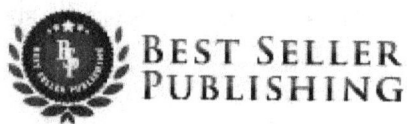
BEST SELLER
PUBLISHING

ISBN-13: 978-1517705084
ISBN-10:1517705088
Library Congress Control number: 2015916689

Learn more informationrmation at:
UniversalEnergyHealing.us Please register Reader's Membership to join readers' discussion and move your knowledge further.

FB: Comprehensive Universal Energy Healing - CHUEH

RICH

&

MEANINGFUL

LIFE

ENJOY ABUNDANCES

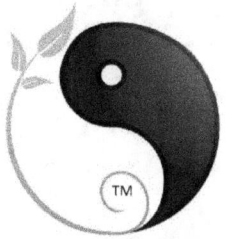

UNIVERSAL ACUPUNCTURE AND TCM CORP.

This is our company's book series to unblock your body, mind, and soul so that you can carry out your life's mission. Meanwhile, enjoy the Universal Abundance.

This is a gift from Frieda's heart as well as from the universe, divine love, and ancestors' wisdom.

THIS BOOK IS PRESENTED TO

FROM:

DATE:

Contents
• • • • • • • • • • • •

CHAPTER FOUR

CHAPTER FIVE

CHAPTER EIGHT

Preface
• • • • • • • • •

I knew Ms. Frieda Mah when I attended the Fourth International Conference of Chinese Medicine and Acupuncture in Los Angeles in July 1992. Pursuit of the cause, a love of life, professional dedication, and sincerity to her friends is a true portrayal of Ms. Frieda. Through Ms. Frieda, I saw many Chinese women living in the United States with a strong, simple, and diligent style.

Ms. Frieda's father was a native of Jinan City, Shandong Province, China. But she was born in Taiwan.

In June 1972, she graduated from the Department of Industrial Engineering at Chung Yuan Christian University in Chung Li City, Taiwan. When I first met her, she was a middle-aged woman with four boys.

Through Frieda's rich life experiences and practices, she has generated great interest in Traditional Chinese Medicine (TCM). She threw herself into the study of TCM, and after more than ten years of hard work and practice, she earned her Master's degree in Acupuncture and Oriental Medicine from Southern California University of Health Sciences in Whittier, California. Soon after, she obtained her California acupuncturist license.

When Ms. Frieda studied at Southern California University of Health Sciences, she was the Dean's assistant. She managed the school's clinic pharmacy and drafted TCM public education manuals. In 2005, she earned the Hua Tuo Award, was on the Dean's List, and achieved the award for Outstanding Proficiency in Clinical Practice. From April 2006 to September 2007, she participated in the South Baylo University's doctoral program.

After graduation, Ms. Frieda worked at sea on international cruise ships for a couple of years. Then, in Southern California, she established Freda Mah, L.Ac. Clinic, Universe Acupuncture, and

TCM Corp. While studying of TCM, Ms. Frieda became familiar with many fundamental, classic TCM books that taught how to combine modern technology with Traditional Chinese Medicine to diagnose and treat disease. She turned many patients' lives around. In clinical practice, Ms. Frieda employs different modalities to enhance her treatment's effectiveness. She earned the National Guild of Hypnotists' (NGH) hypnotherapist and instructor certificate and was a presenter at the NGH August 2014 international convention.

Ms. Frieda is skilled at combining integrated Traditional Chinese Medicine with modern thoughts, psychology, and the notion of longevity. She created the "Comprehensive Universal Energy Healing" method that could be applied to many medical arenas—especially those dealing with pain, stress, and insomnia—and achieve effective treatment results. These are covered in her first book.

After six months of working hard both day and night—equivalent to nearly twenty months' of normal working hours— and referring to more than a hundred references as she practiced Comprehensive Universal Energy Healing applications, she was finally ready to share her method with readers. In June 2014, Ms. Frieda held her first Comprehensive Universal Energy Healing continuing education class at South Baylo University in Anaheim, California (sponsored by SBUEAA—South Baylo University English Program Alumni Association).

Although clinical trials should be done to extend the applications of Comprehensive Universal Energy Healing, the author's dedication and tireless pursuit of TCM professional development and health care improvement is worthy of praise and admiration.

Ms. Frieda's professional goals are lofty. She wants "to be a medical therapy innovator to raise everyone's life quality and prevent sickness" and to "purify everyone's great self to carry out his/her life's mission." Before her first book about Comprehensive Universal Energy Healing of *Your Health Guard, Self-Help for Pain, Stress & Insomnia* was published, Ms. Frieda asked me to write the preface. In fact, I do not deserve to talk about any more than my personal experiences with her. But I will share my medical career's motto:

"Be diligent in pursuing previous discoveries, but do not be limited. Broadly collect formulas and subtract all meaningful essence. Correctly diagnose and treat with accurate prescriptions. Deeply achieve TCM's true meaning."

Chief Physician and Professor Ma, Sheng 2014 Summer at Qing Zhou City, Shandong Province, China

Acknowledgments

Without the following people's involvement, there would have been no way to get this book published. Here, I give them my deepest and most sincere expression of gratitude for their help!

1. Without Stephanie Kimber, L.Ac. and Dan Brown, L.Ac., who hired me to work at sea, I would have never had the chance to learn that the ethnic factor in recovery from sickness is so important. Ms. Kimber and Mr. Brown are pioneers in bringing acupuncture to the sea and helping TCM spread quickly throughout the world. They are the heroes in TCM world history. I am forever grateful for the chance they gave me to grow my acupuncture skills by encouraging my independent thinking and stressing that I always keep the highest standard for my practice.

2. My classmate and one of my best friends—Catherine Lu, L.Ac.—who told me to attend longevitology entry and intermediate level classes. If I hadn't, I might not have had the chance to access the beauty of cosmic energy healing power so early on in my career.

3. Ms. Lin, Zi-Zen who taught us the longevitology we needed in order to use cosmic energy to do healing. Lin, Zi-Hong, L.Ac. and his wife, who helped us to open acupuncture points that are mainly on the governor (Du) *meridian* along the spine.

4. Ms. Stephanie Guiles, Reiki therapist (Reiki therapy is another school of cosmic energy therapy) and also my longevitology classmate, who told me that when she was a child, she used her hands to heal injured animals. It made me notice that my sons, one of my best friends, Ms. Ann Liu, and many other kind people who always help others have cosmic energy naturally in their hands. It led me to discover that we are born with natural healing power! My later chats with many other energy healers in many network events confirmed my conclusion. It was also validated

that my patients can learn from me how to use this healing energy that exists in their hands.

5. I bestow a huge gratitude on my clinical training instructor, Dr. Ni, Hai-Sha, L.Ac. (1954-2012). He taught us Da Zhou Tian[152] and shared his genius in Traditional Chinese Medicine diagnosis and powerful herbal treatments for tough cases. His Da Zhou Tian[152] and diagnoses contributed a lot to this book.

6. During our clinical training at Ni's Acupuncture Center, Merritt Island, Florida in 2010, my classmate Dr. Yang (who was for twenty-three years an MD but after learning Traditional Chinese Medicine started practicing TCM) corrected my Da Zhou Tian[152] practices. In addition, Dr. Yang and Dr. Ma, Sheng did a peer review of my website articles at universaltcm.com. Partial contents from the website are used in this book.

7. My medical school instructor, Dr. Wendy Chen (Wendy Chen, L.Ac., but Doctor was the term of respect for instructors in our medical school), used her pure Chinese medicine practitioner and regular reader's eyesight to do a proofreading of the Chinese book. Also, a classmate in Merritt Island, FL, Mr. Yan Xue, reviewed the Chinese book from the angle of a pharmacist and an active medical therapy explorer.

Dr. Wayne Cheng, who is the DAOM Program Director of The South Baylo University in Anaheim, California proofread my English book. Ms. Judy Stepp—my soul sister and an experienced dream builder coach—also did proofreading and edited a page of my book.

The above serves as peer review for my book.

Ms. Merle Shao, my college roommate had many valuable recommendations from both a writer and a reader's review to criticize my book contents to let me rewrite my manuscript before it submitted to the publisher.

Ms. Lori did a decent job to point out none TCM professionals' questions about my book and allowed me to add more explanations to make the book be more readable for my readers.

Moreover, I am so happy and grateful for Ms. Lori's good question about the 12 strands DNA, which led me a week online research. The excited harvest is that there are more scientific discoveries to be found and explained why the morals and spirits work for healing, enjoying abundance, helps us following the earth orbit moving to a higher dimensional space to communicate with higher dimensional creatures. It also scientifically supports my "Fig 2 Health Relationship for Body, Subconscious and Super-conscious" in Chapter Two.

Ms. Miao Li, the president of Visual Planet Inc., helped me hand-draw acupuncture figures.

I appreciate their dedicated input and priceless recommendations. They eased my mind.

8. Thanks to everyone who wrote testimonials or posted on my websites to bolster potential readers' confidence to practice what they learn from the book. These individuals shared their experiences and the results they attained from Comprehensive Universal Energy Healing. For their unselfishness and willingness to share, I give them the highest respect and appreciation. They have done a good deed to benefit others.

9. I am so lucky that my second son, Michael Chang, bought me a powerful computer on which to write the book. My youngest son, Ted Chang, checks my computer to be sure it functions well.

10. My gratefulness also extends to our loyal dog. No matter how early in the morning or late night, he lies beside my feet and keeps me company. He doesn't allow me to feel lonely while I'm writing. As he sleeps, dreaming his sweet dreams, he lets me think that if this book can help readers and their loved ones sleep soundly, it is worth it for me to have "time out" all day long in front of a computer.

11. I am also grateful that Dr. Ma, Shen wrote the preface for me. He sparked my interest in Chinese medicine when he visited us from China in 1992 and used ear seeds to treat my son. Later, when I practiced on land, we exchanged Chinese medical knowledge and clinical practices from Friday night until China time's midnight.

He always encouraged me to keep moving forward, even in my worst financial years. He pushed me and encouraged me not to give up on my efforts in Chinese medicine and to keep advancing my knowledge and skills.

Dr. Ma was the former President of the Qingzhou Hospital of TCM, Shandong Province, China and the former Chief Executive Officer and currently Chief TCM Physician of Yidu Central Hospital, Weifang, Shandong Province, China. He has made a significant contribution in TCM and to all of his jobs.

More gratitude for my parents who gave me life and encouraged me to write the book. My father and my grandmother on my mother's side are my role models for overcoming life's difficulties.

I am also grateful for my third brother and his wife. They take care of our parents and free the other brothers and sisters to concentrate on our own lives. They never claim credit for taking care of my parents and do not want to be acknowledged in any way. They silently bear the tough job of taking care of them and carry all of the financial burdens. They represent each family's obedient son and daughter-in-law who sacrifice themselves to free the others. Their behavior and spirit is worthy of endless admiration! This book has been baked in the oven of love, gratitude, sharing, and collaboration. It tastes sweet, and I am happy to share it with you!

Frieda Mah, L.Ac., NGH C. Ht, C.I., Energy Healer, Dream Builder Coach and Life Mastery Consultant, January 2014 (year of the horse) writes at Los Angeles, USA

Foreword

●●●●●●●●●●●●●●

I have a pearl. For a long time, it is covered by dust and tiredness. Now, the dust is gone, and it shines lights. It lights up all over the mountains, rivers, and clouds.

Song Dynasty• Cha, Ling Yu Monk

In 2010, I moved my licensed acupuncture practice from cruise ships to dry land. I had been dealing with happy and positively thinking patients at sea. But back on land, I faced severely ill patients—patient on kidney dialysis, young patient with cancer in its terminal stage, cancer migrant patients, medically mistreated patients, patients with heart problems. I felt their pain. I don't think anyone should have to endure this kind suffering. What was the solution to prevent it?

Moreover, there are some people who are always healthy and even more people with pain or illness only because they cannot find a solution—even from health professionals. I figured that every person possessed strong self-healing power. But how could I help individuals find their way back to health through self-healing?

Aside from health concerns, I also saw so many people trapped in their current situations and feeling helpless. Everyone is supposed to be born in abundance with the ability to create a meaningful and healthy life. But a lot of people have discontent and/or belonging problems that stops them from enjoying a satisfying life. Something is missing—somewhere, there is a shortage in their life. How could I help people regain the wealthy life to which they were entitled?

The universe is continually changing and transferring from the four-dimensional world to be in the n-dimensional universe. The only way for people to adapt to this change is to lift their frequency so that it can easily merge into the new universe.

Still, how do we achieve all of the above? After years of research, I created the Comprehensive Universal Energy Healing, a method to transform people's concepts, mindsets, and behavior in order to link with the universe's power and wisdom and guide them away from discomfort and sickness toward an abundant life with health, relationships, vacation, time, money, and freedom.

The transformation starts by unblocking the body, changing the mindset, and purifying the soul to achieve the divine mission and a prosperous life. This book is a start.

Frieda Mah at Los Angeles, California, USA Jan 16, 2015

Introduction to the Energy Healing: Background, Concept, History, and Application Scope
• • • • • • • • • • • • • • • •

Introduction

The book has been written. This article is added at the request of Dr. Sheng Ma. To write a convincing article, I searched a lot of resources—online websites, videos, books in markets and library, dictionaries, and online academic databases.

I devoted my days and nights for two entire weeks to write, and I finished a thirteen-page masterpiece in Chinese (the current one is twenty-three pages in Chinese). But unfortunately, before I could email it to Dr. Chen for peer review, the word software encountered a problem while I was adding page numbers. All of my two weeks' efforts writing the article was lost. No matter how I tried, I could not get my work back again. It was the first event I had encountered in my life when, due to the fatigue from long hours of writing plus the confusion about why I had lost my original article in the first place, my mind went completely blank. It happened two days before a US holiday when my children came home for a reunion, so I took the opportunity to enjoy a much-needed break from the writing with my family.

But my mind continued to ask, "Could there be a reason my original article disappeared? Am I supposed to rewrite it?"

After the holidays ended, and I dropped my youngest son back off at school, I could focus on rewriting the article. And I found the reason for the rewrite. This time, I found some scientific evidence being dismissed as unfounded. I thought I could use this in my series of books, making them more reliable than ever before. I was excited, but I calmed myself and asked, "What kind of message should I send out?" The next day, there was a clear voice in my head telling me to be honest and tell what I know!

While writing the book, two very close friends—trying to protect me—told me that in order to encourage even skeptical readers to read this book, I must not mention things that are not scientifically defined. And so I had revised it to be very conservative and had therefore deleted many powerful methods—that could save lives in an emergency—simply because are not listed in first aid manuals.

But then there was another persistent whisper in my head: that said, "On the cruise ship, you convinced so many skeptics to accept that acupuncture can treat diseases. So why have you not gone further and pointed out the truth existing in the universe?" The concept of purifying the great self to live in the abundant universe is so important and divine! The voice told me that this is the era of big change, and it was my time to set a moral model and achieve glory by writing for the new world.

If you can purify your soul, health, happiness, universal abundant wisdom and enjoyment are easily achievable. This concept is very important and should be spread widely!

Therefore, the structure and content of the original lost manuscript was much different from this article. The original contents of this book have been rewritten many times, and the originally deleted part will be included in future books because it can truly save lives in critical situations. It will wait, though, until either clinical trials are run or until this series of books gains enough trust and support from readers.

In the meantime, I will also be seeking funding and collaboration to execute the clinical research necessary to substantiate the effectiveness of my emergency aids. In this regard, I hope you can give a helping hand. I would be very grateful.

To start, I should point out the following to the reader who deeply believes that *real* science is a thing that must be seen, heard, and measured.

1. **VISUAL DECEPTION.** There are many examples, please google "optical-illusions-pictures" to see if what your eyes show you is always right.

2. **HEARING CAN BE A BIAS.** The same thing heard by different people can promote different feelings and reactions. Why do these differences exist? It is because each brain accepts the same message but processes it differently depending upon a person's environment, education, and subjective opinions and preferences.

3. **TASTE AND SMELL.** Under hypnosis, people are able to eat a sour lemon and swear to others that the lemon is sweet. This means that taste can be implied and changed.

Is scientific thinking the result of undergoing long-term education and being, in a way, hypnotized? A Harvard University Study found that under the age of two, ninety-eight percent of the population could be classified as genius. But after being "educated" until the age of twenty, those qualifying for the label of gifted was only two to three percent. Isn't that interesting? It's no wonder that many parents would rather "homeschool" their kids. And there are many examples of children who, when allowed to follow and nurture their own talents and interests, achieve much more than when parents or schools interfere and force their expectations onto them.

As far as the sense of smell is concerned, there are some people who want to vomit at the smell of the durian fruit. It's impossible for them put the fruit into their mouths. Durian lovers smell it and get excited, putting the durian without hesitation into their mouths and praising its taste. So it's obvious that smell and taste are extremely subjective and they're linked.

The findings of a study reported that adding artificial odors to a sucrose solution changed people's perception of the taste[46]. The people involved in the test went in blind—not knowing about the artificial odors—and those who had experiences a different taste due to the addition left the study very opinionated and ready to debate the smell and taste of the sucrose solution with the people who did not have the odor added.

Some diseases, such as Alice in Wonderland Syndrome (AIWS)[47] or illnesses causing hallucinations can cause a change in the five senses.

4. SCIENTIFIC DISCOVERIES ARE NOT ALWAYS CORRECT.

For a long time, atoms were thought to be constructed of neutrons, electrons, and protons—they were the smallest particles. But over the last sixty years of the twentieth century, scientists have studied even smaller and more elementary particles—quarks, leptons, gauge bosons, and the Higgs particle[48].

The earth for long time had been considered to be spherical[49]. But the latest conception of the earth is not spherical at all. Instead, its shape is as NASA's pictures show it below.[50]

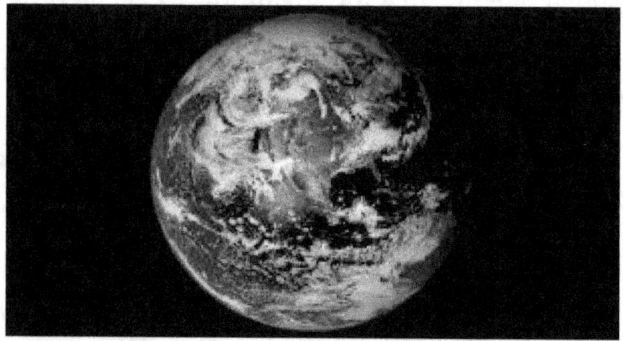

Fig ii Old Earth Shape[49]

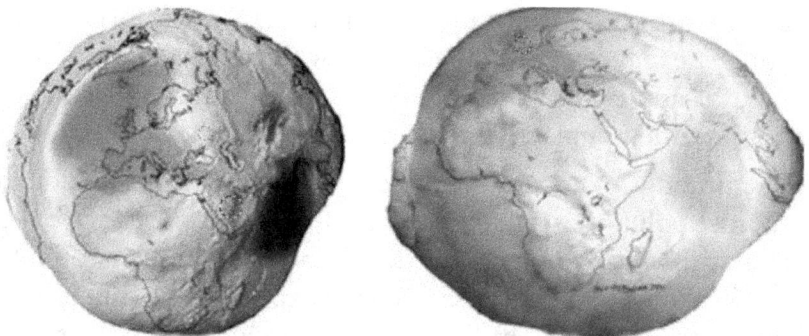

Fig iii The New Earth Shape[50]

A lot of the truth of universal existence is not found by science. The truth cannot be fully revealed because human beings' technology has not yet reached the truth-discovering stage.

It's the bias and/or lack of knowledge that causes fights, attacks, war, and innocent victims. If everyone can learn how to approach things objectively, the world will have a lot more peace, and human civilization will also be accelerated. So without decent research, excluding things that one does not believe in or denying something which is currently unknown is not the appropriate way to go about things.

It is better to take the time to think, to get more exposure, and to verify. You can respect other ideas and hypotheses while still spending time proving your own theories. That way there will be less error.

Even if you spend time studying, you may still be groping in the dark. There may yet be a gap between your understanding and the truth because you didn't spend enough time researching, accessed the wrong information, or didn't have a strong enough desire to prove for certain that your understanding is correct. People in the universe are indeed tiny, but by grace, the human mind is mighty.

Let's get down to business.

Types of Energy Healing

Some sources say that everything can promote the blood circulation or physical vigor known as energy healing. Herbs, herbal diets, health equipment (including machinery and accessories such as magnetic necklaces, bracelets, infrared waist rings, belts, and ankle rings) will not be discussed here.

In the service sector, there is a great difference in the quality of service. Some who serve don't polish themselves and cultivate their morals. But there are others who take the time to provide top-notch service. Without knowing the quality of the service, it is very inappropriate to try to get a bargain on the price.

* **Qi Gong and Breathing**

  Breathing combined with body movement to promote *qi* and blood circulation, improve bodily functions, and increase

Immunity is called qigong. Generally speaking, anyone who dedicates himself to practicing qigong is healthier and has a more youthful appearance the longer he/she cultivates the activity. It's visual—you can see the difference. Qigong is comprised of slow movements, and it can calm people and relieve their stress, making for a more serene existence.

Breathing is a science. Slow, deep breathing can quiet a brain, soothe emotions, and calm thinking. Moreover, it can lead to a stronger and better qi. It improves blood circulation which aids in eliminating body toxins and releasing unnecessary desire(s).

I have a hyperactive friend who could not be still or quiet for even a second. She asked me why, in a yoga class, the instructor had asked her to take continuous deep breaths for fifteen minutes. In her first time doing so, her brain became like a blank piece of paper. She could not remember or think about anything. This was contrary to her usual state where her brain was very active—always thinking it should be doing something.

We should make an effort to take deep breaths to provide the brain with oxygen and qi-transporting nutrients. In this way, the brain will be rejuvenated and can then make the best choices for the beneficial harmonization of the body's functions (i.e. the body's recovery work).

A study pointed out that having students sit up straight and take deep breaths allows them to concentrate, think sharper, and get top grades[90]. Another study pointed out that in emergency situations when a person is in danger, there are increased epinephrine and norepinephrine secretions into the body. They reduce the blood flow to the brain and send more blood to the muscles for use in escape. So in times of crisis, if you can first take five deep breaths to provide the brain with adequate blood supply, your brain will make its best decisions and adopt the most appropriate actions to save your life[91].

Qigong is an active therapy comparable to the exercises used by a physical therapist to help loosen and move the limbs. People's movements generate *yang qi*, and humans must have sufficient yang qi in order to be healthy and live vibrant lives.

High-end qigong requires moral cultivation. It is part of the original requirements of qigong. Unfortunately, today's population often practices only qi gong's form, which is the skill part of qigong—how to make the movements smooth and elegant and thus generate a calm mind. But the spirit of qigong is truly moral cultivation. It raises the qigong level quicker than practicing only the form. It is too often neglected by those who practice it— perhaps the master did not know of moral cultivation or did not have time to teach it.

Qigong is a tool used for longevity initiated by Laozi[67]. According to Mr. Hu Shi's presumption, Laozi was born in approximately 570 B.C.[68].

People who practice qigong can help people to heal. It depends a lot on the healer's qigong gong Fu level and the patient's condition because using qigong to heal can sometimes consume or injure a qigong master's qi.

• Meditation

When meditating, one should always take deep breaths first in order to calm the mind. (You can read more about the benefits of breathing in the previous section.) Meditation has been mentioned in ancient times and in various religions. At the start of meditation, some people cannot stop their *motor mind*, but doing deep breathing can help to break unnecessary thinking. When thinking stills, the mind will clear and act as a hanging mirror—receiving universal wisdom, connecting with the great self, and hearing the small voice of the subconscious.

Like wireless electromagnetic and video waves, there are countless thoughts and ideas running through our minds every day. According to statistics, sixty to eighty thousand ideas a day travel through our minds—how to make big money, how to start a business, how to find the best partner in personal life or business, how to achieve success, new ideas for inventions, how much we miss our parents or relatives and friends, and so on ad infinitum. Naturally, there are also bad ideas and thoughts, but it is only when the mind and our thinking are very quiet—and there is goodness and uprightness present—that we can capture the essence of these ideas.

The benefits of meditation are many. Breathing slowly and evenly without thinking can gradually clear out the blockage in the meridian, allowing the body to be open and receptive to the universal energy. It allows the body do self-repair.

You can use a search engine to search meditation on the Internet. There are many online articles describing its benefits and many videos that teach you how to meditate. You can even find meditation music which will help you eliminate stress or aid you in falling into a deep and productive sleep.

• Acupuncture and Moxibustion

Legend says that Fu Xi invented acupuncture[56]. Fu Xi lived somewhere in the middle or late Paleolithic age[65]. This dates back about 250-260 million years[66].

Acupuncture and/or **moxibustion**—along with an herbal formula used externally—can aid in expelling a body blockage (cold, wind, qi stagnation, dampness, food accumulation, sputum accumulation, blood stasis, edema, inflammation, or tumor), balancing the yin and yang to promote qi and blood circulation, improving body functions, and increasing immunity and vitality.

In the body, stone cases such as gallstone, though the stone has not been eliminated, the pain can be eliminated by soothing the Qi and blood flow. It's due to the stone being pushed into a space that does not cause pain. The small stone can be expelled out of the body.

If write words or read words' sequence in a reverse direction was due to having a severe vomiting that caused the gallbladder twisted. Traditional Chinese medicine using acupuncture or herbs can help to correct the wrong position of the twisted gallbladder by helping expand its size temporary to make it straight out.

Acupuncture and moxibustion can treat common diseases. They can also be used for preventive health care or health maintenance and to slow down or even reverse the aging process. There are many popular cosmetic treatments which use acupuncture—cosmetic rejuvenation, weight loss, and carving the body shape, to name a few. The treatments not only let patients achieve their desired younger appearance but allow the whole body be rejuvenated, organs' functions be recovered and acts younger without having to use commercial cosmetic products every day.

Treatments can also help soothe abnormal and unwanted emotions, promote the growth of damaged nerves in the right direction so that they can connect with other nerves, and treat soft tissues that are either too tight or too loose and many other benefits.

Acupuncture and moxibustion plus my unique external-use herb (see Appendix Eight) can be applied in a broader scope, as well, to include more chronic and severe cases. This will be covered in more detail in other articles in this book. Regarding how acupuncture can balance the body, please follow the link and read "How Traditional Chinese Medicine (TCM) Can Balance the Body?"[96] in Appendix Nine.

The size (length and thickness) of a needle, angle of insertion, and needle technique—as well as the therapist's moral cultivation, knowledge, and willingness to treat the patient—affect the acupuncture treatment results. The acupuncturist's knowledge, skills, diagnosis accuracy, and time/effort/mindset goes into each patient. A good acupuncturist is not only treating visible symptoms but also the root cause(s) as well as doing preventive treatments. It is very important to do more than just eliminate or control the symptoms of the disease.

Manual acupuncture treatment has more advantages than laser acupuncture treatment because of the flexibility to adjust needle length and depth according to an individual patient's needs. Acupuncturists need to be both cautious and brave when needling deeper in some body parts, but the patients do heal sooner and avoid internal disease progression. In addition, manual treatment allows the acupuncturist's qi and expectations for quick recovery to flow through the needles into the patient's body[95]. The added benefits of manual acupuncture cannot be ignored. It helps a patient recover sooner because the healer's power transmits through the needle and enters into the patient's body. There is no doubt that heart-to-heart treatment is one of the best healing tools from nature therapy provides.

The laser pen acupuncture treatment can often reduce pain quickly, and it benefits the performer who does not have an acupuncture license, but for some patients, it is only treating the immediate, lesser symptoms of the disease. The more serious symptoms tend to return rapidly, and the disease then becomes more severe. The disease has more time to proliferate, the later treatments become more troublesome, and the patient must devote additional time and money to further medical treatments.

Patients need to understand that body recovery takes time. The time the needle stays inside the body is necessary to encourage the flowing of the qi and help the body repair itself. Patients with more chronic and severe cases and those with qi or blood deficiencies or a severe blockage in the body take a longer time to treat. Repair involves not only solving the discomfort of the symptom but also fixing the remote cause. Riddance of the symptoms does not necessarily mean the patient has been completely treated. The symptoms are merely the leaves on the illness tree.

Unless we dig out the root, additional problems will grow sooner or later. The speed of recovery depends on the body's vitality, the characteristics of the illness, the method of treatment, and the characteristics of the health care provider.

For blood deficiency, if mild, can use food therapy. If severe, should use herbs to tonify.

Many people blindly seek inexpensive treatments. These cheap charge acupuncture practitioners often do shallower needling* in order to needle more patients in a shorter time period. The patient who seeks this type of medical treatment takes a personal loss. It's possible that the offending disease has already gone deep inside the body and needs to be removed by deeper needling to prevent disease development.

Dong's Acupuncture Theory is an exception.

But the acupuncturist who treats the root problem without reasonable remuneration will surely go out of business quickly. I can never understand why, when patients need to repair their car or their house, they always consider the job quality first and not the price. But when searching for a health care provider, they choose based on the lowest "bargain" price.

Because the needle used for acupuncture is itself very inexpensive, many people mistakenly believe that the treatments should be very cheap as well. This is incorrect. A famous artist and a student painter might use the same pen, pastels, or paints, but the value of their works are not comparable.

It's the same as practicing the Comprehensive Universal Energy Healing by putting hands on or nearby the client's body. It can be so simple and easy if there is no time constraint to do so. Therefore, people are easy to neglect it. By the time constrain, you out to learn more knowledge and skills.

The most value of the CHUEH is taking care the accidents without sequel hassles. You practice it daily as you pay an insurance premium daily.

But, without start to build up your treatment effectiveness now, you may hardly reach the beauty of remote taking care of your loved ones such as your parents who is far away from you by yourself alone at any time when they need your help.

An excellent acupuncturist can treat illness and prevent disease from progressing and worsening so that surgery is needed, quality of life is lost, or even life itself is extinguished. This is so much more important than a painter's painting, but it's easy to see the similarity. An expert acupuncturist can improve a patient's health and quality of life and maybe even prolong a patient's life span. So why do most patients not realize this?

Before I came to the US, I went to a famous outpatient clinic to visit a dentist to have a decayed and infected tooth pulled. An excellent anesthetist came in to numb me. I did not feel any discomfort afterward, and I was able to chat with him as usual. I asked for his information so I could refer patients to him, but he told me he'd be going to the States instead of staying in Taiwan. When I asked why, he said that excellent skill is not enough in Taiwan. He didn't chat with patients or cheer them up, and his performance evaluations were bad as a result. That made him decide to move to the US.

When the dentist pulled out my tooth, I felt no pain. I also did not feel the numbness I'd experienced in other dentists' offices. I don't know where that anesthesiologist is now, but I often wonder if he's being treated better than he was before. I send my blessings to him forever!

TCM's essence is to rid the body of the "root cause" of illness. The acupuncturist puts a lot of effort into doing this, but patients will hardly notice the value because it's not something that can be seen. If the patient only wants to save money, if he only wants the symptoms relieved and no longer desires to seek treatment, if he does not cultivate the morals and change the pathogenic factors such as diet, lifestyle, and exercise, it's like making a playing a game with his life and not realizing it.

There are patients who are not willing to work hard to take care of their own health. They just want a reduced price or free treatments—or maybe even a free but time-consuming consultation where they can get the answers to a lot of their health-related questions. It's not proper behavior—and it's not fair—to take advantage of the kindness of a healthcare provider.

In order to achieve a positive treatment outcome, it's better to read classic books and cases, do active thinking, practice qigong and nourish your qi, and focus on moral cultivation. The effort will gain you no less than the masterpiece of a famous artist or the gold medal of a successful Olympic athlete.

• Light Therapy

There are laser treatments for eye surgery, spinal problems, brain tumors, brain cancer or brain blockage removal, hemorrhoids, and skin diseases. Laser is a method for eliminating the symptoms of a disease. It's fast and has low blood loss, but it does not remove the root cause(s).

I used to use an infrared irradiation lamp with wood lock oil to treat sensitive colleagues at sea whose blood vessels were thin and occurred in higher density. This caused them to experience pain when giving massage therapy to their clients. It generally only treats superficial soft tissue pain. After using the infrared, the surface of the soft tissue and the vascular structures loosen, and it's easier to insert the needle to treat deeper tissue pain.

There is some clothing and jewelry available that uses added negative ions and magnetic elements to improve the efficacy of the infrared radiation therapy. I do not, however, recommend passive health improvement to anyone—except for the elderly or those too weak to do exercise.

Cars that keep running tend to have less trouble than they are static and aren't used. It's the same with our bodies and our health. As animals, only keeping active and maintaining mobility in all parts of our body can help body health.

• Electricity Therapy

There are electric massage chairs and electric heating blankets to promote blood circulation superficially. However, if the user has internal coldness and cannot expel it, electricity therapy is not as potent as infrared radiation—with or without magnet—because it cannot penetrate deeply enough to expel the internal coldness or blockage.

Acupuncturists have an electro-stimulator device to help improve the strength of qi circulation so that a patient's qi flow doesn't drop during an acupuncture session. Some patients need a stronger or weaker stimulation during the treatment. The stimulator cannot be used with a patient with a pacemaker.

When medicine does not work, a gastric electrical stimulator can stimulate the lower part of the stomach. It can control diabetes, mild gastroparesis, or related chronic nausea and vomiting. But there are drawbacks and side effects if used to stimulate often[51].

The portable stimulator can block the pain signals[52] not the actual sickness that might progress toward a worse health situation. A TENS machine only can treat superficial, surface pain and not deep tissue or tendon pain.

There is also electric shock treatment for heart failure, tachycardia (fast heart beat)[53], major depression, schizophrenia, mania, and catatonia[54].

Electrosurgical 200kHz—3.3MHz treats skin cancer. The trend has become more widespread[55], but if not well controlled, it can cause skin ulcers.

• Magnetic Therapy

There are magnetic beads made into jewelry, or you can add infrared or negative ions to improve efficacy.

There are also *yang zai* 陽宅 and *feng shui* 風水. Guo, Pu 郭璞[70] (276-324) in China, Jing Dynasty wrote *Burial Classic*, the earliest book talking about feng shui.

Yang zai and feng shui use natural magnetic fields and the environment to treat diseases, redirect fate, or make personal changes. According to these approaches, maintaining a house with good ventilation, adequate sunshine, and a comfortable, smooth flow of fresh air and energy is enough. I personally disagree. Relying on the feng shui expert who tells you to invest a lot of money to make changes in visible things without putting a large dose self-effort into changing one self's difficulty or doing moral cultivation to earn the pass to a divine life will not enable a person to reach one's dream.

Without moral cultivation, the investment a person makes in feng shui or yang zai could be all wasted. If investing for a grave, the feng shui could be changed or damaged later by another person—intentionally or unintentionally. Perhaps construction will be done, or someone will open the grave to steal the treasures inside, or maybe it will be damaged by war or earthquake or other natural occurrences.

This industry has many people who cheat to make money. Nearly twenty years ago, a female business owner in Taiwan kept losing money and was in severe debt. Still, she invested a lot of money for advice from a feng shui expert who was referred by her friend. The expert told her that her problems were occurring because she lacked a certain precious mineral stone which would improve her feng shui. The expert sold her a NT$50,000 (near US$2,000) stone. In addition to adding more debt, it did not help her bringing in a penny more.

Thirty years ago in Taiwan, there was an IT business owner who did not pay his employees' salaries. Instead, he listened to a feng shui expert who encouraged him to spend a lot of money to move his office to a good feng shui spot and did a big modification for the new office. He designed the man's office door to be tilted with the wall. He told him to place a Buddha statue outside of his office and to worship it every morning and evening—he did that more frequently than he talked to his mother. However, it did not bring any improvements for his business. Instead, it cost him more to buy offerings each day. He was soon out of business because to he hadn't done the right things. He didn't pay his hardworking employees or put effort into running his business.

I had a cousin who lived in Northridge, California during the famous 1987 Southern California Northridge earthquake. A lot of the expensive crystal wares she kept on display in a glass cabinet fell and were broken. Otherwise in her house, there was only a mild crack in a corner of the wall.

I asked her if she had submitted an insurance claim. She replied, "No. I walked around our neighborhood, and most of the houses have fallen down or are partially collapsed. Our family members are all safe, and our house is intact save for cracks in one corner of a wall. We are very grateful. Let the others who've had severe disaster claim their losses first!"

After I heard that, I was convinced that good people live under a blessing. A famous twentieth-century home insurance company left the home insurance market due to having too many claims for this earthquake, the company was out of homeowner insurance business.

There are times when a person's virtues do not provide him with as much as he had expected. There are innumerable cases where people spent money but could not avoid misfortune. Even finding a place with good feng shui does not guarantee that it will pass on to descendants.

Some person's natural life is not long. After completing his life's mission, like my former teacher, Professor Ni, passed away at the age of fifty-nine. He worked too hard with worry too much about bad practices in the medical field and patients who lacked health knowledge and blindly followed information from the wrong authorities. After writing out some of his medical knowledge—enough to correct the mistaken understandings of TCM in the medical field as well as teach some students—he left.

Many of his students are now dedicated to spreading the word of his medical discoveries, even though we would all much rather him be alive to shorten everyone's medical journey to the highest level. However, there is a traditional Chinese saying that goes, "The master can only bring you to enter the right door—the cultivation depends on each student." It means that the master can only guide students to enter a treasure cave. If one does not work adequately, does not catch what the instructor taught, or does not use his brain, he/she could spend a lot of time going through life and never getting the best treasure—or getting not nearly as much as the other students due to giving up too early.

This reminds me of a story from *Think and Grow Rich* by Napoleon Hill. A man found a gold mine. He mined gold until one day he discovered he hadn't found much. So he sold his mine. The new owner hired a professional to do an investigation and discovered that only three feet away, there was an even richer gold store inside. The previous owner learned a lesson never to give up, and that made him very successful in his later business selling insurance.

Some people feel that even desert land is rich in rare metals, including gold and even more precious than that, and it's the best soil for organic agriculture. There is a fortune everywhere—under the ground, on the ground, in the sky. People have the ability to gain abundant wealth, happiness, fun, and joy in amounts more than your brain can create!

Instead of looking for an individual feng shui place, why don't all of us join to create one for all of the people in the world? That can be achieved by purifying all of our minds together. A good feng shui place has an excellent magnetic field. In nature, each individual is a magnetic field. A huge group of people gathered together can form a huge influential magnetic field which has the ability to alter the locality's geographic magnetic field and atmosphere. If you study Chinese history, you will learn that if an emperor was an excellent statesman, or he could fully trust and use an excellent statesman, the whole country was peaceful and happy, and auspicious things like peace and pleasant weather appeared. Otherwise, there were natural disasters and wars with tough weather.

Why do we not work together for everyone's magnetic field by lifting everyone's frequency, making the Earth itself a tremendous magnetic field? The Earth and the universe are dynamic, always changing. But each big change could be maintained for a very long time. Now is the time in the history of humanity for all of us in the world to transform and shine again.

Think and Grow Rich is a great book to help unchain you from limited thinking to realize what the abundant life means—and how you can change your attitude to get it. If you feel that it's hard to change, you can join our coaching programs to transform your concepts and attitude. You're right—it often takes a coach, like the Olympic Gold medal winners hire. Personal coaches correct movement, encourage, and guide you to find feasible ways to keep climbing.

Yes. Guide rather than teach. When people are taught, they don't think. With guidance, you can find the finger to touch the stone and turn it into gold.

It may be that a beloved child dies too soon, allowing his parents to share that love with other children outside their family. It makes me think back years ago to when a group of graduate students took a tour to Las Vegas with their instructor to a famous school in Taiwan. On the way back, the bus tires burst, causing a tragic accident. All of the students were killed because they weren't wearing safety belts.

One student's mother came to the US. She cried and was very sad. Later, after the Tzu Chi Foundation's volunteer spoke words of comfort, she changed her attitude and said it might be that her child had reached his quota for love and had gone. Before, she had put all of her love into that one child. But now, it was time to share her love with the other children.

There's a story about a general who was buried in an excellent feng shui grave, expecting that one of his offspring would one day become the country's leader. His offspring then abused his power and misbehaved, eventually receiving a warning to step back from the presidential election. Otherwise, the general's grave would be damaged and his body would be thrown somewhere without notice. If his offspring's bad behavior dissatisfied other people, the good feng shui would be destroyed. So why not use the money you would otherwise spend on feng shui to do good deeds now to assure your descendants will experience bliss?

Real feng shui masters exist. But they are few in number. And no matter how good a feng shui place you've found, if you do not give your descendants a good family and a good school education, or if one of your descendants turns to bad ways or makes a mistake or was influenced poorly from outside the family, that person can harm the family and the society—even with the influence of good feng shui.

However, a good feng shui expert can teach you how to get a good house to live in or a good commercial building that will bring benefits to the occupants, the business owner, and the customers. But know that in order to get the full benefit from a yang zai, one should live in at the right location inside the house for more than three months.

Some children are born into the world, and are tragically taken away too soon. Their grieving parents are left with the sole purpose of researching whatever it was that took the child's life. Perhaps the parents will start a nonprofit organization to help others in the same situation—like Mothers Against Drunk Driving (MADD).

For example, Ms. Beckie Brown's son Marcus was killed in a drunk driving accident at the age of eighteen. Afterward, Beckie became a tireless advocate for MADD. She realized a lot of lives can be saved by passing laws to prohibit drinking and driving. So Marcus lost his life, but MADD was born out of that loss. Because of this, Marcus' life mission was to have MADD create in order to save lives.

• Heat Therapy

There are many people who use emitted heat or contact heat to treat pain. There was a case on YouTube which used a heated metal rod to treat gastroptosis. Due to heat penetration, power is weak. So one needs to have patience to achieve a long-term result.

Sand therapy is often used in desert areas. People are buried in the sand, and the sun's heat is utilized to expel the coldness and dampness to relieve them of arthritic pain.

• Water Therapy

It's popular in China to use acupuncture injection therapy, where Chinese medicine physicians inject a prescribed herbal liquid into the acupuncture points.[57] The outstanding results are both quick and low cost. This method can be used for pain and/or internal medicine treatments.

Traditional Chinese Medicine has a two-thousand-year history of water therapy—hot water baths, warm water baths, cold water baths, cold and hot water bath with intermediate change, herbal baths, steam therapy, herbal steam therapy. Modern times have used the power of machinery to adjust the flow of the water in treatment.[58]

Europe and America in the nineteenth and twentieth centuries began adopting the Chinese concept of hydrotherapy.[59]

The hot spring bath is a combination of water and heat therapies. It also uses special elements contained in the hot spring to penetrate the body to treat things such as skin diseases, arthritis, and cold-constitution-related diseases. However, the time in the hot spring should be varied according to the individual because some people can experience allergic reactions. The reactions can often be eliminated by intermediate treatment and adjusting the time spent in the hot spring.

Some US companies extract ingredients such as algae, iodine, potassium, calcium, magnesium, and sulfur from sea water and use this to treat cancer, skin diseases, thyroid problems, and many other things. Practitioners in China have patients soak in the seawater for long periods of time to treat pain, fatigue, and a number of skin diseases.

• Cupping

"Fifty-Two Diseases Formula," recorded in a medical book in 168 BC[59], was unearthed from the Ma Wang Dui Silk Book in the No. 3 Han Tomb. It recorded fifty-two diseases and their treatments, including using the horn to treat. At that time, the cupping tool was made from animal horns (Jiao 角). Therefore, it was called Jiao Fa[60] 角法 (Jiao 角—horn, Fa 法 is the method). The cupping tool was made of animal horns until the Sui and Tang Dynasty when bamboo replaced the horns[61].

Cupping uses heat to create a vacuum which suctions a cup to the patient's or body. This method is used to suck out the wind, dampness, coldness, phlegm, dead blood, or pus that is in the body. Some therapists move the cup around, called a moving cupping. By doing so, one can soften tissues and eliminate cellulite on the legs or arms.

Cupping is a widely known Chinese folk therapy. The cup can be anything from which the air can be vacuumed. A baby food jar or any nonplastic container works, but avoid any plastic containers (to avoid melting and the release of toxins) and metal cups (to avoid the cup getting too hot and injuring the skin). Burn a piece of paper or cotton ball, move it inside the cup, and then remove the fire as quickly as possible, allowing the cup to suck onto the patient's skin. The uneven pressure pulls the pathogens out of the body.

Push the skin down near the cup opening to release the cup. It is a powerful method with which to treat chronic pain, dead blood, and pus located at the surface of the body.

• Exercises

There are many different types of exercises—swimming, skating, hiking, all kinds of ball games, dancing, and more. The most popular sport is walking. All of these are active therapies. In addition to providing physical fitness for the individual, some of them require teamwork which helps to develop other skills and gives added benefits. However, all physical activities are likely to cause some type of sports injury, and you must always exercise caution. When an injury does occur, however, the pain therapy methods in this book may come in handy.

If a patient is deficient (weak), has poor balance, is injured, or is recovering from surgery or illness and cannot participate in exercise, he/she can employ a physical therapist help to move the limbs of the body. This is called passive exercise. Although it is better than no exercise at all, it isn't as good as getting a good amount of active exercise. In general, Traditional Chinese Medicine has better treatment results in patients with a deficiency or poor balance.

An experiment run on Olympic athletes concluded that it didn't matter whether athletes practiced physically at the playground or in their imagination, the results were all the same. The subconscious cannot distinguish between real and not real—it only recognizes the repeated visual appearance and performs accordingly. It is this basis that allows patients to conquer diseases. It sounds easy, but there are many factors and skills behind it. You'd better hire a coach or repeatedly read this book to acquire all of the knowledge and techniques.

I urge all family members and physical therapists to do their best to push the patient—except in cases of mentally ill and memory loss patients—to do exercises often in his imagination, even during sleep time. Let the patient imagine the happiness and freedom of mobility after recovery. It will speed up the rehabilitation process and help the patient recover quickly. The happy vision is what the patient's subconscious should help him attain. Skipping the practice part in the imagination and repeatedly playing only the happy visual won't work to help the patient achieve the results that he wants.

I used to read classic medical books. There are higher level skills needed to process the information in these books. Some of the other acupuncturists used to complain that the classic books were difficult to understand. *How can I conquer this material?* They'd ask me.

I grew accustomed to sharing my studying techniques:

1. Start with a classic book that has higher-level wisdom inside. If you start at an advanced point, it will be easier to reach the end.

2. If it's hard, repeat it and read it a thousand times. Its real meaning will flow out eventually. The shortcut is to record it and repeatedly play it during sleep. Many students use this method to pass tests. I used it to pass my TOEFL. Before taking the test, I was far too busy to study. I was grateful to one of my college roommates for giving me all of her TOEFL audio review tapes before she left for Taiwan. I practiced the sample tests nightly during my sleep.

    This might be a way to help mentally handicapped children to learn. Do not, however, use the whole night—whether it's you or anyone else. Your brain needs time to rest. Without enough time off, its reaction will slow down.

3. If you looked at a picture from the side of an animal, and that was the first time you'd seen that animal, you'd be totally dumbfounded when you saw it from another angle. The best way to know and understand that animal is to get as many books as possible that illustrate it in words or in pictures—

and from all views. Then you have a complete picture. This is the study method I use the most. I look at the same thing from more than a thousand angles if I have to. If one studies in this way, how can one not master the knowledge?

4. Classic literature, no matter whether in Chinese medicine or by authors such as Shakespeare, can lead the learner to a higher level of learning.

It's the same with music—classical music is better, no matter if it be Eastern or Western music. Listening to it repeatedly when young can help you learn better.

My trick to help my kids learn was to use multiple learning stimulation tools coupled with much encouragement and compliments. When kids move ahead of their classmates, they feel proud of themselves and want to hold on to that feeling. That is the key to keeping them wanting to succeed. It also built up their confidence to overcome difficulties. The best teachers have an abundance of tools for this, and kids learn problem-solving skills they can apply to their daily life forever. Kids learn that there is always a way to solve a problem if they can just calm themselves down, focus, and be creative enough to think of a solution. There is nothing that cannot be solved.

This doesn't mean increasing kids' stress by requiring that everything they learn be difficult material. Instead, let them learn interesting things, and hire the best teacher you can find to teach them. The tuition will most times cost you more, but the payback arrives sooner than with an instructor of lower quality. The investment revenue is for the kids.

We often see that successful people are the ones who invest in themselves by searching for quality instructors. They provide the instructor with high pay, show respect, and work hard, enabling the instructor move them further along as quickly as possible. Life is too short to waste time.

However, most people are unwilling to pay high prices to learn. They bargain, show no respect for the knowledge and effort of other people, and do not work hard themselves. The loss is their own—it is the loss of their potential growth.

In general, for a patient—or anyone, for that matter—to do one thing as a habit, they must do it every day and continue to do it for more than twenty-one days. After a person practices an exercise for more than twenty-one days, that person will have a sense of loss if it's not done. He/she must do it to feel comfortable.

Exercise is not only participating in sports in a gym or on a field or on a golf course. Some people do manual labor on the job every day. Their physical abilities are most likely better than those of many professional athletes. And keep in mind that there is probably more carbon dioxide in a gym's air due to the number of people confined in the small space at once. It's not as fresh as the air in the morning in a park. So doing exercise outside is always preferred.

Exercising at the gym is not nearly as beneficial as spending time helping the wife with the mopping or vacuuming or yard work. In helping his wife, the husband gives her more time to rest. It's like using one stone to kill two birds. The benefit is that both people are exercising while at the same time promoting family harmony. Exercise is something you should do to increase self-health.

• Spiritual Therapy

Spiritual and mental health are the two major factors in human health. Unfortunately, these have been overlooked by medical school education. General public school education also ignores this, instead encouraging things residing on the yardstick of success—money, social rank, power, material enjoyment, and academic rank.

Money has the power that can raise one's social rank, buy material enjoyment, or hire coaches and tutors to lift academic rank. Today, money drives businesses without concern about health, a clean environment for later generations to live, and so on.

The shortcomings are obvious. Most people are suffering. Finding a simple diet without the effects of pollution is difficult. Strange diseases came into existence. Medical costs are increasing, but people's health and life satisfaction are plummeting. When it hits the extremes, it will reverse. Now is the time for returning to simplicity.

Qian Zao Du 乾鑿度[122] said that the visible things are generated from invisibles. Therefore, there are the times of tai yi 太易→ tai chu 太初→ tai shi 太始→ tai su 太素→ muddle 渾淪→earth formed 天地→ all Creatures 萬物[63].

- In tai yi, even the qi was not formed. That is the most ancient of times.

- Tai chu was the beginning time of the qi. In the tai chu period, the universe generated qi.

- Tai shi was the beginning of shapes being formed. At that time, both qi and shapes* existed in the universe.

  * Like clouds and water—they have shape but do not have a fixed form.

- Tai shu was the beginning of materials*. During that time, there were both form and materials. Shu means materials.[62]

  *The materials have fixed forms.

- *Zhou Yi Qian Zao Du* 《周易乾鑿度》 is one chapter of the **Wei (Latitude) Shu** 緯書 Yi Wei 《易緯》 published (B.C.90-68)[203,204,205,205] in the late Western Han. It is also referred to as *Qian Zao Du*. It is one of the most complete and preserved philosophical works. It proposed the systematic Universe Generation. The order of the universe is generated from tai yi to all creatures in the world 萬物[63].

From the above, we learn that the invisible was the beginning of the visible. Therefore, the invisible dominates all things visible. There are invisible laws which regulate the visible material world. The invisible deeply influences the perfectness of the shape of physical existence. We as humans are very small visible things in this huge material world.

People discovered natural law theory[122]. It's been called the nature law, the nature law of ethics, or the law of ethics. All morally correct acts are defined as following this law of ethics.

But if we do our research, we can see there is a misuse of this natural law for survival's sake. Is it morally right? If a restaurant chooses to use chemical additives, and another one follows, justifying it as a necessity for survival, does that make it right? No! There is the choice to change the tools used to survive. In this case, the person could opt to run an organic food restaurant with higher prices for menu items instead of adding chemicals to their foods which will in turn shorten their customers' lives.

From the above, you can learn the focus of your life. There is nothing in the world that can harm the invisible. But the invisible has the ability to form *anything* later in time in the visible world. Yes, that includes the materials you need to serve your dream. There is a formula that we can teach you through our training programs to let you live your dream life sooner. Or you can choose to learn from our books if you are a good self-learner.

Clouds and water have varied forms, but aside from changing their form, nothing can destroy their existence. Some people simulate the characteristics of water, trying to fit themselves into any situation. It's not the time or place to debate here the rightness of that. Sometimes carrying out a dream or a new concept or a new way to achieve a thing requires being bold and creative.

The lowest capability in the world in the Chinese cultural concept are the materials that we call devices—qi 器 in Chinese. Please do not confuse this with the functional energy qi (氣) that flows in a living person's body. The devices are not only visible, but most of them have forms, colors, and fixed shapes and sizes (except for the expandable ones that were still made from parts of a fixed size and shape). They are easily damaged and destroyed. Their life is the shortest among the invisible forms and devices.

Therefore, the top intelligent people like to think and study the invisible world and convert it to be feasible visible projects which benefit the world and help them achieve their dreams and goals.

Huang Di Nei Jing 黃帝內經 *(Yellow Emperor)* • *Su Wen* 素問 *(Plain Ask)* • *Shang Gu Tian Zhen Lun Pian Di Yi* 上古天真論篇 第一*(Chapter One The Ancient Time Naive Theory)*:

The former Yellow Emperor was born very smart. When he was young, he was good at talking. During his childhood, he could understand things around him very quickly. When he was growing up, he was not only honest and sincere but also diligent. In his adulthood, he became the emperor of the ancient China.

He spoke to his Health Minister Qi Bo. "I heard that the ancient people's age could be more than a hundred years. Their mobility did not show aging. Now people who are just past the age of fifty show debilitating weakness and no strength. Is it caused simply because of the different times? Or is it because people today do not know how to nourish their lives*? "

Nourishing life means extending life and be healthy.

Qi Bo replied, "In ancient times, people knew how to nourish life. They could adopt the universal yin and yang, adapt to natural changes, harmonize with life mysteries, set restraints for their diet, regulate schedules and avoid overworking themselves for no true life meaning, also avoid excessive sexual intercourse. Therefore, both their shape and **shen** were flourishing. They could end their natural life past the age of one hundred."

This is not the case today. People treat wine as broth, absurdity as normal behavior, and have sexual intercourse when drunk. Their excessive sexuality empties their essence and literally dries up their **zhen qi** 真气. Moreover, they do not know how to maintain the fullness of their zhen qi, and they are not good at governing their shen. Because of this, they weaken themselves by the time they are fifty years old.

The ancient sages taught their people to avoid the deficiency pathogen and the evil wind at the pertinent time. If they are calm and cheerful without distraction, and they allow their zhen qi to follow and keep within the spirit, how could they get sick? When willpower flows easily with fewer desires (with focus), when the mind is calm without fear, when the body is laboring but does not feel tired, the qi follows smoothly—and behavior follows accordingly. Everyone passes through their desires and carries out their wishes.

So they would enjoy their own foods, be satisfied with their dress, and be happy with their customs. No matter whether their social rank was high or low, they wouldn't look at each other with jealousy or desire. People would be simple and unadorned, and improper desires would not catch their attention. Depraved, iniquitous thoughts wouldn't confuse their minds. These individuals would fit the principle of nourishing life. This is why they'd live to be older than one hundred.

They had high moral standards and better character than most normal people. Because of their good morals, there was nothing that could hurt their health. From this, we can see that morals and health have a very important relationship.

Now, let's look at the Western records:

1. There are more spiritual therapies in private sectors than in the academic researches. The biological and psychological mechanisms of spiritual therapy have long been neglected by academia.

   Take, for instance, twelve cases of breast cancer patients who have had long-term hormone therapy. Spiritual therapy reduced the side effects of their original treatments, increased their energy levels, enhanced their sense of health and emotional relaxation, and reinvolved them in their pre-cancer activities[64].

2. A study of breast cancer patients concluded that cancer patients with a higher level of gratitude experience milder symptoms than patients with less gratitude[72].

3. For patients with chronic or terminal illness, mental exercises such as praying and thanksgiving have been proven to improve the patients' health and quality of life[73].

4. Forgiveness and gratitude have benefits on health[74].

5. Religion improves the mental health and social functioning of elderly people who are living alone, thereby improving their quality of life[88].

From the above, we can see that the morals of thanksgiving are also related to health. Whether it is one's immorality causing the emotional problems or being noble but still worrying about social problems, emotional problems are finding their way directly into internal organs and injuring them. For the emotional problem and its concomitant injured organ, please refer to Table 1 Five Elements.

If you worry that the world's moral behavior is low, why don't you stand up and do something to fix it? You can write speech or set up a behavior model for merit. If you fear there are too many things that you don't know how to do, or if you think you do not know what to do, please do not worry and feel fear. This book series and my coaching programs can help you. After you have learned all of what I teach you here and have been diligent in practicing it, your health and soul will be enhanced, and your eyes will be opened.

If you desire to improve even more rapidly, I have many training programs that will help you transform and open up the blockage in your body, mind, and soul. Please visit Comprehensive Universal Energy Healing at universalenergyealing.us to find Training Programs to unblock your body, or go to NBAARC at nbaarc.com to find dream builders, life mastery, and hypnosis training programs to meet your needs.

- ## Cosmic Energy Therapy

The acupuncture points on human bodies allow their connection with the outside universe. Therefore, a human's health is closely related to the universe. A study showed that the Swan planet emits cosmic energy that is changing all Earth beings' DNA[40]. Cosmic energy therapy has both a broad and narrow sense.

The broad aspect includes both the receiver and the healer's own virtue cultivation (i.e. spiritual therapy). This book focuses on broad cosmic energy healing. It uses cosmic radiation energies to unlock bodily energy and release blood flow blockages—and it all starts with doing daily moral acts. From there, you can open the divine universe and enjoy the abundant life of health, happiness, life achievements, wealth, freedom of time, as well as close and reliable friendships. It includes soul and spiritual therapy.

Narrow cosmic energy therapy does not include soul and spiritual therapy. It uses only the cosmic tangible tiny floating space particles and cosmic radiation to do the therapy. The universe is fulfilled with photons, gamma rays, electromagnetic waves, microwaves, and so on. These energies supply the power for growth and repair of all of Earth's living creatures.

Photons are the basic particles that transmit electro and magnetic interactions. Their rest mass is zero. In space, their speed is the velocity of light[83].

The gamma ray's energy is between 1 PeV ~ 100 PeV[41]. eV[125] "is the electronvolt, a unit of energy equal to approximately 1.6×10^{-19} joules (symbol J). An ultra-high-energy (UHE) cosmic ray (CRs), its energy can be measured up to 100 EEV[87].

Between 1987 and 2008, near Earth's orbit, the energy of the rays of the sun was in the range of 10-100 trillion electronic voltages (10-100MeV) as an integrated proton spectrum. A radio pulse's peak flux value S is between 9 and 15 thousand trillion Hz (9-15GHz). High frequency radio spectrums are (FM≈30 thousand trillion Hz)[42].

From the above stated, you can learn that there are rich and strong cosmic energies that are far more powerful than a human being's to be used for health problem's healing.

The universe appears to be empty, but there are various elements floating in space[75]. These elements are respired by humans, animals, and plants to help each particular organism's growth and survival. The simplest example is the essential breathing of oxygen.

There are nutrient particles in the air. This explains how some practitioners who do not even eat or drink can still survive. Their intelligence and lives are linked with the universal abundances. They live very calm and simplified lives.

Seeds can be dried in the air or dried in machines, and both types of seeds can grow the same plant—Eucalyptus Regnans—but the air-dried, trees planted in forest soil grow better[44]. Those trees— and those practitioners—are able to absorb the universe's essence (pure nutrition) to feed their nutritional needs, even including water from the moisture in the air.

H + 3 was observed in the interstellar boundary in the galaxy. Dense clouds of cosmic-ray ionization rate ($\zeta 2$) were low. It was due to the low energy protons (several MeV MeV) penetrating the clouds[71]. The high or low of the cosmic-ray energy level and the cosmic ray ionization rate impacts the clouds density and also affects the nitrogen, hydrogen, and ammonia chemical changes in the air[43].

- ## Comprehensive Therapy

  Some physicians and therapists integrate two or more of the above therapies in their treatments. This book recommends the same. It combines qigong, cosmic energy, spirit therapy, meditation, self-hypnosis, and Chinese medicine/theory/ diagnosis/treatments—all enhanced by my clinical experiences and the dream builder coach/life mastery consultant skills derived through Comprehensive Universal Energy Healing.

The Background of Cosmic Energy Therapy

The complexity and frequency of ancient people's material life, recreational exploits, and interpersonal contacts were fewer and less involved than those of today's population. The people were closer to the nature of the universe than those of modern days. In ancient times, there were many wise men of high intelligence and great spirit who observed nature. Their wisdom communicated directly with that of space, the Earth, and the universe. They deciphered many mysteries of the universe, and their discoveries were a lot more impressive than modern man's discoveries with expensive equipment.

Many ancient cultures of the "mystery" knowledge inherit and executive persons need to have higher virtue and wisdom to understand.

Feng Shui was not a mystery originally. Chinese respect elderly and ancestor. Therefore, study the place for grave, to avoid water, merge the body, insects bit the body, etc. Eventually, people discovered that the magnet field and the atmosphere around the grave can influence descendant's personality and fortune. Such as can let descendants be emperor, musician, physician, etc. It's especially true for the personality due to ancient time, male child should live besides the parent's grave for three years.

It also can be approved from one of my TCM instructors. His grandfather hired a feng shui expert to look for a place for him to bury after he died. One year later, the expert back and reported to him: "I cannot find a good place for a high level government officer. But, I found a place for a famous doctor." So my instructor was the famous doctor who corrected more than two hundred years of misleading information about TCM.

His life mission was to teach the correct TCM to let it go back to the traditional route. I am so lucky to be his student. He wrote books and taught many students. After he finished his life mission, he passed away at the age of fifty-nine. He studied hard, worked hard for his patients and was worried and angry about the results from Eastern and Western medicine. As his students, we have the responsibility to transfer his discoveries to the world. I use his basic skeleton but I dress it up with energy healing.

Because of feng shui's huge benefits, and in order for the emperor and his descendants to remain stable at the emperor's chair, feng shui was covered as a mystery. We should avoid a bad person using it to rule the country. Books were filled with incorrect information, and the transmission of the knowledge became an underground activity.

Some people were selfish and deliberately spread false knowledge, leading us to lose those national treasures. It is a pity.

Many ancient cultures have long neglected their treasures, and they have deteriorated. In recent years, however, their value has increased. The Western world is eager to learn from India. The

Chinese Jing Kong Master 淨空法師 lectures in the US, Australia, and Southeast Asia. China has a great desire to teach Di Zi Gui 弟子規, which sets regulations for interpersonal relationships.

In modern times, many highly educated people devote themselves to doing scientific research, gradually picking up and utilizing some pieces of lost civilizations. Meanwhile, because they use these ancient treasures in their research, they endow the discoveries with scientific proof and explanation.

During this long time mistraced the secret of the universe, people began acting for self, and this led to extreme individualism. Materialism caused people to ignore public health, led to incredible environmental pollution, and destroyed the harmony of the natural world. The kindness of humankind was being oppressed or lost.

The communication of and through spiritual awareness and cosmic wisdom was pushed to the wayside as people began to assert that the only scientific and true results were those deemed so by technology. People began to dismiss spiritual awareness as absurd.

Fortunately, when things reach extremes, they often turn in the opposite direction. People began to feel their higher spirit awakening and set to work to spread the light. This awakening comes from contact with other persons, or from studying ancient books, or—like I found it—because of winning the universe's fortunate favor.

Thus, ancient civilizations have been researched more and more by determined and qualified people. For example, Western neurologists are now analyzing handprints and brains, sorting out a set of data, and connecting them with the person's life mission[78].

The Meaning of the Cosmic Energy Therapy Appearance

Virtuous ancient Chinese leaders and thinkers paid attention to *metaphysical science*. Metaphysical science is invisible. Due to its invisibility, it is not limited by changes and it cannot be changed. It can adapt to any changes. Because of its invisibility, it is long-lasting without damage. Metaphysical science represents the invisible universal norms of "morals" and "energy" as well as the superior statecraft, which governs the country, life skills, and the science of healing. This is true regardless of how things change with the centuries. The morality is constantly being reaffirmed. It's why the emperors of ancient culture must read classic materials to learn the essence of true wisdom.

Under the invisible is the visible. Visible shape can be changed.

Under the visible are the devices. If it is a device, it can be broken.

Once people have material things, they put too much emphasis on forms and the pursuit of such. This causes people to show off and become more materialistic. They start to notice the possession of devices. And in this era of valuing and owning devices, wisdom has become solely dependent on having measurable scientific statistics or appropriate criterion for the assessment. That's why there is now a significant lack of great statesmen and thinkers. They have been replaced by blind followers.

The Comprehensive Universal Energy Healing that we want to spread uses invisible morals and universal energy to purify the human body and spirit to improve the frequency and the wisdom of humans. They then can obtain metaphysical knowledge and enter the metaphysical world.

Do you notice that ingesting longevity herbs for a long time causes the body to become lighter? The description of an immortality-enlightened practitioner is light and buoyant. This comes from having a light body with no blockage of waste. Emotion and desire are unblocked by immoral thoughts of competition, stealing, cheating, putting down others, or fear and many other negative things.

When entering the metaphysical world, a person's wisdom is highly unpredictable. Einstein, by merely grasping a pen, could describe the knowledge of the universe. He pushed human science and technology forward, and most important is his contribution to promoting human knowledge.

Everyone who comes into the world is born as a spiritual being. Our nature and instincts are much stronger than our cognition. Please take a look at Ms. Helen Keller, or Boddy Martin from Dayton, Ohio who has no legs and is the homecoming king, or Vinod Thakur who is a legless hip-hop dancer in India. Through their efforts, they tell the world that everyone is a genius, no matter what! A noble spirit can help one conquer any difficulty.

There is a Chinese saying that goes, "There is no species for the general and the prime minister. A man should be self-reliant to create it." A person moves from nonexistence, to being alive, to death, back to nature, and returns to nothingness again. Everything starts and ends from emptiness. The entire life experience that we can count on and give to future generations is not the wealth, possessions, power, and status, but the morals and the merit that warms people's hearts.

Character cannot be developed in ease and quiet. Only through the experience of trial and suffering can the soul be strengthened, ambition inspired, and success achieved.

—Helen Keller

The universe as a whole is being transformed. The Earth is being promoted from the four dimensions to even higher dimensions, gradually connecting with the other universal n-dimensional planets that have high moral characters and high-tech standards and interact with their biological creatures.

Human beings' spiritual elevation and physical load (the summary of weight, disease, and mind setting) should be enhanced to be as light as possible. If you have questions, you can watch Videos[140] of Lifting[141]:

1. Video 1[142] is the universe's cause and laws.
2. Video 2[143] is the dimensions of the universe.
3. Video 3[144] is the hidden truth of brain and mind.
4. Video 4[145] is related to conscious education.
5. Video 5[146] is to shape a new you!

You can also use search engines to key in your question or "n dimensions of the universe."

How to meet the requirements? Diligent practice in the universal codes mentioned in the book and in Comprehensive Universal Energy Healing to converge into the divine universe. Please note that the kindness and diversity of the universe allows many ways to access it. This book series is only one of many. However, you do not need to do trial and error. This book gives you a ready-made, feasible structure, proven and supported by 250-million-year-old theories, experiences, and evidence for you to follow. It's a lot easier to understand than ancient literature or Sanskrit.

In addition, I must remind you that the days are shrinking due to the expansion of the universe and the increase of the planet's rotations. Human life is too short! Blink an eye, and your life is here. But within another blink, the pages of your life will be turned to the end. What do you want to see recorded in your life's book? What kind comments do you want people make about your life's journey? It's all up to you!

Do you want to leave something as a gift that can be passed on from generation to generation in your family? Would you like your friends or family to be involved in creating a better environment for your descendants to live in?

Maybe your answer is yes, but you do not know how to do it. This book will teach you how to find your talents, unleash your desires and dreams, and make them real. There is nothing good that is impossible. Believe me, and believe yourself —**YOU CAN!** You need only a person who can teach you how to build a staircase to walk to the heaven in your mind.

I'm reminded of a time in 1984, five years after I left RCA Taiwan. I went back there from the US to look for my best friend's help because my husband was diagnosed with cancer. We went back to the US on an emergency flight ticket. A female clerk in RCA saw me and walked along with me. Would you like to know what she told me?

"Frieda, I am so envious of you that since you've worked here, you've always had something going on that got a lot people talking about you."

I said, "It's cancer this time. How do you feel about that?"

"It's better than my life. Every day is the same," she said.

Have you ever noticed that even in the bad times, there are still people who envy you and your position in life? You have the ability to grow stronger and smarter from the bad times and learn to deal with difficulties so that you can ride on the top of a higher wave later in life. I wish I'd had a dream builder coach certificate at that time. Maybe I could have helped my coworker's life to be more colorful.

So do you just want to play around, or do you want to wake up early enough to complete your life's mission? You can do meditation and listen to your subconscious talk to you, and I can advise you and send you in the right direction. As a transforming educator, I can guide you down the correct path for your life's journey, and if you join one of my programs and allow me walk with you, I can be by your side. But your final destination is decided only by you.

Let's carry out a dream together to shape a better future for the world.

The Basic Concept of the Cosmic Energy Therapy

The basic concept of health is to have smooth qi and blood circulation, a smooth mind, and positive thinking. It's so easy and simple—no mysteries. The greatest way is the simplest one. Today's medical schools teach a lot of complicated knowledge instead of giving students a synoptic health concept. If everyone could understand this, life could be a lot simpler.

Let me give you another example to use simplification to combat the complication that imbeds in the TCM treatment methods: A pile of spoiled food attracts flies, insects, roaches, mice, spiders. Instead of investigating the attracted species and matching the needed killing pesticide, TCM removes the spoiled food and cleanses the area. All of the attracted species then run away. So there is no blood test in the TCM practice.

From previously described, we know that the cosmic radiations are very high in energy. We can use this energy to help us clear the blockage within our body. But the premise is that we need to find a way to open the body's switch(es) in order to allow the cosmic energy to enter into the body.

Then we can use its power to lift the body's frequency and enhance the qi and blood circulation to remove physical blockages. However, if we do not cultivate the psychology, thinking, and emotions, the body will still be blocked.

In addition, if we psychologically reject Comprehensive Universal Energy Healing, it sets up a strong obstruction which rejects the universal energy trying to enter the body. Eager for a quick and immediate result, it also adds a layer of obstacles to the effectiveness of Comprehensive Universal Energy Healing.

The soothing of mind and mood and smooth, positive thinking and emotions can be achieved through virtue. There are a lot of ways to achieve it. We can start with love, gratitude, sharing, and collaboration. Depending on the severity of the congestion, sometimes a change of mind, setting, thinking, and emotion, will remove the physical blockage. But sometimes it doesn't, and then we can use narrow cosmic energy therapy. If more severe, we can use acupuncture and moxibustion, herbs, or other therapies of hypnosis in conjunction with Comprehensive Universal Energy Healing.

If a body has a severe blockage such as too much coldness, blood stasis, sticky phlegm, blood deficiency, or essence deficiency then one can use a combination of acupuncture and moxibustion, herbs, or other therapies such as hypnosis or a dream builder coach to treat. Sometimes people get sick because they've been obstructed from carrying out their dreams. Dream building coaches can provide encouragement and guidance that helps them get past any obstructions that might cause them to give up.

But the best and most effective way to maintain your health is to use Comprehensive Universal Energy Healing often—every night before falling asleep, during meetings, while chatting or watching TV or a movie. You can do self-healing by following the instructions to put hands on the necessary places to improve your health and raise your body frequency.

Use the four universal codes to clear away what is causing the body blockage and raise up the soul, mind, and body frequency. By doing so, you can connect to the universal energy's resources and wisdom. You will also have better and closer interpersonal relationships.

Cosmic Energy Therapy History

New and Old Testament Bible readers remember that Jesus used his hands on a person to remove that person's pain or sickness. Why? Because Jesus had high virtue, and thus he had high energy in his body which passed through his hands to the patient. His powerful energy opened up the patient's body, allowing energy to flow and relieving the patient's pain and illness. It has been more than two thousand years of history.

In the East, Islam and Buddhism believers' chanting and improved health is a kind of spiritual and mental therapy. Buddhism was founded in the sixth century BC by Sakyamuni Buddha and has more than 2600 years of history[89]. Islam appeared in the seventh century.

Chinese culture emphasizes shen and the metaphysical knowledge that is called "above the forms" (xing er shang 形而上). It's similar to western metaphysics. The ancient Chinese studied existing theories of yin and yang and the invisible becoming visible. Ethics were valued as the number one success rule. That's the real science, and it is a lot more advanced than the so-called Western science. The next lower in level to the invisible of the metaphysics is the forms. The lowest level is the devices that are touchable.

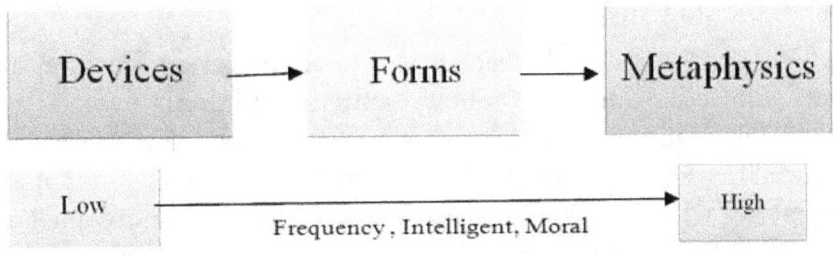

Fig iv Devices, Forms, and Metaphysics Relative Frequency

Unfortunately, ancient Chinese scholars may have knowledge of the ancient Chinese books and the treasures inside, but if their language translation skills are not good, they cannot write those things down in other languages. There is no time to translate them from Chinese into a foreign language. So let me again give thanks to Dr. Ma, Sheng, who encouraged me to write this article when the previous one was lost. Rewriting this one gave me the chance to discover that the Nobel physics prize should be given to China's ancient thinkers, such as Lao Zi, the author of the *Zhou Yi • Qian Zao Dou*[122]. They are the ones who mentioned the visible coming from the invisible—thousands of years ago.

Everyone has high intelligence, but it has always unknowingly been confined to the devices-type of education. Not daring to go beyond. This is the main cause of today's disease and the disharmonized social phenomena. The root problem is due to not thinking beyond to control the finite situation and not searching for a way to get free from the "as is" lock. Instead, the majority of people stay trapped in their current situations, worrying and fearing but afraid to move out. This is the basic way that schools deny genius—the main school education model does not use their device-measurement methods to measure a genius metaphysical talent. That is what forced the Einstein and many other geniuses to drop out of their schools.

It reminds me that one of my sons was in a GATE class since he was a fourth grader. His fifth grade teacher was a great teacher for pulling out the kids' genius. She threw out questions and let students discuss them, welcoming all kinds of opinions and criticisms coming out of the students' mouths.

My son's sixth grade teacher was totally different, however. She only allowed students to follow—and the children's voices were squelched. One month after his sixth grade school year started, I noticed my son's personality was changing. He was losing his appetite no matter what I cooked. He also became more and more quiet and didn't chat with me. Later, he spent more time sitting alone with a drooped head or blank eyes staring at a spot for a long time.

Eventually, he opened his mouth and said, "Mom, we were used to discussing things with our fifth grade teacher. The sixth grade teacher doesn't allow us to do so. I like to listen to one of my classmates. He's very smart. But every time he talks, he gets a check mark from the teacher. There are so many things that were allowed in the fifth grade teacher's class that aren't allowed now, and everyone has many check marks."

It caught my attention, and I did not know how to make a change because the sixth grade teacher was a star teacher in the elementary school. She had a record for a high entrance rate for students in a number one school among all of the local high schools, and even out of all in the entire state of California.

One day, my son handed me his textbook and asked me to redo the wrapping in a paper bag from the grocery store instead of wrapping it in a copy paper bag cover. My son got a check mark due to not following his teacher's instruction. At that time, if you wanted a paper bag at the grocery store, you needed to make a special request of the supermarket cashier. Everyone everywhere was talking about saving trees by saving paper. I wrote a letter to my son's teacher and asked for an appointment.

The fifth grade and the sixth grade teachers both attended the meeting because the fifth grade teacher was the school's GATE education mentor. I used an article—"Thinking like a Genius"— from *Future Society* magazine as a tool to challenge the teacher. I won my case by talking about achieving the purpose of protecting the textbook with a cover while by reusing the copy paper cover and saving me a trip to the grocery store for a paper bag—and having to doing extra shopping to get one. My son recovered his appetite and good humor soon after the appointment.

Fu, Xi 伏羲[65] relied on his virtue. He made the innate eight trigrams and the **Xiang Tian Yi** 先天易. He taught people how to make a net for fishing and hunting and how to farm animals, advocated the marriage system, stopped the consanguinity marriage to avoid the consanguineous marriage and replaced it with the etiquette and kinship exogamy, made writing characters to replace the previous rope knots to express things, created music and songs and brought them into people's lives, divided and ruled his territory in geographical regions, appointed officials to manage societies that supplied a model for the future community management[65]. These achievements all came from his excellent virtue. He solved his people's problems and was good at adopting the universal natural laws. As a ruler in China, Fu, Xi ruled China for one hundred and ten years. You can image how long his life was!

Huang Di Nei Jing 黃帝內經 • *Su Wen* 素問 *(Plain Ask)* • *Chapter 13—Yi Jing Bian Qi Lun* 移精變氣論 *(The Theory of Essence and Qi Changes)*

The Huang Di (Yellow Emperor) asked, "I heard that the ancient time treated diseases only by using the *Zhu You Shu* 祝由術. That was enough. Why today do we treat diseases with toxic drugs* to treat the inside and acupuncture to treat the outside. Why can some diseases can be cured, but some cannot?"

> *   In Chinese medicine, there is a saying: "Once it is a medicine, it is 30% toxins." It does not mean that there is some toxic ingredient in there that the FDA can extract. It means that besides the natural toxins, overindulgence in good stuff is also toxic to the body. Health is a state of homeostasis. If we get too much of anything, it breaks the balance, and it is toxic to the body. Therefore, the dosage and controlling the amount is important.

In Chinese culture, everything in moderation is better. It's wise to control everything and is improper to overindulge in enjoyments. Just as a Prince exchanged his clothing with a beggar, many businesses and successful people own all kinds of fancy things but still feel something is missing. Too much of a good thing does not create happiness.

Qi Bo replied, "The ancients living among animals, they moved to avoid cold, lived in the shade to avoid the summer heat, had no concern to bind with the twilight internally, and did not appear to pursue expanding positions externally. In this tranquil world, pathogens could not invade the body too deeply. So the toxic medicine could not treat them inside, and the acupuncture could not treat them outside. Only Zhu You Shu changing the essence (spirit) to treat was enough.

However, today's society does not like that. People worry about hardship internally. They overwork and hurt their outlook, do not follow the four seasons to make needed changes to protect their health, go against the proper ways to deal with the cold and summer heat, and always allow the wind and pathogens to invade their body and lower their immunity. It causes external pathogens to attack the deficient body and enter deeply into the organs, even inside the bone marrow. Externally, it hurts the skin, muscle, and pores. Thus a mild disease becomes severe, and a severe disease becomes death. The Zhu Yu Shu could not treat them well."

The above shows that the ancients maintained their health, but there was no way to retroact when they started. Before 2600 BC, the Huang Di (Yellow Emperor)[10] had set thirteen health departments, including Zhu Yu Shu, to increase a patient's emotions and will and strengthen his physical health against pathogens. From this, you can see some trace of the cosmic energy therapy.

Today, worry and desire for position have made diseases even more severe. The desire for material things is much higher than it was even thirty years ago.

"*Huang Di Nei Jing*" that was complete between 221 BC to 221 BC already clearly pointed out that" worry the hardship internally............. a mild disease becomes severe and a serious disease becomes death...... ." This is still true now and the severity is even were than that time.

Cancer cases and rarely seen diseases are becoming more and more common today and are at history's highest point. This challenge of the medical world cannot be addressed by needles and medicines only. It must return to morals and humanity and kindness to solve these problems.

Using the cosmic energy wave to do healing is something that we can learn from a lot of ancient literature and the Chinese martial arts (Wu Xia Xiao Shuo 武俠小說) novel that said, "The practitioners absorb the universal essences from the air and treat patients." It has been a long-standing method of healing. So far the earliest record for the Chinese martial arts novel can be traced back to Xi Han Dynasty Si Ma, Qian西漢司馬遷 who wrote *Shi Ji* 史記[131]. It's from around 145-90 BC[132]. The actual application of cosmic energy to treat disease was even earlier.

Introduction to the Cosmic Energy Therapy Schools

The **Conception Vessel (Ren meridian)** and the **Governor Vessel (Du meridian)** are closely related to our body's organs, no matter whether they are solid or hollow organs. Therefore, many cosmic energy therapy schools' opening or treating points are located at these two meridians. Meanwhile, all schools use the TCM (Traditional Chinese Medicine) meridians as the basic cosmic energy traveling channel to treat diseases.

Some acupuncture points can promote qi and blood circulation to the whole body from a specific area more effectively than others. We are used to opening our hands to make adjustments because they are easy to move, and they have the flexibility to be angled or flipped over. Plus the hands are directly connected to our heart and can transmit our willpower.

Everyone has an innate healing power, and cosmic energy therapy is one of them. As inserting an acupuncture needle into our body, it promotes qi circulation. The qi brings away metabolic waste and stasis-blocking substances such as sputum, blood, qi, and coldness, and brings in nutrients, hormones, neurotransmitters, immune cells, and all the things needed to repair cells. It can help to repair a wound or damaged cells or tissues or organs.

Anything we take in—no matter whether food or water—and all substances that circulate inside our body are in the form of electrolytes. The electrically charged channels on a cell membrane control whether the nutrients, hormones, or neurotransmitters are allowed enter the cell or not. The natural food after digestion produces larger nutrition particles. When the cell needs the nutrient, the cell will send a signal asking the body to secrete a specific enzyme to slice it into smaller particles so it can pass through the channel on the cell membrane.

However, Western drugs and a lot of things sold in health food stores are refined—they are very small particles. Regardless of whether the cells need them or not, they can penetrate the cell membrane and directly enter the cells. This fills the cells with excess nutrients, and they eventually become unhealthy toxins in the body.

Electrolyte-rich qi circulates as a current within the body. That current produces a magnetic field, and thus the human body can be measured as an electromagnetic field. This means a person can be easily influenced by the outside environment. And on the contrary, many of the same kind of people gathered together can affect the environment.

Many people suffering from physical, emotional, and spiritual illness do not feel comfortable or soothed, This blocks the qi flowing in the body meridians and makes their natural healing power gradually disappear. Many people lose it on a conscious level due to not believing it exists and dismissing it as nonsense. They do not understand the theories behind it. This book will uncover the secrets and mysteries for them.

Many of the founders of various cosmic energy therapy schools discovered the therapy by accident. Some of them derived their ability from academic theory, like what I do now. But no matter how they found it, they all attempt to spread this affordable and very beneficial therapy. Discovering cosmic energy therapy and knowing how to teach it is a wonderful gift. One should not be reluctant to teach what he knows so that it can be carried forward and promoted.

There is a time sequence, though, to learn a concept, and there is no limitation on who can own the most complete knowledge first. I hope you as a reader can use your wisdom and good morals to master it and make it even better so that it can be passed down and shared with more people. Then, as an author, I can feel some comfort from your divine contribution.

We are highly expecting all of the Comprehensive Universal Energy Healers' morals and wisdom to enhance the general public's long-term benefits and guide the communities and the whole world to a harmonious and prosperous realm. Here, I give you my most sincere gratitude.

Everyone is born with unlimited potential. As long as you have good will, sincerity, persistence, and perseverance, you have the chance to be successful—or even to be a sage.

Good or bad exists only in the mindset of the people who are involved or using something. If you invent something against the norm, you are often rejected or called crazy. But history will give you quite a list of those who did not give up—the Wright brothers, Henry Ford, and Steve Jobs, to name a few.

"First they ignore you, then they laugh at you, then they fight you, then you win."

—Gandhi.

I have met many individuals who, when they found their own hands had energy, and they could help people heal, stopped doing volunteer healing and charged money, using it to make a living. They did not teach and did not form their own school. So cosmic energy therapy has many varieties. It's not our focus, however, to list their differences. Hope that there will be more researchers for the cosmic energy healing to spread the low cost cosmic energy healing broadly.

We'd simply like to introduce you to some famous schools.

• Yoga

Yoga came from the ancient Indian culture. In 300 BC, the famous sage Patanjali created the "Yoga Sutra". He combined theory and knowledge with the original Indian yoga and formed a complete theoretical and practice system[19]. Yoga has four big branches:

- Raja Yoga, also known as the "Royal Yoga." It includes eight limbs or eight steps through meditation to control the mind to be steady and calm.

- Jnana Yoga talks about the intuitive or luminous knowledge of the yoga. The Brahma Sutras" is the main text of the Jnana Yoga[133].

- Bhakti Yoga uses love to reach the ultimate. It's the path of devotion[134].

- Karma Yoga asks yogis to treat others' pain as their own pain and do their best to help others to relieve the pain in order to perfect the yogis' humanity[135].

Gandhi's "My life is my message" is the best description[135].

The above four are more popular on websites than the earlier yoga.

Many new yoga varieties have come out as well.

Mantra Yoga uses seed sounds to vibrate the body, mind and spirit to their divine level in different regions (i.e. in the different chakras). It goes through more than one thousand repeated chants. The repeated chanting can be used in learning, too. If you cannot understand something in a book, you can repeat it one thousand times, and you will pierce through the meaning barrier.

That's a Chinese study skill listed at the *Di Zi Gui* 弟子規: 書讀千遍，其意自現。 It means if you read one thousand times, the meaning comes out automatically. In other words, when you focus on something that is invisible to you, if you do not give up and hold it long enough to practice one thousand times— which means many times, and not necessarily exactly one thousand— then you break through the invisible obstruction of understanding. It's also one of the secrets of gold medal winners, who practice innumerable times to win. Inventors invent a pattern, and big thinkers spread their thoughts.

Tantra Yoga, also called Ritual Yoga, summarizes ancient and modern knowledge through exercise forms to cultivate life energy and reach a moral realm beyond that of regular people.

I am not familiar with yoga, we are not here to teach or learn it, so let's stop here. But if you have any input, please let us know. It is highly appreciated because we are all coming from the same divine source.

• The Human Bio-Electrical Energy

Human Bio-Electrical Energy was created by a Ceylon philosopher, Dr. Dasira Narada, in the nineteenth century. It requires people to be self-cultivated and combine with the cosmic electromagnetic therapy. However, practitioners need their masters to open their body points (i.e. acupuncture points).

Since its discovery in the nineteenth century, it has become widely distributed throughout the world. Learning is divided into fifteen levels[80]. It can be used to treat humans, animals, and plants. There are touching, short distance, and remote distance therapies available.

• Reiki

In 1920, Japanese Mikao Usui Sensei rediscovered the ancient meridian healing energy[76]. He climbed Mt. Kurama, and he fasted and did penance there. On the 21st day, he felt the Reiki energy and discovered the therapy method known as Usui Reiki (The Usui Spiritual Energy Healing System[14]). Later, in April of 1922, he moved to Aoyama Harajuku, Tokyo and founded an institution in which to teach Reiki[136].

Reiki therapists must go through training. Basically, there are six levels. Some branches even divide to become nine levels[78]. Each learner must have moral cultivation and therapy experience before moving to the next learning class. The student starts with self-healing first. Then moves on to helping others. Then he does group therapy. After that, the student can begin teaching. Each level uses different symbols to do treatments[77].

Reiki therapy can treat humans, animals, and plants. There are touching, short distance, and remote distance therapies available.

With Reiki spreading around the world, its forms have diversified greatly. Some have even claimed their own name[78]. If you are interested, you can follow the reference materials.

- ## Johrei Healing[31]

Johrei Healing was founded by Japanese Mokichi Okada in the 1930s. It uses light to active the body's immunity, regeneration, and detoxification capacities in order to achieve self-healing. Johrei Healing absorbs light into the body to clear its toxins[85].

Purification via intensive praying, love, and light transmission causes a spiritual vibration to generate mental, psychological, and physical reactions. That creates the best personal qualities of the spirit, and the spiritual pollution, chemical additives, drugs, and other poisons are eliminated from the spiritual body. The toxins in the body are resolved and expelled[86].

During the treatment session, the therapist and the clients sit and facing each other. The therapist uses his palms facing the client and scans the forehead, chest, and abdomen for about ten minutes. The client then turns around with his back to the therapist. Then the healer uses his palms to scan the client from the back of the head to the shoulders and down to the tail bone. The client then returns to his original posture, and both of them join together to pray with gratitude[34].

Johrei Healing has a research institute. Therefore, there have been clinical trials at the hospital[32,33,34,35].

- ## Longevitology

Longevitology is a branch of Human Bio-Electrical Energy. It was founded by Linzi Hong, L.Ac. 林子洪中醫師, his sibling Ms. Lin, Zi Zhen Lin 林子珍老師, and her husband Mr. Wei, Yu-Feng 魏裕峰老師 about twenty-six years ago. Learners need someone to open the six acupuncture points on their Governor Vessel. There are classes for beginners and intermediate levels as well advanced classes. They claim to use the light of the cosmic energy.

Longevitology is a nonprofit organization.

Longevitology encourages students to do meditation and adjust other people.

Longevitology can be used for human, animals, and plants. It covers touch, short distance, and long distance adjustments.

• Network Spinal Analysis or NSA

Network Spinal Analysis was founded by a chiropractor named Dr. Donald Epstein around twenty five years ago. The therapy has evidence-based clinical research.

Through consultation, the Network Spinal Analysis therapist asks the patient to awaken her spirit stress and release it. The therapist uses a gentle touch to activate the patient's brain waves, awakening her health and body consciousness. Two unique healing waves spontaneously release the patient's spinal cord and life stress, allowing the spinal cord to realign, enhancing health. The treatment has a total of twelve stages[81]. The most important thing is to find out the differences from before the onset of symptoms and after the onset[82]. It also requires the patient to collaborate cognitively in order to achieve the desired effect.

NSA can be used for people, animals, and plants. The treatment includes light touching therapy.

• Reconnective Healing[9]

Reconnective Healing was discovered in August 1993 by Dr. Eric Pearl, a California chiropractor. Energy flowed through his hands and into his patients. His patients could see an angel, or hear someone talking to them. Dr. Pearl saw miraculous results[15]. Later, many chiropractors joined him in doing research and discovered his therapy was unique. It's different from Reiki and the other cosmic energy therapies.

During a Reconnective Healing session, an EEG scan confirms that significant changes are triggered in the brain and in the cardiac activities of both the doctor and the patient[16]. During the treatment session, both of the therapist and the patient absorb gamma rays and radiate low frequency gamma rays. The therapist radiates light, and the electromagnetic field that surrounds the therapist increases in both the amplitude and oscillation[16].

In laboratory studies, the energy therapy caused measurable gene (DNA) changes and helped repair damage in plants[16].

Reconnective Healing is good for human, animals, and plants. Both short distance and remote distance treatments are available.

- ## Comprehensive Universal Energy Healing (CHUEH)

In October 2012, I began to combine the universal codes of love, gratitude, sharing, and collaboration with the universal energy to create the broader Comprehensive Universal Energy Healing. Cosmic energy includes any form of energy that is available on the Earth. It includes the measurable light waves, electromagnetic waves, gamma rays, and radio waves—plus the universal wisdom also showing as an energy wave. The varying forms of energy have always been interchangeable.

Energy can enter into the body from any acupuncture point and also can be emitted from any part of the body. Another important point to note is that the wei qi guards the outside of the body and eliminates—as much as possible according to each persons strength of immunity to avoid—all hazardous substances entering the body. The stronger and thicker the wei qi, the more power it has against the pathogens invading the body. Of course, positive thinking and a positive mindset can also help expel the negative, sick psychology and help defend against the pathogens invading the body.

January 2013, I began to teach people to practice **Da Zhou Tian**[152] without having anyone help open the acupuncture points, allowing the learners to have the power of universal energy on their hands. If some people were able to sense heat on their hands, they could do self-healing even without practicing Da Zhou Tian. The energy from different people could connect together and synergize the transferred energy. A patient would be able to put his hands on himself during healing and achieve a satisfactory synergistic effect. I also invented many different techniques to enhance the results, and you can learn them later in the book.

CHUEH can treat people, animals, and plants. It can do touch, short distance, and remote treatments. This book, however, will only cover touch and short distance treatments.

In addition to cosmic energy, CHUEH also integrates hand application techniques, Eastern/Western moralities, Traditional Chinese Medicine, Chinese and Western cultural essence and wisdom, meditation, hypnosis, and Dream Builder Coaching and Life Mastery Consultant skills. The Eastern/Western moralities are basically the same, but they express themselves in different ways.

The CHUEH will adopt both profit and nonprofit systems.

Cosmic Energy Therapy Application Scope

Because there is no extensive collection of academic researchers in the academic research database—and also a lack of thorough academic research—there is no detailed description. But we will point out that there is currently a vast field in which to do research. It is worthy of the investment of time and funds to gather data and do a comparison of all of the cosmic energy therapies so that we can expand the application of this economic and successful therapy.

Additional applications are posted on my website universalenergyhealing.us. You can also add your adjustment experiences and results to the readers discussion[137]. The data will be gathered to do an analysis to facilitate CHUEH application, so if you post, you do something to benefit others. Continue to do so to accumulate your merits.

The Other Schools of Cosmic Energy Therapy

They are all applicable to humans, animals, and plants. There was even an instance when a radio's sound recovered— it needed electromagnetic energy to support its function properly[45].

The majority of therapies can do touch treatments, short-range treatments, and remote treatments.

Application scope of disease:

1. Pain (the most basic and common application)
2. Body deformations
3. Internal medicine
4. Tumors[9] and cancers
5. Diseases of spiritual, emotional, or mental illness[31]
6. Five sensory organ problems
7. Spirit possession (very common for many cosmic energy therapy schools)

The Comprehensive Universal Energy Healing Application Scope

It is used for people, animals, and plants.

It covers touch treatments, short-range treatments, and remote treatments.

Application scope of disease:

1. **PAIN SYNDROMES:** There are many cases in clinics that involve commonly seen pain syndromes. For severe pain caused by severe blockages—extra coldness accumulation, blood stagnation, and cancer—clinical trials are still necessary to validate the effectiveness of CHUEH treatments. Please refer to the power of the CHUEH[147] and Pain Relief[148].

2. **BODY DEFORMITIES:** Pop-up Veins[149], protruding thoracic vertebrae bones, chest and rib deformities.

3. **INTERNAL MEDICINE:** heart disease, diabetes, high blood pressure, insomnia, Cold and Flu[150], cough, nonstop nasal discharge, constant drooling, sputum in the lungs, nasal congestion, difficulty swallowing, sore throat, thirst, stomach pain, abdominal pain, menstrual pain, liver area pain, vomiting, stop bleeding[151], etc.

4. **TUMOR:** A uterine tumor patient improved, but she had already arranged a surgery for a couple days later.

5. **SPIRITUAL, EMOTIONAL, AND MENTAL DISORDERS:** depression, anxiety, unhappiness, irritability, easily gets mad, sadness, fear, stress, inability to concentrate.

6. **DISORDERS OF THE FIVE SENSORY ORGANS:** blurry vision, dry eyes, deafness due to kidney yang Qi deficiency, lost smell due to a stuffy nose, runny nose, dry mouth, etc.

7. **ADDICTIONS:** Alcohol and smoking.

In January 2013, I started to teach people how to do self-healing. As time passed, the treatment scope and results increased quickly.

After gaining some experience in self-healing, you can then start to adjust others. It's better to do self-healing first. That way, when you adjust others, it will be easier for you to understand their feelings. It will also be easier for you to answer their questions during your adjustments. For remote adjustments, that means the client will be in another room or perhaps far away on the other side of the Earth. It requires great concentration without any distractions in your mind. You will be taught later until it improves your moral and physical health and lifts your frequency, which will help you transmit your healing energy with or without any medium.

Note:

My Dream Builder Coach and Master Life Consultant were both certified by Ms. Mary Morrissey. Mary is a famous spiritual leader of the world. For more than thirty years, her formula for success has helped thousands of people to succeed and live their dream lives. Her students have had a huge impact on the world and have contributed by creating groups like the Unstoppable Foundation.

Ms. Mary Morrissey, the Dalai Lama, and some other spiritual leaders were invited to the National Union to discuss how to promote world peace.

CHAPTER ONE
Introduction
• • • • • • • • • • • • • • • • •

All life is dignified!
Universal Divine Echoes

Why Write This Book?

Since practicing on land in 2010, my severely ill patients, who reside in neighborhoods within a twenty-five mile radius of my clinic, are considered to be from non-wealthy families. In order to rescue the patients from physical and mental suffering and help them to improve quickly, I taught them exercise, diet, and a healthy lifestyle. I have been polishing my knowledge and treatment skills since that time, looking for low- or no-cost treatments for both my patients and myself. I invested in hefty tuitions to learn from a multitude of instructors, mentors, and coaches.

I had been ashamed of being an acupuncturist instead of a Western medical physician. I hadn't realized that I could turn my patients' life around. Until then, all I saw was my immature view of Western medicine. But I was very surprised to discover that everyone has a natural self-healing power. I realized then the true power of universal abundant love and miracles. We are so accustomed to using costly approaches toward to diseases and health maintenance, but in order to reduce our future generations' medical burden, I think that everyone must accept the responsibility to maintain their own health. We all have the ability to do so.

Some of my patients could not pay for their medical expenses. Some with severe diseases suffered through painful Western medicine treatments that reduced their quality of life. Some patients had unnecessary surgery. Some women had young children and were too busy to take care themselves. Most of my business network members were too busy to visit healthcare providers until they got sick and literally collapsed onto the bed to get some rest.

These people made me feel the urgency to write this book. I hope to plant the concept of preventive health care in the general public's mind in order to cut down on the expensive medical treatments that eat up our younger generation's educational costs and almost everyone's meager fortune. Wouldn't it be nice to spend those exorbitant medical fees on much more useful and meaningful items?

For those patients who encountered diseases and suffered, and for those who died innocently, you are the motivation that drove me to write this book. There are times when I would have enjoyed doing something other than writing, but then I would think that each moment my book wasn't published would mean more lives lost and more innocent patients suffering unnecessarily.

I wrote this book, too, for the numerous patients suffering through chemotherapy, radiation therapy, and avoidable surgeries. I had to smile when I faced patients, but my insides were bleeding. When a patient lost his life, I mourned his unnecessary death and unworthy fate. I deeply feel that **it's better to teach people how to use self-healing to avoid severe diseases**. Therefore, I worked hard to learn how to write, and I sat down and did just that.

Teaching self-healing will let people know how to maintain their own health. It can help more people than I can by using my two hands to treat patients. Even if I worked for twenty-four hours a day without sleep or rest, I could only treat a limited number of patients in a day—or in my life.

I hope that you can heal the people you know and even show them the power of Comprehensive Universal Energy Healing. Encourage them to join our preventive healthcare angel team. We want only happiness and longevity without sickness.

The Benefits of Comprehensive Universal Energy Healing and Self-Healing

1. Universal energy is inexhaustible, and there is no worry about a shortage. We can withdraw in unlimited amounts without paying any usage fees.

2. It is green and environmentally friendly that produces no waste product.

3. There is no need for any medical materials, machinery, or equipment. There are no inventory or cost problems.

4. When encountering a disaster or thunderstorm with electro-magnetic disturbance, medical devices could be affected and have a severe impact on health. In these situations, if there is no medical equipment or device, it's safe.

5. Everyone can learn. You don't need many years of education, and it's easy to learn. If you forget about how to practice Da Zhou Tian[152], go to Appendix Nine References to find the online video or Chapter Five to read the steps so you can remember how to do it.

   The feedback from practicing Da Zhou Tian is your daily improved health. One day in the computer repair lab class, a classmate asked me excitedly to look at his lips. In only one week of practice, his lips had turned from dark to pink in color. Lips represent the health status of the spleen. This classmate had diabetes. He told me that he felt so much better after practicing Da Zhou Tian[152].

   I had another classmate who had a work injury and had quit his job. His worker's compensation had already stopped his medical payments. He learned how to use Comprehensive Universal Energy Healing, and I treated him in three minutes. Thereafter, he practiced Da Zhou Tian[152] and did self-healing every day. He told me his pain was subsiding and that he hoped go back to work soon when his pain was completely gone.

6. There is almost no limitation for places to practice. There's no need to go to a clinic or make an appointment to get healed.

No matter what the discomfort, at any time, you can open your hands for a couple of minutes and can help the person get some relaxation. Please remember, though, that I mentioned earlier that this book does not cover patients with mental disorders.

7. CHUEH is convenient. It can be used at almost any time and in any place.

One time, by accident, I stepped on our dog's tail. He howled painfully and withdrew his tail. It made me fall down on the kitchen's tile floor. The back of my head hit the wall, and I sat down forcefully onto the floor. My eyes were full of stars. I put one hand on top of my head (U3 position) and the other hand at the back of my skull to avoid blood stasis at the striking point. When my headache was gone, I put hands on my hip where it hit the floor. It felt like mild bone fracture pain. After continuously using Comprehensive Universal Energy Healing for a couple of days, the hip pain went away.

A couple of months prior to this accident, I had lunch with friends at an open-air restaurant on a hill. There was beautiful scenery. We enjoyed the breeze, the pretty view, and chatting with young people. I was reveling in the ecstasy happiness, forgetting my age.

After lunch, we took a stroll and reached a place where we might take a detour. If I could jump a couple feet downward, it could save me a couple of minutes walking. I forgot I was over sixty years old, and I jumped down to the road. I hit a stone that was covered by a thin layer of soil, and the impact fractured one of my foot bones.

After several more hours of walking, the pain deepened. Later, I used self-hypnosis to alleviate the pain. It was completely removed for the moment, but when I squatted to the ground that bent my injured foot, the pain came back. After the pain had continued for more than a month, I realized that my self-hypnosis was not the solution in and of itself. I decided to use herbs to treat myself. The pain was completely healed.

8. You are ready to help others at any time. If your friends or relatives have any mild, uncomfortable ailments, you can immediately use your hands to help their problem, purely to help them without charge. Surely, your interpersonal relationships should improve. The healing is especially good for older people who need more services. In addition, they have accumulated a lot of life wisdom. If they give you any advice as feedback, it will benefit you a lot.

9. There are many other benefits…the treasures await you!

The Differences between Comprehensive Universal Energy Healing and Other Cosmic Energy Therapies

1. It includes more than two hundred fifty million years of the wisdom of Traditional Chinese Medicine. It helps you to diagnose and use healing skills in order to get faster and better results. In addition, you learn how to treat your root problems. That is not usually included in the other cosmic energy healing schools.

2. It is developed from TCM, and TCM can explain a lot of it. Therefore, it will not fall within the scope of metaphysics.

3. Its application is different from the other schools where you need to spend a lot of money or take a lot of time to learn. Though mastering the CHUEH takes time, you can soon start treating simple discomfort and health issues. As time passes, you can gradually heal more complicated and severe situations.

4. It does not need to open acupuncture points. So you do not need to rely on others to help you start to do healing.

5. It will not generate any hallucination or fear (at least up until now, it hasn't occurred) as some other cosmic schools have done. Part of it is due to its strong positive energy and expelled negative energy.

6. It's easy to learn. If you learn only Chapter Five, you can start to do healing. However, we highly recommend that you learn more to avoid situations in which you may feel helpless and not know what to do.

7. If its application abounds with the universal codes of love, gratitude, sharing, and collaboration, its powerful effectiveness will be seen sooner, and it will also open the door for your life luck, allowing you to access and absorb abundant universal resources. When these universal codes are combined with self-healing, they will complement each other to achieve synergistic healing effects.

   A person's ethics are directly related to his physical health, whether he is sick or not. Please read Chapter Two for more information.

   I use specific moral characters to guide you to moral cultivation rather than using a broad cultivation without specific guidance. You can follow my books to learn gradually and build up the character of a successful person. Eventually, they will become a habit and will be yours permanently.

8. There is no conflict with any religion. Anyone can keep his faith and still practice Comprehensive Universal Energy Healing.

9. It has gone through peer review from a variety of medical professionals.

10. My broad TCM treatment experiences include tough cases. As a member of the medical profession, I know the limitation of CHUEH and will advise you not to delay a client's professional treatments when necessary.

    It's common to hear that people attended other kinds of healing classes for months without improvement and then gave up. With my CHUEH book(s), you will learn how to make the impossible becomes possible through cultivating your morals, doing good deeds, and practicing what you learned. You will be surprised at what you can do!

The Difference between Comprehensive Universal Energy Healing and Formal Traditional Treatments

CHUEH utilizes universal energy rather than the therapist's personal energy to do healing. The power of universal energy is far greater than any mortal individual's power can be. It benefits both the healer and the client during the healing sessions.

CHUEH includes universal codes that can treat problems of the mind and soul. A lot of sickness today is due to problem(s) in the mind and soul, and those things are not included in the scope of traditional medical treatments. Patients often lose confidence in the medical fields and think they are stuck in in a painful existence. Actually, with a small conceptual mindset change and gratitude for what one has instead of what one does not have, life can be turned around very quickly.

For example, a former patient's mind was full of memories of abuse spanning from childhood to adulthood. She was in constant pain throughout her body, complained a lot, and even had a mobility problem. CHUEH healing and chatting recommended that she empty the garbage from her memory and replace it with a treasure box full of good memories—the fact that her deceased husband left her extra money so that she can enjoy life with financial freedom and without financial worry. For this single thing, she should feel gratitude every day.

Within twenty minutes of using CHUEH, at the mention of her deceased husband, she smiled beautifully, feeling gratitude instead of complaining. Later, she could stand up quickly without the aid of her cane. She even walked briskly with her cane in her hand. Isn't it amazing the kind of power a little mindset change can have?

What are the Limitations of Comprehensive Universal Energy Healing?

It does not cover severe blockage, infection, injury and blood deficiency. Other than that, the limitation is set only by the healer and the client's individual factors.

The Expectations of the Medical Field

Comprehensive Universal Energy Healing does have remarkable healing effectiveness. I first noticed my uniqueness when practicing at sea. I didn't know about cosmic energy healing then, but I discovered my treatments were more powerful than a lot of acupuncturists' treatments on land. I was able to well treat health problems that my patients had had for decades, and even those for which they'd regularly visited acupuncturists. If you want information yourself about my medical history and knowledge, please visit universaltcm. com and follow the links to my other websites to read my testimonials and articles.

If you are in the medical profession, please do not speak against CHUEH. It may be able to assist you with your own health or your business. When you lie down on the bed, you can put your hands on your body to do self-healing, or when you have a patient who can't afford your services, aside from referring them elsewhere, you can use the Comprehensive Universal Energy Healing as an auxiliary tool to speed up that patient's recovery. You can offer the book in your clinic or hold group healing classes to increase your income while at the same time reducing the patient's visit charge. It can be a good thing for you. My hope is that there will be rigorous clinical trials performed in Comprehensive Universal Energy Healing so that its benefits will spread quickly across all disciplines.

The Comprehensive Universal Energy Healer's training is a lot easier and less expensive than a regular medical health care provider such as an MD, nurse, or acupuncturist. It can save a lot of medical costs for governments and insurance companies. In our new era, elderly care is a huge economic issue. Da Zhou Tian[152] is an easy exercise.

There isn't a high cost to build a special exercise room. Patients can simply lie down on a bed or sit on a chair to do it. Teaching patients to help each other do Comprehensive Universal Energy Healing together with universal codes can shorten hospitalization periods. It's something worth considering.

Which Items Are Not Covered In This Book?

Universal energy can penetrate clothes or comforters to do healing. This book does not discuss long-distance healing. Long-distance healing will be covered in more advanced books in the future. This book doesn't cover patients with mental disorders, especially those who are bipolar.

We strongly recommend that you apply Comprehensive Universal Energy Healing to your family members and/or the persons that you already know well in order to avoid adjusting someone who may have severe repercussions during the healing process which you may not know how to handle. The biggest thing you want to avoid is a delay in someone's emergency care, causing severe problems that no one can fix.

How to Study This Book

If you want to own self-healing power immediately, please turn to Chapter Five—"How to Get The Universal Energy to Improve Health." It will teach how to apply Da Zhou Tian[152].

However, if you have the patience to read chapter by chapter, you will gain much more than you will by jumping to Chapter Five directly.

To better help people, please follow through this book series to grow your knowledge and skills. Put your heart into accepting the messages here and study carefully. If you have any questions or ideas to share, please join us and go to the proper readers' discussion[137] website for the chapter of the book you're reading and join the discussion!

All words/word groups in bold and italic are explained in the Appendix Two Glossary.

When you see a small Arabic number in the upper right corner of a word or phrase, please refer to Appendix Nine References, to view the original source material. We express gratitude and give appreciation to the original author's hard work and contribution to the subject matter.

At the end of each chapter, you will find an Investment Revenue Exercise. This is provided to help you in understanding and implementing what you learned in the chapter to increase the value you receive from this book. The exercise will require you to be involved, practice, and participate to consolidate what you have learned and put it into action!

We remind you to pay attention to your body's signals and your feelings. Listen to the still, small voice that your inner great self uses to speak to you. Your inner great self offers the best wisdom and advice.

Why Should We Promote Self-Healing?

It is a common scenario in clinical practices—patients often ignore their body's alarming warning signals. Because of this, the right time to take care of the diseases is ignored, and healing is delayed. When it finally gets to the point where the patient notices, it has already become an emergency or a case for hospitalization. This often leads to regret as irreversible diseases like terminal stage cancer or gangrene have set in.

One day, I had just entered my computer repair classroom and sat down when I asked a twenty-year-old classmate of mine, "What's wrong?"

"I only slept three hours," he told me.

"Why is that?"

"My uncle died last night. Only forty-seven years old. Pneumonia. It's such a shock!"

I explained the relationship of phlegm in the lungs and pneumonia. I also told him that as young as he was, he also had phlegm in his lungs. I touched his hands, and they were warm. Because he usually loved helping classmates, and helping me to solve problems, I taught him to put his hands on his chest, and when the lower part of his hands grew warmer, to wave his hands down. He felt a lot of comfort in his chest. He agreed that if his uncle had been able to use universal energy self-healing early on in his illness, perhaps he would not have died.

If everyone treated preventive health care as important and maintained their health at the highest level, paying attention to moral cultivation, it could save a country's resources so they would not be wasted in the health care system. We could use the money saved on health care to provide free parental education to educate future parents on how to have a healthy baby, giving couples the best health scenario before pregnancy and teaching them how to maintain a healthy and happy pregnant woman. After birth, the newborn would be healthy and smart with a lovely personality. Doing this would create a true win at the starting point of a new life.

Another benefit is that, in many cases, the power of Comprehensive Universal Energy Healing has better and faster effects than acupuncture treatments because the cosmic energy is much stronger than a human's qi. Moreover, it enhances the patient's personality, speeding up recovery and avoiding potential sickness later. It goes well beyond what acupuncture and medical treatments can do.

Except for cases involving cancer, chronic or severe blood stasis, blood deficiency, sticky sputum, chronic scarring, and extra coldness entering the body, CHUEH is successful in healing many health issues. I treat all of the aforementioned conditions with a combination of acupuncture and moxibustion—with or without my unique external herbal formula—and gain exceptional results.

For my herbal formula, please refer to Appendix Eight for more detailed information. It has successfully helped many patients. Two acupuncturists, each with more than forty years' experience, tried my sample and successfully extended their cancer patients' lives.

Universal Expressing

Do you like to watch the clouds and the sunshine? Do you enjoy the beautiful fragrance of flowers? This is the universe's silent way of telling us to be a part of the universe, not an exception. Each person's life is so colorful, rich, and abundant!

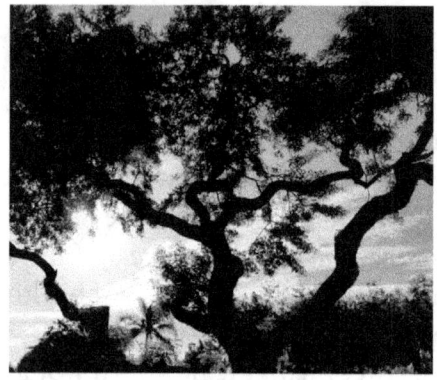

Pic 1 A Peaceful Moment

Pic 2 Colorful Sunshine

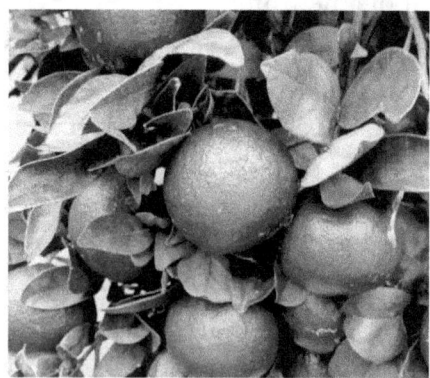

Pic 3 Abundance

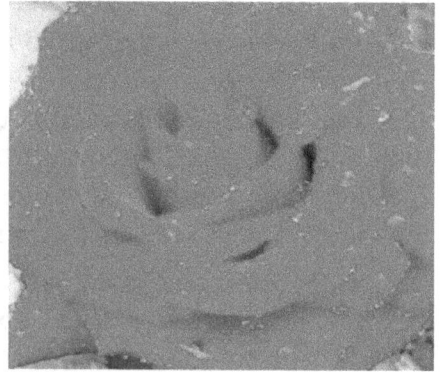

Pic 4 Rose

If you and all of your family members are healthy, congratulations! You belong to a select group. If you want to develop your own or your child's talent, wealth, or anything else in order to have a more glorious life, please contact Natural Born Abundant Ability Recovery Center[162].

Some people think that in growing older, it's normal and expected to have difficulty swallowing, to have to accept pain as a loyal friend (my father's words), to have blurry vision, tinnitus, limp when walking—and the list goes on. This mindset is the result of closed thinking, the thinking of those who have not found the key to good health and have no knowledge of longevity and no one to execute longevity activities. "Aging" is not an inevitable process, and all of the ailments and annoyances listed above don't have to be byproducts of growing older. Thus, I encourage friends, relatives, and colleagues to take care of each other and form a trend to break free from this helpless dilemma. Follow this series' books to feel secure and enjoy life's happiness, abundance, colors, and diversities.

I accompanied my friend to visit two elderly women. For the elderly, especially those with poor mobility living alone at home, Comprehensive Universal Energy Healing is very practical.

One of the women was unable to stand up after sitting down. She had body chills and abdominal pain. She experienced immediate improvement after using Comprehensive Universal Energy Healing. Her children also learned the Da Zhou Tian[152] exercise and joined in the healing. It provided a convenient option for them to care for their aging mother and reduced the inconvenience and the chances of having to bring her to a clinic.

The other elderly woman stayed by herself in the daytime on weekdays while her son was at work. She was deaf in one ear and had blurry vision. She improved immediately from using Comprehensive Universal Energy Healing. Since she needed a cane when standing, I taught her how to practice the Da Zhou Tian[152] while sitting and how to continue use of Comprehensive Universal Energy Healing to maintain the results by herself. Clear vision was especially important to her because the floor of her house was not flat, and she walked with a cane and had poor balance. Because my friend had to move on to her next appointment, I did not have time to help her with her balance problem. However, continuing CHUEH would have been beneficial.

If you want to learn about the scope and quality of our services, please check Appendix Seven Our Websites.

The Purpose of This Book

This book is mainly for preventive health care. It can also be used for the healing of mild diseases or as an adjunctive therapy for severe diseases and disorders.

It also can delay or prevent the problems associated with aging. If, before you're sick and/or experiencing organ degeneration, you do the Da Zhou Tian[152] (which you will learn in Chapter Five) in combination with Comprehensive Universal Energy Healing every day, you can avoid the aging of your organs and body. It can slow down and/or reverse the aging process.

I expect—through the four universal codes of love, gratitude, sharing, and collaboration—to raise your awareness of spirituality and open your pair of love hands to improve each other's health and build closer interpersonal relationships. I hope to purify reader's heart and promote a harmonious society where love floods the earth.

If there is someone nearby who needs help, and you—or they—the application of Comprehensive Universal Energy Healing can reduce your worry and stress. In emergency situations, such as an elderly person falling down or having heart discomfort, it might save many lives and ease the sorrow and regret family feels about being unable to take care of faraway relatives and friends.

The recognition of universal abundant love and having tolerance for all can expand your limited thinking. It will release you from the shackles of a narrow and confined reality and allow you to move bravely towards your merit, your achievement, and ultimately a worry-free life. Let's connect our behaviors, intentions, and motivations with the universe's abundant supply of richness and harmony. Let them forever coexist and prosper together.

Precautions

Though I am a licensed acupuncturist in California, this book cannot and should not replace professional medical services. A licensed acupuncturist in California is equivalent to a Chinese medical physician on mainland China or Taiwan. But in the US, the law does not allow acupuncturists to adjust bones or treat cancer—it only allows acupuncturists *after* chemotherapy and surgery to treat the sequel as well as tonify and balance patient's body.

No matter at what the situation that caused a patient to visit an acupuncturist, after balancing the patient's body, his immunity is boosted. His body's internal environment is no longer fit for bacteria, viruses, tumors, or cancer cells to survive.

As a reader, you may not be a medical professional or a physician. Please note, in the comments of each disease, under what circumstances you should refer the patient to seek professional medical services to avoid delay of treatment or cause irreparable health damage. If, after two to three Comprehensive Universal Energy Healing adjustments, the patient does not improve or can maintain the healing effect only for a very short time, please seek professional medical services immediately.

Note:

When the uncomfortable symptoms disappear, it does not mean everything is okay. For example, if lungs or both the lungs and kidneys have a functional deficiency, there will be symptoms of a cold or flu. You may eliminate the symptoms, but a little while later, the client may be exposed to cold wind and get the cold or flu again. It's not due to a failure in healing.

It's because the root cause was not eliminated. Once the lung and kidney functions have been restored to a larger degree, the client will not easily regain an illness. Therefore, we must eliminate the root cause in the client in order to prevent the health issue(s) from coming back too quickly.

The basic principles of acupuncture treatment and Comprehensive Universal Energy Healing are the same. The following are frequently asked questions in an acupuncture clinic. Please click and read all of the articles listed below for further information:

1. How can I know that I am well healed? Please refer to How do I know that I am well treated?[156].

2. When can I stop the healing adjustment? Please refer to When can I stop my treatments?[157]. If Comprehensive Universal Energy Healing is restricted and must be stopped, the client can spend five minutes a day practicing Da Zhou Tian[152] to allow the qi and blood to flow smoothly. Meanwhile, use the available time to do self-healing.

3. How long should I wait to do the next healing? Please refer to How often should I get treated?[158].

4. How long for each healing session? Please refer to How long do you keep the happy pins (needles) in?[159]

The universal energy's power is stronger than the insertion of needles (happy pins), and its transmission (heat and light) is faster than human invented pins can induce qi flow. But it encounters more severe blockage, and its penetration ability depends on the hardness and/or the thickness of the blockage.

If you are a novice universal energy healer, you can use several things as units of measuring—ten minutes, or when your client tells you that he/she feels better, or when you feel the energy penetrating to the opposite side of the client's body. These are referred to as a healing units. Of course, the latter two are more practical and are of more benefit to the client. The time unit of ten minutes means that you can then move your hands to another site on the client's body.

My patients love to call my needles "happy pins" because the pins truly give instant happiness and help to remove the symptoms and uncomfortable sensations from the body. Moreover, they remove the root causes of a patient's disease.

A happy pin induces qi flow because the qi is made of energy (the yang part or the function part of the qi) and electrolytes of all kinds of particles (the yin part of the qi). The needle is made of a metal that attracts the electrolytes, thus causing the qi to flow.

Acupuncture treatment and Comprehensive Universal Energy Healing cause the qi to flow because qi is composed of both yin and yang. The yin part of the qi is the material contents of the qi—nutrients, water, hormones, neurotransmitters, immunity substances metabolism waste. They exist in the body in the form of electrolytes.

Comprehensive Universal Energy Healing and acupuncture treatment share the same principle. They encourage the qi inside the body to flow more forcefully and in greater amounts.

Once the acupuncturist follows Traditional Chinese Medicine treatment principals to balance your body's yin and yang and the five internal organs, your qi and blood circulation become smooth and balanced, and the functions of the organs are restored. This results in **strong yang (strong immunity)** internal bodily environment that has no room for any disease and/or cancer cells to exist. Unless you or the outside environment shatter this balance, you will remain healthy. If things become out of balance, you will get sick.

A Lament to Today's Medical Field

For more than 2.5 billion years[65], Chinese medicine has been developing into a natural remedy that does not cause harm to the patient. All energy healing methods are within the TCM (Traditional Chinese Medicine) scope.

Huang Di Nei Jing • Su Wen Chapter Seventy-Five:

"...If one has knowledge of astronomy, geography, and medicine, then a person's treatment results can be long-lasting and expand the life span. The practitioner can then teach the general public without any doubts. Medical theories can be passed on to future generations and valued as a treasure...."

From the above, we can know that classic Traditional Chinese Medicine has a wide breadth. Its scope encompasses astronomy to geography and divides into three arts—Tian, Di, and Ren. Tian deals with astronomy. Di relates to geography. Ren has to do with medical things that human beings can do. These three parts are equally powerful.

Modern Chinese medicine does not depend on the abandoned sectors of astronomy and geography, but only discusses the human side. It does not completely cover many important aspects such as hypnosis, moral education, and the four Chinese medicine treasure books—*Huang Di Nei Jing*[113] (Some translated it as "*Yellow Emperor*"), *Shen Long Ben Cao Jing*[114], *Shang Han Lun*[115] and *Jin Gui Yao Lue*[115]. Plus the newly discovered *Huang Di Wai Jing*[116]. These are not taught today in Chinese medical schools.

The teaching of *Shang Han Lun* is limited in schools, but it is needed. Unfortunately, the necessary hours are many, and the available hours are too few.

After graduation, however, there are some students who dedicate themselves to studying or learning from a senior Chinese medical physician who studied and practiced it well. But usually, the majority of acupuncturists rely on continuing education courses, and they are not nearly enough to be able to practice competently.

So modern Chinese medical schools teach less than one third of the classic TCM scope, and the treatment effectiveness is thus far less powerful than that of classic TCM practitioners.

Some of Western medicine's invasive diagnostic methods and treatments cause irreparable damage to the human body. In contrast, in the history of more than two hundred and fifty million years, Traditional Chinese Medicine (TCM) has been implemented in many high moral physicians' hands, such as Shen Long, Fu Xi, Huang Di, Qi Bo, Hua Tou, Bian Que, Zhong Jing Zhang, recent Professor Hai-Sha Ni and many other famous physicians. It comprises a monumental humanitarian medicine system that is the most complete one in the world.

In the time of Spring and Autumn* in the Chinese history • Lao Ran "*Dao De Jing*"[3] said, "The greatest way is the simplest one." If medical schools taught how to achieve health while emphasizing moral education, medical education could be tremendously simplified instead of being so complicated. Additionally, it would prevent innumerable physicians and researchers from investing decades—even lifetimes—only to remain groping in the dark. Medical costs today—medical equipment, facilities, professional expenses—are exorbitant. It would be beneficial to medical schools, institutions, and legislators to invest more time in this issue to benefit the public and cut back on costs for everyone.

In this context, Spring and Autumn do not refer to the seasons. Rather, it refers to a period of war in Chinese history that occurred in the seventh to fourth century B.C. Like the European Renaissance of the 14th–17th centuries. There were many great statemen, politicians thinkers and physicians born.

A Contemplation of Today's World

Ancient people's lives were a lot simpler than those of modern people. They were closer to nature and not as greedy.

Advances in technology bring conveniences. But rapid change in technology also brings a rapid accumulation of environmental waste. How do we recycle the waste so that those living in financially disadvantaged areas don't have to live amid health hazards?

People need to study and solve these problems. A Japanese individual invented a small machine to recycle used plastic and turn it into gasoline. He solved a big problem. Please watch the video "Man invents machine to convert plastic into oil[161]" at youtube.com.

Moral education was very important in ancient China. However, it's not as important now. The yardstick for success includes money, reputation, and social rank. It is focused more on self-interest and making more money than the health of others. Today, there is a downgraded social morality and a poor mindset that is leading humanity to a state of lonely callousness.

If everyone could calm down and think rather than blindly believing the statistical data, things would be a lot better. Statistical data comes from privately funded research by interest groups for their products. We need to think more. We need to not only look at the data but also know the real theories behind them. Perhaps then, today's general public would not be misled so easily!

This book will teach you to practice the Da Zhou Tian[152], do meditation, and use Comprehensive Universal Energy Healing to unblock your body, mind, and soul. The end result is that you will be calm enough to obtain the true wisdom of the universe.

Especially so if people do not mess up science and technology*. Acupuncturists (Chinese Medicine physicians) operate among the mainstream Western medicine, mainly treating its failed cases or cases that have continued for a long time without improvement. This prevents acupuncturists from doing longevity, preventive health, but doing treatments for severe cases or rare diseases. It caused many acupuncturists like me to always feel painful and sad that patients' situations are so bad!

*What is science and what is technology? Science is truth, and it does not change as time passes by. Traditional Chinese Medicine has already passed a 250 million years' test of time. It still exists, and it has been proven to works even when modern therapy fails. Modern technology looks fancy on the surface but can be phased out quickly.

Upon meeting a new patient who has already been through formal medical treatments but has experienced an increase in the severity of the disease, the pain in a physician's heart is sometimes worse than a knife stab to the heart. The acupuncturist knows how to achieve longevity, but the public must be educated about self-health and other options.

Any imperfection or deficiency in a health care system, substandard education, or lack of interpersonal skills can eventually cause physical or mental diseases, and then people look for a health care professional's help. The basic problem is that if the patient's mindset or skills for handling things and relationships is not right or not good enough or social value is deviated from ethic, how can a health care professional relieve the sickness? It's out of the formal medical school teaching scope. Patients need transforming programs to correct concepts, fear, mindset with a broad needs.

Chinese medicine has more than two hundred and fifty million years of experience in fighting diseases, and countless caring physicians have studied and verified many theories. It has been used to treat many diseases that Western Medicine could not conquer— diseases like SARS, auto-immune diseases, and blood diseases. In addition, Chinese Medicine is the crystal of humanity's wisdom that uses minimal surgery and avoids painful physical tests. All this is replaced by simply reading the body's signs for diagnosis.

There are many knowledgeable medical researchers. One should understand that knowledge and wisdom are not entirely equal. Much knowledge is only a part of the truth. However, wisdom is comprehensive and has wide applicability. Ancient Chinese medicine has evolved from the book of Yi Jing. It is metaphysical. It has convincing power.

Why Should You Study This Book?

1. Anyone who wants to keep his health top-notch, maintain face and body in the most attractive state, does not want to suffer pain, and wants to ward away physical and mental illness should study this book. Aging and being out of shape are signs of disease and substandard health.

2. Anyone who wants to keep productivity at the highest level should study this book in order to achieve their best performance.

3. Anyone who is suffering from pain or emotional disturbance, insomnia should study this book.

4. Anyone who has loved ones who have pain or any other physical or mental health disorders—insomnia or mental stress, unhappiness, anger, motor mind, heart palpitations—should study this book, both to express your concerns to them and help them feel better,

5. Anyone who enjoys helping others should study this book. If a colleague has discomfort, you will have the ability to mentally soothe his emotions to calm him down and let him feel better physically.

6. Any Reiki healer, energy healer, or person in a medical profession who wants to learn Chinese medicine diagnosis or learn how to treat root problems should study this book in order to know the wisdom of Chinese medicine.

Who Should Buy This Book?

1. If you want to express your concern for health and happiness to your loved ones on Mother's Day, Father's Day, birthdays, Thanksgiving, New Year or any other day worth giving a gift, this book is the best choice.

2. Employers should buy this book to give as a gift to their employees. It will ultimately give them physically and mentally healthy employees, save on their employees' health insurance premiums, improve their employee's productivity and life satisfaction, meanwhile cut down on employee turnover rate, sick leaves, accident insurance premiums, disability insurance, worker's compensation cases and legal proceedings.

3. Organizations and religious groups can give this book to their members, clients, and supporters.

4. Anyone who lives in the countryside or a remote area where it is not convenient to visit a doctor, this book is a must to have, and you ought to study it thoroughly.

5. Hospitals that would like their patients to recover quicker and discharge promptly should not only purchase this book but offer Comprehensive Universal Energy Healing classes to their patients and patients' family members or caregivers.

What Benefits Can You Get From This Book?

1. By practicing Da Zhou Tian[152], you open the body's acupuncture points to receiving universal energy. The acupuncture point is the channel of our body that communicates with the outside world. Acupuncture points accept the universal energy entering the body to enhance our body's energy.

2. Your body's energy will increase, which means that your energy frequency increases as well. Both your physical and emotional health improve as a result.

3. Meditation opens your wisdom and your third eye as well as lifts your spirit level so that you can more easily receive universal

energy. Meanwhile, it creates the path by which you can achieve your life, career, and academic success. It gives you peace of mind so that you can be more alert to the people and things around you as well as the things that could happen soon.

4. *Huang Di Nei Jing • Su Wen • Chapter Three—Alive Qi Connects with the Universe*

   "If universal energy is clear and clean, then your will and intention are under control. If you follow it, the yang qi is anchored. Even if there is evil (pathogen) existing, it cannot do harm..." If a person follows the nature qi, then this person's qi can be balanced and stabilized. Even when there is outside pathogens invading, it cannot harm the person. The natural qi offers indispensable nutrients and nourishment to a human being's organs.

5. When you practice the universal codes, you open the door to the richness of the divine universe.

6. When you practice the universal codes, you open the gate to your heart. That increases your life satisfaction and increases your value. You will be more respected and welcome.

7. Practicing the universal code of sharing makes you emerge in the world of the givers' happiness. You can share a smile, a greeting, an encouraging word to soothe a person's loneliness. You also can share your knowledge by writing a book or post a blog to benefit people without their hard working money, be cheated or whatever. When you do things benefit the others or meaningful, you enoy a giver's happiness.

8. When healing another person, the universal energy goes through us to transmit into the other person. Therefore, our body also gets the universal energy to do healing and improve our own health.

9. By helping others, you have accumulated good deeds that can help either you or your loved ones find reward and avoid bad luck.

10. Investment Revenue Exercises give you back the cost of this book ten or a hundred or thousand times.

Learn the advantages of Traditional Chinese Medicine, but also understand why and how it treats diseases. Treat TCM knowledge as a part of your daily common sense, and use it to maintain your own health rather than blindly following the wrong messages given in commercials on television.

The Perceptions of Medical Life in Recent Years

It's already been a few years since I returned from the cruise ships to dry land to practice. I had profound feelings that the medical field was a mess, so I temporarily gave up my clinic to write this book. My hope is that everyone can have greater health and more medical understanding. Many people have fear and lack self-confidence, but they have no idea of their great potential and infinite creativity. They can create opportunities.

People forget what they own and only see what others have. Their inner selves feel poverty and are greedy without satisfaction. They are insatiable and ungrateful. They are selfish and have no concern for others. They don't share and never cooperate. Please read Raise Up Your Energy Frequency to Avoid Sickness[160].

1. Because of greed and because food industries fear losing business and profits, they ignore their clients' health by adding chemical flavorings. It is bad for the descendants and it pollutes the environment. People feel helpless and say, "I go to the supermarket, and I don't know what to buy." Natural, organic food is not easily accessible.

    It is not only causing medical costs to soar, but it's also triggering natural and manmade disasters. We are losing our serene, happy society and our lives.

2. The entertainment industry has a saying "Ten years' hard work for one minute on stage." As a health care provider, sometimes we want to treat a disease, but it may take a decade of hard work and a lot of money to learn from others. Unfortunately, many people do not understand this concept.

3. Before, when people got sick, it was usually a physical illnesses. In recent years, when people get sick, it is often mindset disease. This has caused a deepening of the practice the cosmic energy healing plus using the universal codes to do self-healing and helping others to heal in order to raise frequency, the total frequency of body, mind, and spirit. Through practice, you can raise your energy healing scope and level. This will lead to spiritual healing and will allow you to conquer diseases.

Investment Revenue Exercise

Think of yourself, your loved ones, your best friends, and your colleagues who have health issues. After learning some healing skills from this book, you will be able to help them.

Adding the names and the corresponding health issues for each one on the list can increase your enthusiasm to learn. Later, you can easily find a target from the table on whom to practice your Comprehensive Universal Energy Healing. You can design your own form or copy the form provided for you below. As you learn more, you can gradually add more people so the table below will grow longer and longer.

You can fill in the last column of "I Discovered Issues" after you read the fourth and the eleventh chapter of the book. It will help you decide where you should put your hands.

Name	Health Issues Waiting for Improving	I Discovered Issues

CHAPTER TWO

The Root of Health and Wealth

● ●

Know what is within you,
even if others can't see it.[118]

Michael Jordan

Once upon a time, a yellow cat asked a young boy, "Where can I find a wealth of foods and enjoyment without having to do any work?"

The boy replied, "It's all within one of your tail hairs." From that moment on, the yellow cat spent his entire life chasing his tail when he should have been looking for food to alleviate his hunger. There were plenty of creatures that the yellow cat could have hunted to feed himself. But he gave up trying to catch them by himself.

The black cat, however, did not hear the conversation between the boy and the yellow cat. So he hunted for his food and enjoyed a lot of free time to play and enjoy sleeping in the sunshine.

Actually, there was food available for the yellow cat to obtain without too much hard work. But he worked his life away chasing his tail hairs without any true enjoyment. It's the same with most people today— they listen to the wrong messages and waste their lives chasing their tail hairs in search of wealth and riches instead of doing as the black cat did by relying on his natural ability to hunt for food and enjoy life.

This story is commonly played out in contemporary society. People forget the abundances of nature in the universe.. They rely on the wrong messages to make decisions and but waste their whole lives chasing after money and material things. The yellow cat was not using his head by chasing his tail. A smart cat like the black cat always lets his tail follow his head and is therefore never short on food or the pleasures of life.

There is no need to chase after wealth. Let wealth chase you once you have the skill and knowledge that everyone desires and needs. Keep polishing your profession. Be persistent. Believe in yourself, for what you have is better than anything else!

In 1965, a Korean student went to Cambridge University to study psychology[165]. During afternoon tea time, he often went to the school coffee shop for a cup of coffee and listened to some of the conversations between successful people—Nobel laureates, academic authorities in a number of fields, and others of that ilk. They declared that their successes were very natural and logical.

When in Korea, this student had been misled by some locally successful people. In order cut competition, they tried make new entrepreneurs quit. They exaggerated their entrepreneurial hardships and used their own success stories to frighten those who were not successful. As a psychology student, he believed it was necessary to study the mentality of the successful people in Korea.

In 1970, he submitted his thesis "Success is Not as Hard as You Thought" to the founder of modern economics psychology professor, Mr. Will Braden. Professor Braden read his thesis and was very excited. He thought it was a new discovery, although the phenomenon was prevalent throughout the world and even more in the East. But there was no one who had yet so boldly proposed and studied it.

He wrote to his Cambridge alumni, the President of South Korea—Mr. Park Chung Hee. He stated in his letter that he couldn't say how much this thesis would help Mr. Park, but he was sure it could produce an influence more than any one of Mr. Park's decrees. The thesis ended up being a factor in South Korea's rise in economy.

Later, this student became a successful businessman and then the President of KIA Motors Corporation in South Korea.

Sometimes success comes from more than hard work and struggling through extreme hardships. Sometimes it comes from seeing things from a new perspective. If you have an interest in a career, be bold and stick with it, and you will succeed. You have more than enough time and wisdom to accomplish your dream.

It's not because a thing is difficult that we don't dare to do it, it's not daring to do it that makes it difficult. In other words, those who are capable dare to do things naturally. We all have the ability to solve tough problems if we make the decision to do so—and never give up until we find the needed solution.

Let us now return to our main topic and learn some basic knowledge that will help us to gain our natural self-healing power.

What Is Qi?

In Chinese medicine, qi is one of the circulatory systems in our body.

Qi has yin and yang parts. The yang maintains body functions and is the energy part of qi. The yin circulates materials—nutrients, water, hormones, neurotransmitters, metabolism waste, and lymph fluid. All exist in the form of electrolytes. That's why inserting acupuncture needles can start the qi flowing.

1. Qi moves materials through the body to deliver nutrients, detoxify, and expel blockages. Therefore, it controls blood, lymph, and fluid circulation, sperm production, and endocrine secretion. It governs body growth, reproductive functions, and all organs' normal functions as well as stabilizing the nervous system and emotions.

2. Qi warms up the body and adjusts the body temperature to maintain the optimal environment for the body.

3. Qi defends against coldness, wind, dampness, dryness, summer heat, and fire. Inside our body, it controls the body's immune system.

4. Qi consolidates (some books call it an astringent function) and governs all body fluids, including storing them and keeping fluids such as blood flowing through blood vessels. It also keeps all organs and tissues in the right place, keeps their shape, and ensures that nerves and blood vessels grow in the right direction.

5. Qi vaporizing transforms material and energy. It also connects body and spirit. It controls and binds the soul and body, and it controls the state of water inside the body (such as absorbing water from the large intestine or vaporizing water and sending it to the lungs to distribute to the skins). When a person dies, his soul leaves his body. Therefore, raising his spirit can improve his health. On the other hand, it controls qi, blood, essence, and fluid. It also controls different material states of mutual transforms i.e. control body metabolism.

Smooth Qi Circulation And Healthy Relationships

The root of health in life is the smooth flowing of the qi. When the qi can flow free and unimpeded in our bodies, this, coupled with having good mental and physical health, would mean there would be virtually no disease.

The Fundamentals of Health and Wealth

We have the body, the subconscious, and the super-conscious (soul). They are mutually influenced. They are also closely related to our health and wealth. Please refer to the following chart.

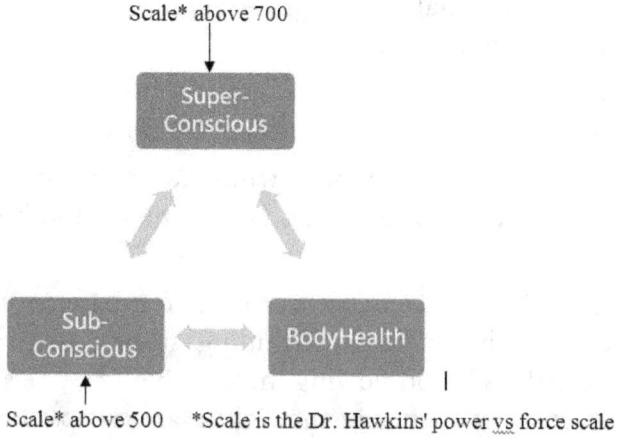

Fig 1 The Dr. Hawkins' score for opening the subconscious and super-conscious

The body maintains our daily activities. Less blockage of qi and blood flow makes for better health—and thus there is more enjoyment of life.

The subconscious controls our health, our shape, our talents, our ability, and our wealth. The subconscious never rests. It even works for what you want—such as your desires or dreams or eliminating your worry—while you are resting. If you can connect with it and activate it, it helps you create what you want and has a magical efficiency. The key to doing it is to let your frequency match the job that you want it to accomplish. The bigger the dream is, the higher the frequency needed.

The super-conscious links us to the universal abundances. It can heal us physically and mentally if we sincerely ask it to do so from the heart. The super-conscious allows us to harmonize with the universe.

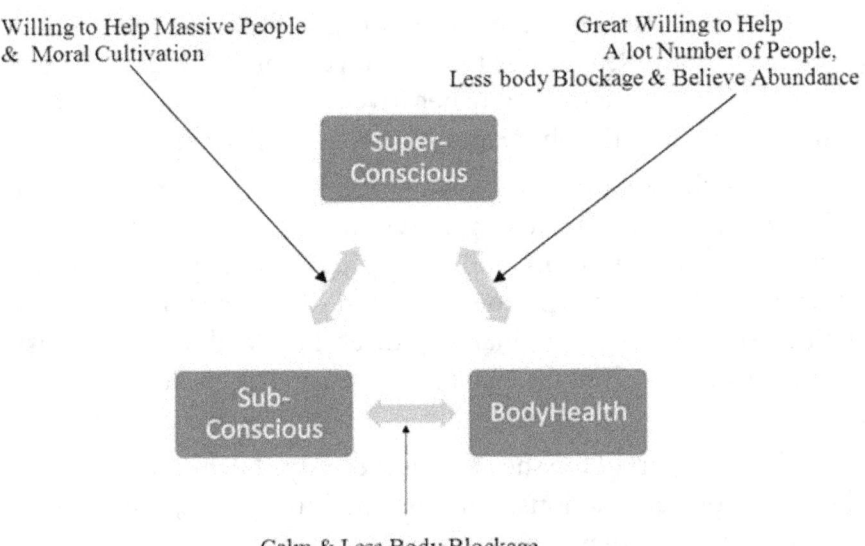

Fig 2 Health Relationship for Body, Subconscious, and Super-conscious

From the above chart, it's important to realize that body blockage can block our access to the benefits of health, wealth, universal abundances, and even happiness. Therefore, the book series starts with unblocking body blockage by applying Comprehensive Universal

Energy Healing. Through practice, the universal codes will also help to improve your health. If you learn the benefits of practicing the universal codes, you will gradually open your subconscious.

Later, after you open your body blockage, we will guide you in accessing your subconscious and super-conscious.

In Chinese medicine, the heart is the monarch of all the organs. It maintains body temperature and circulation to maintain metabolism and body functions. It hosts the shen 神 that includes one's virtue, the wisdom showing in the eyes and the vitality of the whole body and body health.

The invisible part of the shen is the bridge which connects us with the divinity of the universe. The invisible shen is the Western culture's concept of mind and soul. If the heart is healthy, the shen can reside within, and the person will be happy and joyous.

In Chinese medicine, any deviant organ function will show the organ's emotion. Please refer to Appendix Four Basic TCM Theory. The prolonged existence of any negative emotion will go right to the heart, altering it to the abnormal emotion of unhappiness.

It is much like a country—when the people in the country are sick, and their mindset is wrong, the county is turbulent, the monarch is full of worry and unhappiness, and gradually the country's prosperity goes down. The country could divide, change ruler, or be subjugated—unless the monarch himself has wisdom, or at least a wise statesman, can put trust and braveness in the wisdom to help get the country back to normal.

The visible part of the shen shows the body's health, shape, vitality, alertness, correct reactions, emotion, mobility range, and speed. A healthy heart can guard the body organs' health and maintain their highest functioning status. In order to achieve this state, it needs not only a healthy heart but also healthy organs. This means if any organ function is deviated, it should be fixed as soon as possible.

Our body has a very strong healing ability. When the pathogen(s) or emotional hit or accident is so strong that it exceeds our body's self-healing ability, we start to feel discomfort and need to seek help to fix it as soon as possible.

It's a transformational process, and you need to take action and practice what you learned from the book in order to be transformed and enjoy the benefits. Otherwise, you will hardly see a big improvement. If you need a training program or need to hire a coach to help you transform faster so as not to delay your healthy and wealthy life, please visit our website at universalenergyhealing. us/events.

It is important to know that achieving your dream life is like entering a locked room. Your key should match the lock exactly. To live a richer life, depend on your skill. Turn your frequency (skill) high enough to match that necessary to achieve a high income. But don't be afraid to take the necessary actions to make that kind money.

Otherwise, you may still live a less wealthy life—even with your precious skills. That could mean you never attain your dream life—or you reach it at a much later time in life.

We Are Abundant

We are all born with a wealth of abilities. One of the most important abilities is self-healing. It helps us live longer, healthier, happier, and better lives.

Here are some important things to keep in mind:

1. A Harvard University study showed that 98% of two to three-year-old children are geniuses. But only two percent are geniuses at twenty years of age. This report has shown that everyone is born with abundant talent. Due to family, school, and society's education, children's talents are limited by a fixed frame and lose their genius. There are ways, however, to reeducate to recover the natural born talents.

   We have far more talents than we can imagine. There are many ways you can excavate and develop these talents. Education and training, including meditation and hypnosis, are feasible ways to develop the ability in your subconscious.

2. Our lives should be full of love and happiness. Once a person owns health and has a healthy heart, a sense of happiness and

joy will naturally exude from the heart. True inner beauty will be exposed, and the person will love his life and count every day as a blessing. This is the most natural, real, and valuable human beauty—and it's available without spending any extra money for makeup!

One of my patients had experienced a few decades of abuse. She often woke up from nightmares in the night. After my treatments had restored her health, she asked me why her life was so full of joy—she always wanted to smile. I told her, "This is our true nature—to naturally emit a smile from the heart, just like a baby."

3. The level of the truly happy life is far richer than our finite minds can imagine. Based on your current situation and unique talents, through successful modeling and applying feasible methods, you will be successful in transforming your thoughts and behavior patterns. Continue your transformation with your coach's guidance and encouragement, and own the health, wealth, relationship, time, and money you deserve. These methods have helped thousands of people successfully achieve their dreams. They live in their dream life, continuously improving and expanding.

We offer related courses. Please visit Natural Born Abundant Ability Recovery Center[162] to learn about them and register for the classes that best fit your needs. The most important business of the Natural Born Abundant Ability Recovery Center is to transform your thoughts, attitudes, and behavior so that you can gradually explore your talents and eventually peer into your great self.

The Key To Opening Universal Abundance

There are keys which allow you entrance into the universe of infinite love, joy, talent, and wealth. The tools to getting the first key are the universal codes of love, gratitude, sharing, and collaboration. In later chapters, we will teach you how to use these universal codes during your energy healing or meditation.

The route to abundance is regulated by four laws—the law of ethics, the law of service, the law of standstill, and the law of sacrifice. These laws have regulated and helped to create many great people in human history as evidence of their existence.

A proverb says, "People feel joy when there is a happy event!" Whenever there is love, there is joy or surprise. When one falls in love, one can think and learn faster with higher productivity.

Sharing with another is better than going it alone. Why can we not use it to open the door to success? One who shares can get more feedback and live a more colorful and rich life. The development of universal energy healing as a self-healing method is my way of sharing my medical knowledge and skills with you. It will bring innumerable benefits and will enhance your health, happiness, productivity, and satisfaction. It will reduce health care costs and simplify health care complications. It opens up a needle-free and drug-free territory in the medical field. It is a product of Traditional Chinese Medicine theories, universal energy healing, hypnosis, dream building, and life mastery.

We also know that if goes to a big influence activity or a big project, only go through team work to collaborate different expert be easier to achieve the desired result.

Modern Pitfalls

Many people put one hundred percent their health in their health care providers' hands. But this not only ignores the power of self-healing but also loses the concept of self-care. They are not taking responsibility for their own health but are instead allowing health care professionals and the community to bear the burden of their medical care. This choice affects both their health, as they must bear the pain and suffering of their diseases, and their purses.

Why not use self-healing power to keep their youth and save money on healthcare?

In the today's materialistic world, people so often compare their possessions with those of others. This not only leads to the loss of human simplicity, but it also discards the key you need to enter into universal abundance. People think that to make money, they must neglect morality. Thus, they trap themselves in their manmade scourge.

What Will You Get If You Practice What You Learn From This Book?

If you follow the guidelines in this book and do your homework every day to put the method into action, you will notice the universe giving you a lot of inspiration, joy, and early warnings. You will gradually enjoy life in satisfaction and abundance. You can avoid disasters and move continually toward good fortune as early as possible.

If you follow the book and do Da Zhou Tian[152] and self-healing, you will have health and joy. It helps you keep alert, make quick responses, feel energetic, make smarter choices, keep a youthful appearance, and maintain good body shape. You will be able to naturally express your gratitude and life satisfaction without unneeded worries and fear. You will respect and love others as well as be loved and have good interpersonal relationships.

If you can save the money you would normally spend visiting a doctor, you are already richer than before. In addition, the appearance of more joy will bring you unexpected good fortune and opportunities for wealth.

Investment Revenue Exercise

In the table below, list five people you like who have had the most influence in your life. You can list more if you like, and if you're young and don't have a long list of influential people, you can list fewer. But be sure to write at least one person's name. Write their names, their relationship to you, and the impact that the person had on you. If you can remember, please also put down how old you were at the time.

Name	The Influence to Me	My Age at That Time

1. Do meditation—Choose one person from the above list and give your gratitude to that person.

   - Take a deep breath.
   - Slowly inhale through the nose, and then slowly exhale through the nose or a slightly open mouth.
   - Slowly inhale through the nose, hold your breath three to five seconds, and then slowly exhale.
   - Repeat three to five times.
   - Slowly close your eyes.
   - Clear everything from your brain. Empty it and do not think about anything.
   - Relax the skin on your skull. Relax the facial muscles and the neck muscles.
   - Relax your spine from the top of the neck. Relax it section by section until you reach the last section of the tailbone.
   - Relax your chest muscles and upper back muscles.
   - Relax your abdominal muscles, your waist, and your lower back muscles.
   - Relax your shoulders, upper arms, elbows, forearms, wrists, and hands until you reach your fingertips.

- Relax your hips, upper legs, knees, lower legs, ankles, and feet to the tips of your toes.

- Set your internal time machine back to the past, to the happiest time with your benefactor. Meanwhile, express your maximum gratitude to this person. You can also chat with him.

- Write down his reaction and your feeling.

2. Share your experience and your feeling of meeting your benefactor with anyone you trust and are willing to share with. Alternatively, you can go to the comments column of the book's website Chapter Two and write down your comfortable feeling to share with the other readers.

3. Every day, choose a different person from the list in your table, and repeat steps 2 and 3 until you have given your gratitude to everyone.

CHAPTER THREE
Introduction to Healing Cases
• • • • • • • • • • • • • • • • • • • •

Heart stashes spirit, lungs stash qi, liver stashes blood, spleen stashes muscle, kidneys stash will, and thus they form the outer shape. When the will and intention are connected, internally connected with bone marrow, they form the body shape and five solid organs. The five organs essential to circulation are all coming out through their channels in order to deliver blood and qi. Blood and qi are not harmonized, and it causes all kinds of diseases. Therefore, treating diseases should tune the channels to ensure smooth flowing.

《*Huang Di Nei Jing·Su Wen • Chapter Sixty Two Theory for Tuning Meridians*》

As a therapist, I like to test and study the water flow ahead of time before deciding to get into the water or not. But the majority of people like to jump into the water first to decide whether or not to stay in the water.

Well, the water that is this book has already been studied and tested for more than two years by me. So I am going to share with you now some fun cases that were hidden in the water. But I advise you to keep the table for later reference.

CHUEH Application Cases

Below pictures were taken after the original treatments by using a model. So please do not worry that the gender is different from the case. Thank you for your understanding.

1. A new friend who sat beside me in a workshop was holding his head. He told me he had a headache. During break time, I put one hand on his top of his head at the **Baihui** (Baihui is an acupuncture point.) and another hand on his right head migrant painful side. Five minutes later, he thanked me—he felt fine already.

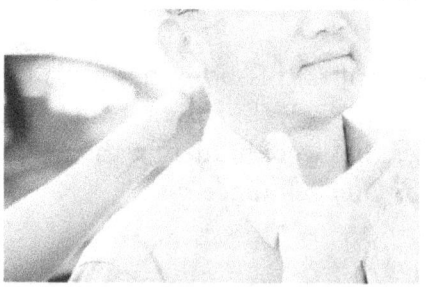

Pic 5 U3 (Baihui) and Migrant Painful side

2. At a health fair event, a booth owner came to try my Comprehensive Universal Energy Healing for his neck pain. I put my hands on his front and back neck. Nine minutes later, the booth owner stood up and told me that his pain was gone.

Pic 6 Neck (Front and Back)

3. One day, during lunch time, a classmate of mine complained about his neck and shoulder pain. I put one hand on his Baihui and another hand on his neck until he said that his neck pain was gone. Then I moved my hands to the center of each shoulder until he said the pain had gone. The total time used was only twenty-five minutes.

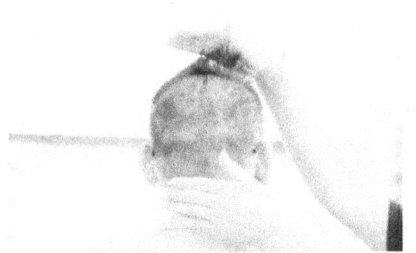 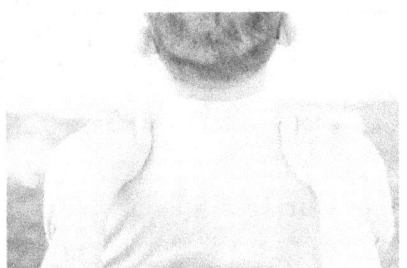

Pic 7 Baihui and Neck (B*)   Pic 8 Shoulders
       *B: Back.

4. During a break between two sessions of a workshop, the person in the seat next to me talked about her left shoulder and upper back pain. I discovered that her upper left back ribs were a little bit deformed. I told her what I had found and said that she should not to put too many heavy things in her purse. I then put one hand on her left shoulder and one hand on her left scapula (shoulder blade). Fifteen minutes later, she happily told me that her pain was gone.

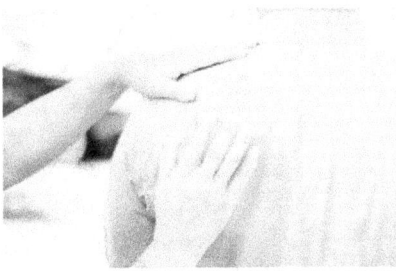

Pic 9 Left Shoulder and Scapula

5. A workshop attendant came to me to ask for help with his chest distention. I put one hand on his back heart area and another hand on his right upper back in the lung area. Ten minutes later, he showed gratitude for his chest distention not existing anymore.

Pic 10   Heart and Lungs (B)

6.   During a fifteen-minute break from a workshop, I went to the restroom. After I had returned to my seat, a young girl came from across the room and told me that the person sitting next to her had suggested she come to me to ask for help with her back pain. After asking permission, I touched her upper spine and discovered that her sixth theoretic vertebra bone protruded backward. I looked at the clock on the wall and saw there were only ten minutes left in our break.

I told her that I would give it a try, but it might be not enough time to fix her pain. I put hands on her Baihui and T6. Surprisingly, before break time was over, the girl told me that she was fine. I asked permission to check her spine again. All of her theoretic vertebra bones were aligned well. For T6 on the spine, I put my hand right above the lower edge of the scapula (shoulder blade).

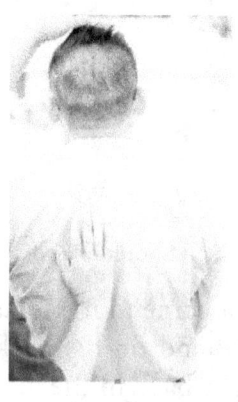

Pic 11   Baihui and T6

During the adjustment, I could feel that the energy flowing on her spine was strong, so I asked her if she helped people a lot. She said yes, she helps street musicians to post their songs on the Internet. When the young girl returned to her seat, break time was not yet over. I thought to myself then that the power of Comprehensive Universal Energy Healing is unbeatable.

7. A classmate came to me during lunch hour and asked for help for her lower back pain and soreness. I put my hands on her Baihui and L2 until I felt the qi flowing smoothly in her spine. I then moved my hands to both kidneys until all of her discomfort was gone. It took around twenty minutes.

L2 is on the spine, two discs above the level of the upper edge of the illiac bone (hipbone). It's the location of the acupuncture point Mingmen. It controls both kidneys' functions. The kidney controls lower limb circulation. Strong kidneys can prevent lower back pain and/or soreness.

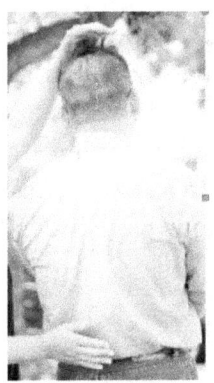

Pic 12   Baihui and L2

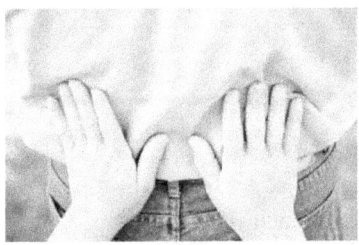

Pic 13   Both Kidneys (B)

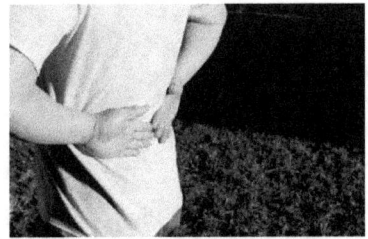

Pic 14   Both Kidneys (B)

8. A friend came to my hotel room. She lay on the bed and asked if I could offer any help for her that her hip that was sprained the night before because of the soft mattress on her bed. I asked permission to do a touching diagnosis and discovered that only part of her hip muscle was tight. In Chinese medicine, the spleen controls the muscles. So I put one hand on my friend's spleen area and another hand to her painful hip area. Ten minutes later, my friend jumped up and said, "Let's go for dinner!"

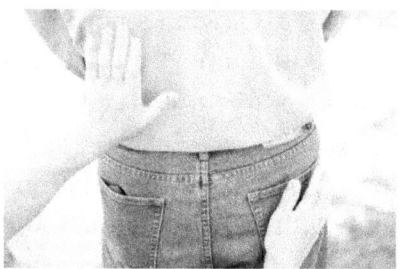

Pic 15   Spleen (B) and Hip Painful Area

9. While visiting a friend, as soon as I entered the door, she ran to the bathroom and vomited. She came out but still felt nausea, so I put one hand at Baihui and the other on her stomach area until I felt her energy flowing on her head. Then I moved my hand from the Baihui to her liver area. Twenty minutes later, she felt fine and told me that her emotions were much better.

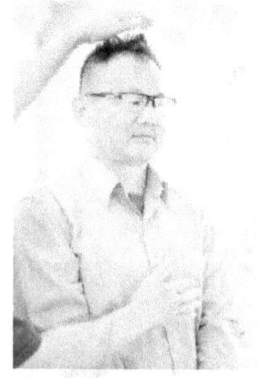

Pic 16   Baihui and Stomach (F*)
*F is the Front

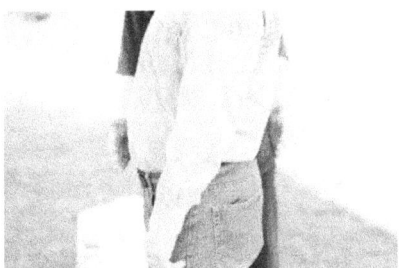

Pic 17 Stomach (F) and Liver (B)

10. After class had ended, a classmate came and asked for help with her abdominal bloating. I put one hand on her Baihui and one hand on her lower abdomen. After feeling the heat moving on her head, I moved my hand from her head the back of her abdomen until she felt no bloating sensation there. It took fifteen minutes.

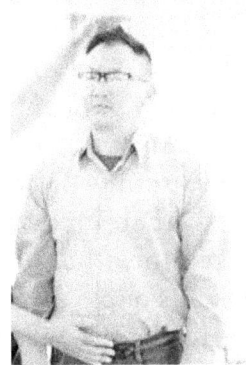

Pic 18   Baihui & Lower Abdomen (F)

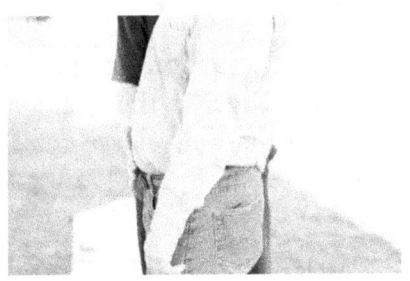

Pic 19   Abdomen (F & B)

11. A workshop attendant came to me and told me that his right elbow and right wrist were in pain. I put one hand around his right elbow and the other over his right wrist. Fifteen minutes later, he was pain free.

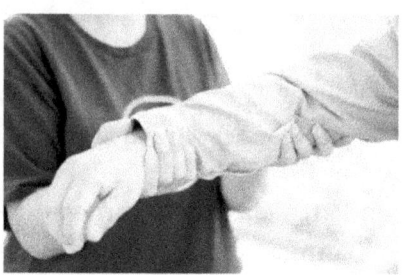

Pic 20 Right Elbow and Wrist for pain
between elbow and wrist

12. After the end of a workshop, two female attendants still sat on chairs after everyone else had left, I approached them and asked if they needed any help. One told me that her right knee was hurt, her right ankle was very swollen, and it would be difficult for her to drive from LA back to San Diego. I sat down with them and put my hands around the woman's right knee until she felt her pain relieved. Then I moved my hands to her front of her heart area* and put the other hand at T5. The total time was thirty-five minutes. A couple of men came in and told us that the room needed to be cleaned out and readied for an evening event. At that time, the swelling had been reduced by fifty percent. The woman told me that as long as she could bend her ankle, she would be able to drive back. So the adjustment stopped, and we left.

For the majority of people, T5 is on the spine locates two thoracic bones above the lower edge of the scapula (shoulder blade). For more detailed information, please refer to Appendix Five Locations for Important Acupuncture Points and Organs.

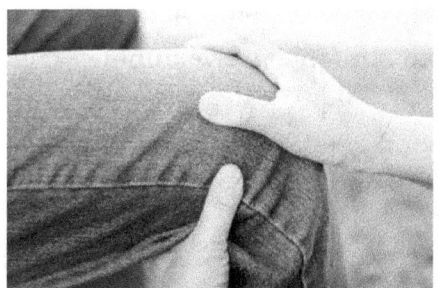

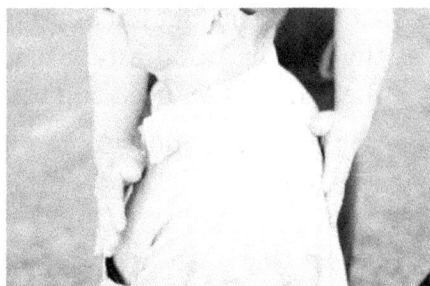

Pic 21 Around the knee   Pic 22 Heart (F) and T5 (B)

* Poor heart function can cause ankles to swell. Heart problems are the number one killer in the US, so we will teach you how to diagnose those problems in our book about heart and blood vessel issues.

On a side note, I recently encountered some friends' parents who were either sick or had fallen. It made elderly care a high priority on my list. Please go to new book content recommendation[166] Chapter Three[167] to make suggestions about other things you would like to learn. If a number of people request the same thing, I will write and publish earlier.

13. A lady came to me and asked for help with her right leg and ankle that were swollen, painful, and numb. I put one hand on her left knee and one hand under her left ankle. Twelve minutes later, the pain and numbness had gone and the swelling was reduced.

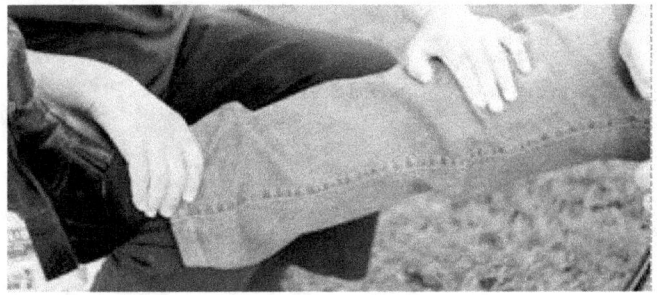

Pic 23 Right Knee and Ankle

14. At lunch, a woman sat beside me complaining about right lower leg and Achilles' tendon pain. She asked for help, so I put one

hand on her right knee and one hand around her right ankle. By the time our food was brought to our table twelve minutes later, the pain had reduced and was very mild. We started to eat.

The Achilles' tendon is the tendon right above the back of the heel bone.

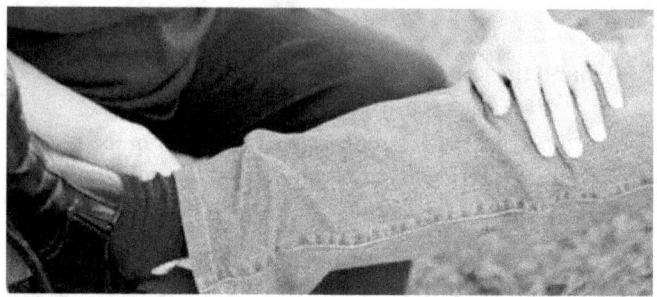

Pic 24 Right Ankle (Achilles' Tendon) and Right Knee

15. A lady complained about right upper leg pain and soreness. I put one hand on her right knee and one hand on her lower hip at the level of the hip joint. Twenty minutes later, she felt fine and was smiling.

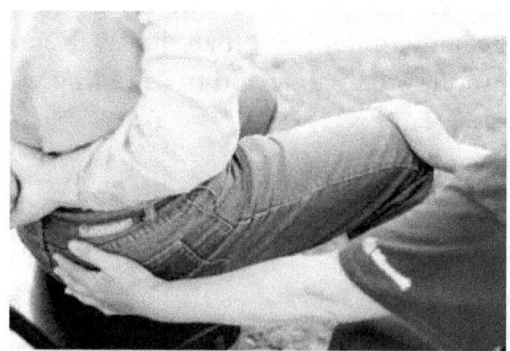

Pic 25 Right Hip Joint and the Right Knee

16. A woman told me that her lower limbs felt cold. I put my hands on her lower back. One covered her L2 (the second lumbar spinal bone), and other hand covered her tailbone at S5 to help her

lower leg circulation. Ten minutes later, she told me that she was comfortable, and her legs and toes were warm.

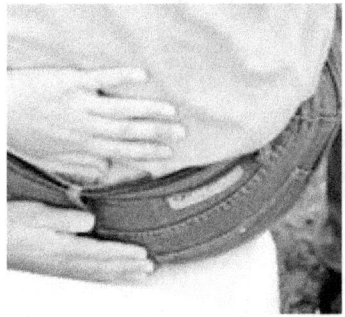 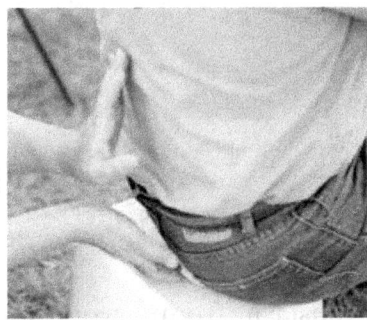

Pic 26 Hands on L2 and S5   Pic 27 Hands on L2 and S5

17. A speaker chatted with me at the end of her workshop. She mentioned her stress from traveling. She also complained about neck and lower back pain from long hours sitting in a car or plane. I put one hand at her Baihui and one hand on her forehead. The speaker felt a calmness that she had not experienced in a long time. Then I moved my hands to cover the back of her lower head just above the lower edge of the skull and T5 (the 5th theoretic spinal bone). When she told me that she felt happier, I moved my hands to her painful lower back area. The total time was fifteen minutes, and the speaker left with a calmness, happiness, and no pain.

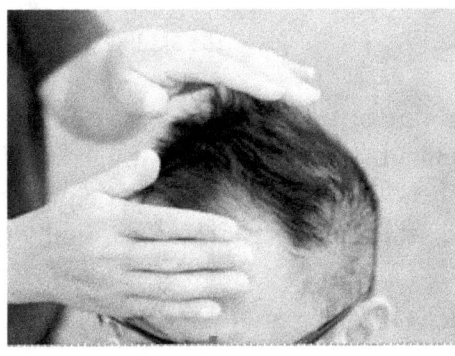 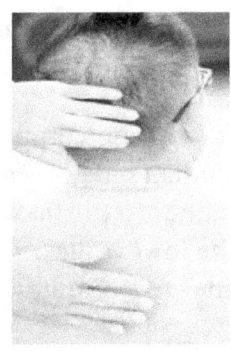

Pic 28 Baihui and Forehead   Pic29 Lower Edge of the
Skull & T5

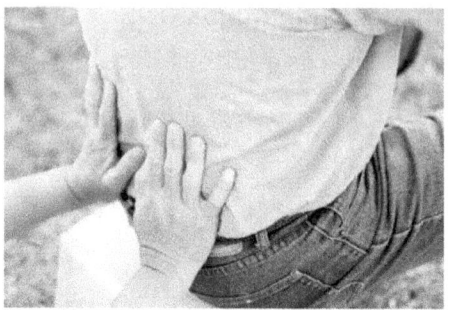

Pic 30 Low Back Painful Area

18. A musician from a workshop asked me to relieve his stress. I put one hand at his Baihui and one hand on his forehead. The musician felt calm. Then I moved my hands to cover the back of his lower head just above the lower edge of the skull and T5. Only three minutes later, the musician claimed that he felt no stress and was calm and happy.

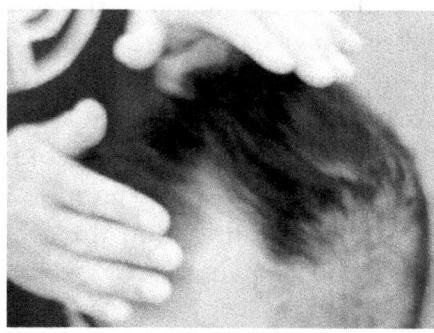

Pic 31 Baihui and Forehead

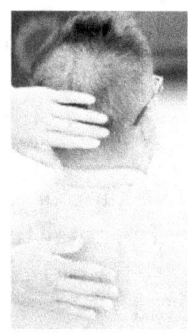

Pic 32 Lower Edge of the Skull & T5

19. A student complained about stress. I put my hands on the student's Baihui and forehead. Later, I moved my hand from Baihui to the back of her head with the pinky finger right above the lower edge of the student's skull. Her stress was totally gone after five minutes.

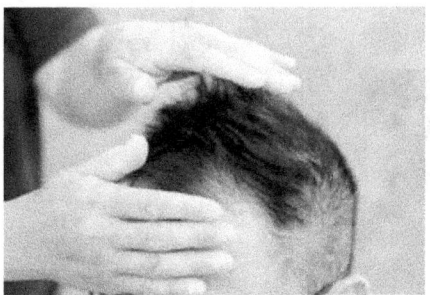
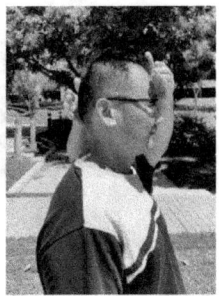

Pic 33 Baihui and Forehead

Pic 34 Forehead and
above the Skull

20. A female entrepreneur friend told me that her stress level was high due to traveling more. I put hands on her Baihui and forehead. Later, I moved my hand from Baihui to the back of her head with the pinky finger right above the lower edge of her skull. Six minutes later, she felt calm and could enjoy the network event.

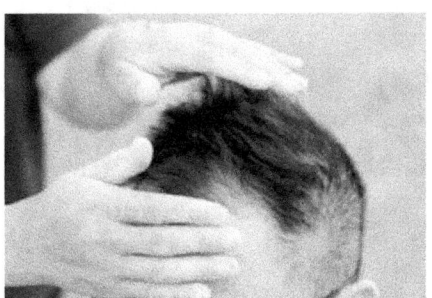
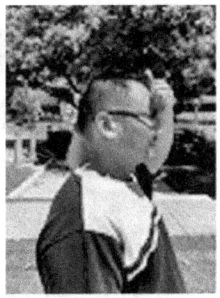

Pic 35 Baihui and Forehead

Pic 36 Forehead and
above the Skull

21. A female business friend felt stress and sadness. I put hands on her Baihui and forehead. Then, I moved the hand from Baihui to her back head with the pinky finger right above the lower edge of her skull and gave her some comforting words. Twenty minutes later, she felt no sadness and was happy.

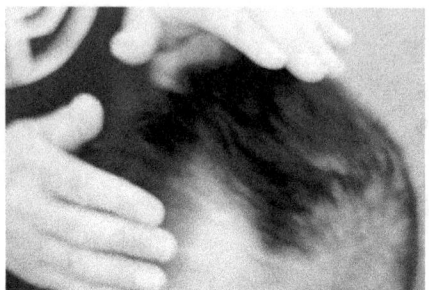

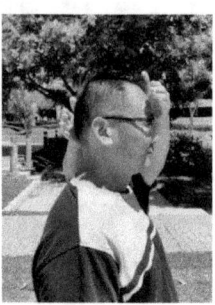

Pic 37 Baihui and Forehead

Pic 38 Forehead &
Above Skull (B)

22. A classmate felt stress and had no energy. I put hands on his Baihui and forehead. Later, I moved my hand from Baihui to the back of his head with the pinky finger right above the lower edge of his skull. Then I moved my hands to his back on his heart and liver areas to boost his energy and further relieve his stress. Fifteen minutes later, he felt happy and energetic.

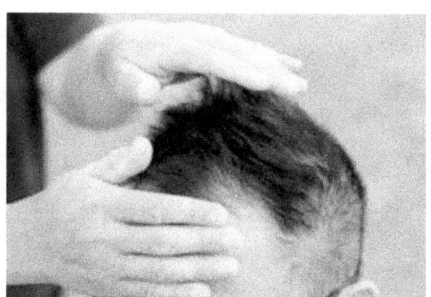

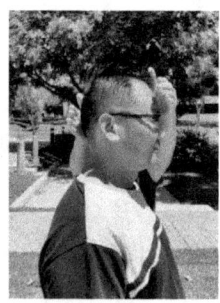

Pic 39 Baihui and Forehead

Pic 40 Forehead and
Above Skull

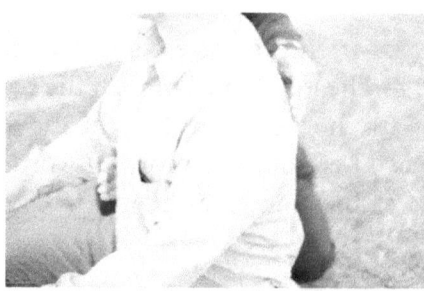

Pic 41 Liver (F) and Heart (B)

23. At a volunteer center, a woman had high stress and insomnia. I put hands on her Baihui and forehead. Later, I moved my hand from Baihui to the back of her head with the pinky finger right above the lower edge of her skull. Next, I moved my hands to her back on her heart and liver areas to further relieve her stress and allow her to sleep. Total time spent was forty minutes. In following up the next week, I learned that she felt happier and was sleeping better.

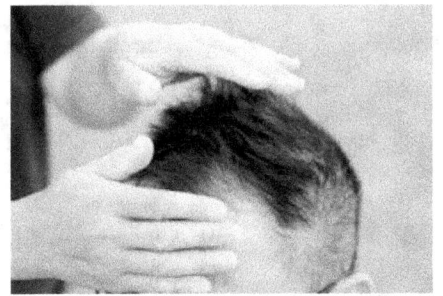 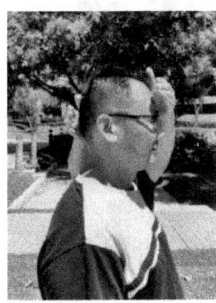

Pic 42 Baihui and Forehead

Pic 43 Forehead and Above Skull

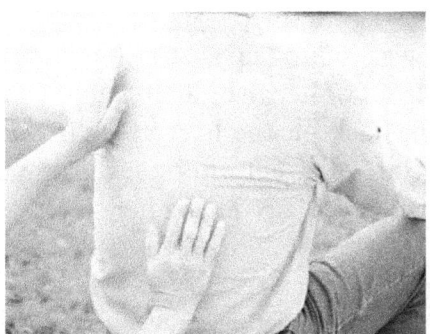

Pic 44 Heart (B, L), Liver (B, R)   L: Left   R: Right

24. At a volunteer center, a man woke up daily between 4 and 5:00 a.m. I put my hands on his Baihui and above the back of his skull. Then I moved my hands to the center of his lungs in both of the front and back. I next moved my hands to his liver area on both of the front and back sides. Total time used was forty-

five minutes. He did not come the next week due to no more insomnia according to his friend's feedback.

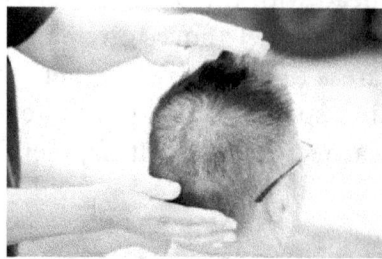
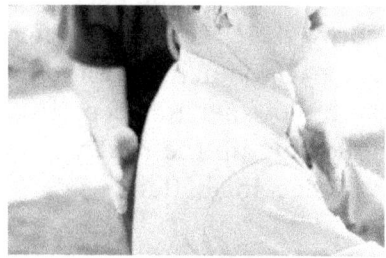

Pic 45 Baihui and Back of the Skull   Pic 46 In the Center of Lungs B & F

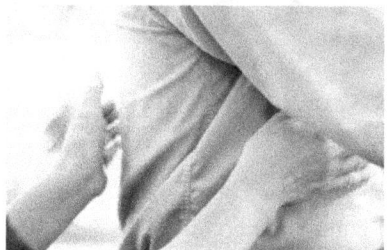

Pic 47 Both sides of the Liver

25. A classmate was waking up at 3:00 a.m. I put hands on her Baihui and on the front of her liver area. Later, I moved the hand from Baihui to her back on the liver area. This was done during the class break time of twenty minutes. The next day, she told me that she did not wake up during her sleep.

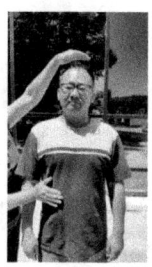
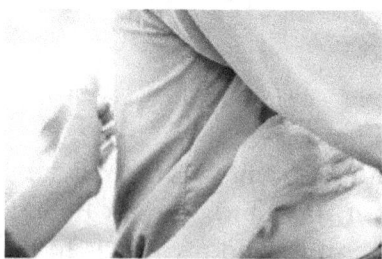

Pic 48 Baihui &   Pic 49 Liver Front and Back
Liver (F)

26. I had a meeting with my friend. She was experiencing restless and shallow sleep. I put hands on my friend's Baihui and a lower back skull. Later, I moved my hands to her back on the liver and heart area for a total of twenty-five minutes. The friend called me the next day and said that she had slept through the night comfortably without waking up and was fully charged that morning.

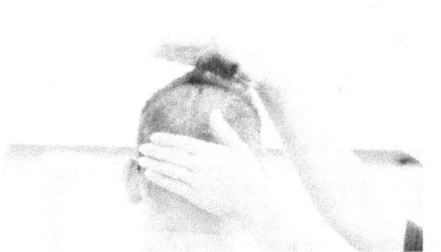
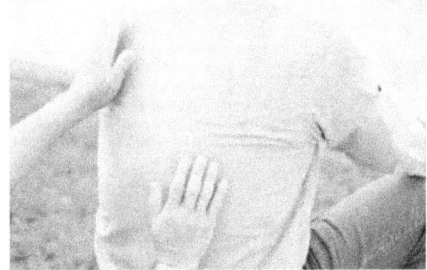

Pic 50 Baihui & Back of the Skull   Pic 51 Heart (B, L), Liver (B, R)

27. At a volunteer center, a young man could not sleep at all during the night due to nightmares. Two volunteers adjusted him, one focusing on his head to do the adjustment. I put my hands on his heart and liver as well as both of his kidneys for a total seventy minutes. The next week I met with him, and he said that he could sleep until 4:00 or 5:00 a.m. without waking up.

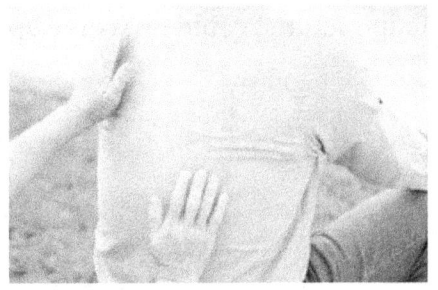
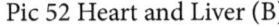
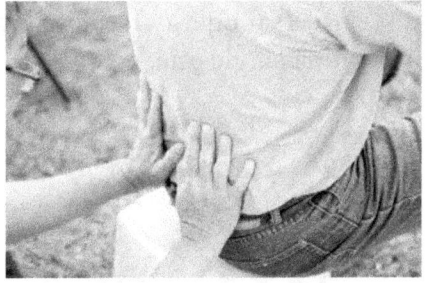

Pic 52 Heart and Liver (B)   Pic 53 Both kidneys at back

28. A banker felt fatigue and was sleepy at the end of the day. He wanted to get a cup of coffee in order to drive without falling asleep when trapped in traffic. I asked him to try my Comprehensive

Universal Energy Healing. He agreed. I put hands on his Baihui and a couple of inches away from his body in front of his heart area for three minutes. The banker was so surprised that it was quicker and better than a cup of coffee. He felt calm and happy and had good energy.

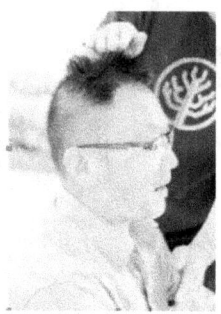

Pic 54 Baihui and Heart (F)

29. An MD from China, who held an acupuncturist license in the US, had heard about my energy healing. He wanted to give it a try. I put my hands on his Baihui and forehead, then at Baihui and above the back of his skull. Later, I put one hand a couple of inches away from his heart in his front and one hand on his T5 as well as playing universal codes with him. Within five minutes, he felt calm and relaxed. I asked him to give me the name of a drug or herb that could have the same effectiveness as my Comprehensive Universal Energy Healing. The acupuncturist could not come up with a single one.

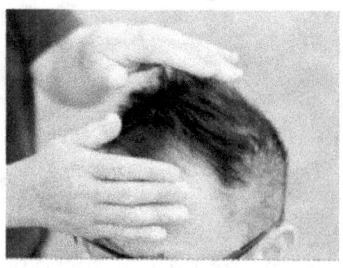

Pic 55 Baihui and Forehead

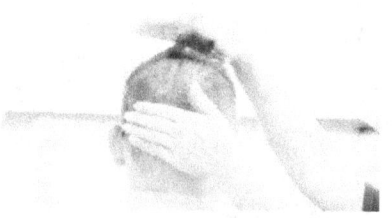

Pic 56 Back of Skull and Bai-Hui

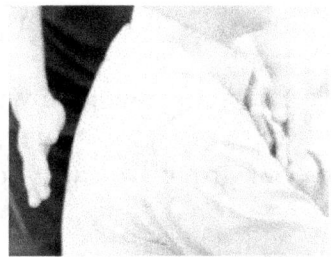

Pic 57 T5 and Heart (F)

30. A friend of mine was wondering if Comprehensive Universal Energy Healing could do anything good for him if he was already healthy, so I put my hands on his Baihui and C8, and then Baihui and T5. I next moved to T5 and S5. After ten minutes, my friend felt comfort throughout his whole body. It did make him feel better.

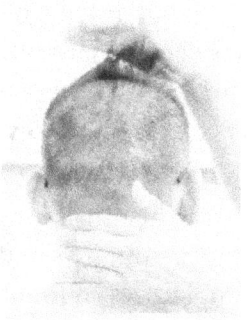
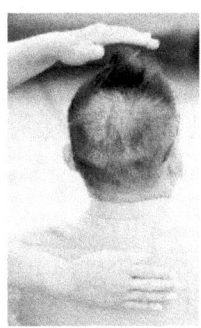

Pic 58 Baihui and C8   Pic 59 Baihui and T5

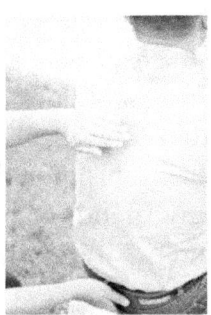

Pic 60 Heart/T5 and S5

The above are commonly seen situations listed here for your reference. Once you learn how to use Comprehensive Universal Energy Healing to help yourself, your family members, your loved ones, your friends, and your colleagues, you will be one of the most in-demand persons in your group. You will be surrounded by love and gratitude.

If you want to read about more cases, you can visit universalenergyhealing.us for an update.

If you are an entrepreneur, you know the potential value of Comprehensive Universal Energy Healing. You know what it can mean to you, your business, your employees, and your company's healthcare premiums.

Below are some brief introductions to Comprehensive Universal Energy Healing applications for your reference to increase your willingness to learn.

The healing effectiveness of combining universal energy and universal codes is often better than that of acupuncture treatments. It also overcomes the limitations of acupuncture—the requirement of a treating bed, the inconvenience of carrying needles to visit patients, and the cost of herbs.

For many patients who have pain and health issues but cannot pay medical expenses, universal energy healing provides a simple method by which they can restore health. However, for some patients with severe blockage, the efficacy of acupuncture is much faster. Adding the herbal formula mentioned in Appendix Eight can speed up recovery by two to six times.

If Comprehensive Universal Energy Healing can make me—with more than twenty years' experience in Chinese medicine and treatments—decide to invest a lot of time in writing a series of books, you should be able to see that it is a healing method that cannot be ignored and is worthy of being promoted. I am pleased to be able to offer this book to help my friends to learn more from my skills. When you read the book and put the methods into practice, you will immediately notice the benefits.

Please read How Does TCM (Traditional Chinese Medicine) view diseases?[139] to understand why it is so important not to delay treatment if you are sick. It is just like a car or a house— you should always address small problems as early as possible to prevent them from becoming big problems and costing more to fix. But it is so odd that for the most valuable asset in life—your health—most people do not apply this rule. Moreover, patients are much more reluctant to pay more for quality and effective services.

Treatment Items

Head & Neck

Headaches, migraines, dizziness, tinnitus, deafness and other auditory problems, visual impairment, pain, red eyes with pain, nasal congestion (cold/flu), runny nose, drooling, sore throat, neck pain, difficulty swallowing, fatigue, and inability to concentrate.

A three-year-old girl with a congenital brain injury could not lift her head. Her neck was soft. The ribs on her right side were deformed and higher than those on her left side. Nothing stopped her nasal discharge, saliva, phlegm, wheezing, and difficulty breathing. After a twenty- to thirty-minute adjustment, her neck could support her head, the part of her ribs that had been covered by my healing hand became a normal shape, and her other symptoms disappeared. She could breathe normally without noise.

Shoulder

Frozen shoulder, shoulder pain and soreness.

Upper body

Upper back pain, chest pain, heart discomfort, palpitations, unhappiness or irritability, phlegm in the lungs (after an adjustment, breathing is easier and lung capacity is increased), protruding thoracic spine bone, pediatric ribs on the right side were higher than the left side (could be adjusted to be the same height).

Lower body

Lumbar disc stenosis, pinched nerve, inflammation and pain after hip replacement surgery, hip sprain, lower back pain.

Upper abdomen

Stomach ache, upset stomach, depressive mood, nausea, loss of appetite, vomiting.

Lower abdomen

Abdominal pain, bloating, discomfort due to uterine tumor, menstrual pain.

Upper limbs

Arm, elbow, forearm, wrist pain, vascular protrusion of hand and forearm.

Lower limbs

Swollen legs, swollen ankles, leg pain, knee pain, foot pain, varicose veins on leg, poor blood circulation, and inability to stand up after sitting.

Others

Insomnia, poor energy, fatigue, fear, cold/flu, heart palpitations, high blood pressure, mental stress, motor mind.

Below is a table of adjustment examples for pain, stress, and insomnia based on the cases at the beginning of this chapter. It is a quick reference for your adjustment providing information on condition, time period involved, and placement of hands. This is just a guide, however, so please bear in mind that there are many ways to place your hands, and the adjustment time can vary from case to case. Even the weather, the environmental temperature, or emotions can influence the time needed and the adjustment results.

Summary of Adjusted Cases

No	Physical Conditions	Position of Hands	Min.	Result
1	Right side migraine	Top of head, migraine location	5	No pain
2	Neck pain	Front and back of the neck	9	No pain
3	Neck/shoulder pain	Top of head/neck, both shoulders	25	No pain
4	Left shoulder and upper back	Left shoulder and scapula	15	No pain
5	Chest distention	Heart and lungs	10	No feeling of distention
6	T6 protruded and pain	Top of head/T6	9	T6 got back to its position and no pain
7	Lower back pain and soreness	Top of head/L2, both kidneys	20	No pain and soreness
8	Hip pain due to sprain	Spleen and painful area on hip	10	No pain
9	Nausea and vomiting	Top of head/ stomach, liver/ stomach	20	No symptoms and emotions improved
10	Abdominal bloating	Top of head/lower abdomen, front and back of lower abdomen	15	No bloating sensation in abdomen
11	Right forearm and hand pain	Right elbow, right wrist	15	No pain
12	Right knee pain, right ankle swollen and painful	Right knee front/ back, heart/T5	35	No pain, reduced fifty percent of swelling

13	Right leg and ankle swollen, numbness and pain	Right knee, right ankle	12	Swelling reduced and no pain/numbness
14	Right lower leg and Achilles tendon pain	Right knee/Achilles tendon	12	Pain reduced to very mild
15	Right upper leg pain and soreness	Right knee and right lower hip	20	No soreness and pain
16	Cold lower limbs	L2/S5	10	Legs and toes felt warm
17	Stress, neck and lower back pain	Forehead/top of head, T5/back of lower head, lower back pain area	15	No pain or stress, felt happy and calm
18	Stress	Forehead/top of head, back of lower head/T5, T5 and heart	3	No stress and calm
19	Stress	Forehead/top of head, back of lower head	5	Calm
20	Stress	Forehead/top of head, back of lower head	6	Calm
21	Stress, sadness	Forehead/top of head, back of lower head, heart/liver	20	No sadness, happy
22	Stress with poor energy	Forehead/top of head, back of lower head, heart/liver	15	Happy with energy
23	Stress with insomnia	Forehead/top of head, back of lower head, heart/liver	40	Happy and insomnia improved

24	Waking up between 4:00 and 5:00 a.m.	Top of head/back of lower head, front and back of lungs, liver	45	Not waking up early
25	Waking up at 3:00 a.m.	Top of head/liver, front and back of liver	20	Not waking up early
26	Shallow sleep	Top of head/back of lower head, heart/liver	25	Sleeping comfortably through the night
27	No sleep overnight due to feeling threatened (Two persons do adjustment)	One person adjusts head, another one adjusts heart, liver and kidney	70	Could sleep until 4:00 or 5:00 a.m.
28	Fatigue and sleepiness	Top of head/heart	3	Good energy
29	Curiosity to try	Forehead/top of head, top of head/back lower head, T5/heart	5	Calm and relaxed
30	General health maintenance	Top of head/C8 and T5/S5	10	Whole body felt comfortable

Note:

1. Due to the time constraints, there was not always enough time to completely solve each problem.

2. If your hands are large, do your best to cover as many points as possible. For example, cover U1/U2 or U2/U3 or U5/U6 or U5/Heart.

3. The above adjustments were done in the earlier stages of CHUEH practice without inviting the client to participate (i.e. only one person did the adjustment without collaboration). Records for

pain level were not kept. At that time, I was not thinking about writing a book.

Investment Revenue Exercise

- Do meditation.
- Take a deep breath.

  Slowly inhale through the nose, and then slowly exhale (exhale through the nose or slightly open mouth to exhale).

  Slowly inhale through the nose, hold your breath three to five seconds, and then slowly exhale. Repeat three to five times or until the brain calms down.

- Slightly close eyes.
- Clear your mind without thinking anything.
- Relax skull, relax facial muscles, and relax the neck.
- Relax the chest and upper back.
- Relax abdomen, waist, and lower back.
- Relax shoulders, upper arms, elbows, forearms, wrists, hands, fingers, and fingertips.
- Relax hips, upper legs, knees, lower legs, ankles, feet, toes up to the tips.
- Pull the time backward to your most healthy and happy moments, or meditate in the health and happiness of your dream scene. Try to enjoy and remember this pleasant feeling.
- Compare your current health status and the ideal health that you visualized in your meditation. Write them in the following table and decide which health item(s) need improvement. Learn ways to improve without delay.

My Health Situation		
Ideal Health Situation	My Current Situation	Item(s) Needing Improvement and How to Improve

CHAPTER FOUR

The Causes of Sickness, Pain, Degeneration, and Aging

• •

"If the righteousness qi is not deficient, there is no pathogen can do (harm)."

Huang Di Nei Jing • Su Wen Lost Chapter • Needling Method Theory

How Does TCM Views Health

A healthy person's body is balanced in yin and yang, qi and blood, zang and fu organs. The person's qi and blood flows smoothly, and he/she feels happy and thinks positively. If this doesn't happen, sickness occurs.

A healthy person is agile, thinks quickly, possesses an optimistic personality, is just and considerate, does not give himself a hard time (can tolerate a small loss but not a big one), is alert and generous, and can both give love and accept it.

A healthy person has good moral character. Unhealthy attitude and behavior is not only an expression of poor performance but is also one of the root causes of damaged health. If a person is selfish and greedy and say negative things behind someone's back, he will lose popularity and get unpleasant feelings in response. And sooner or later, he will be sick.

How Does TCM (Traditional Chinese Medicine) View Diseases?

In TCM internal medicine, we treat diseases as seeds that cause sickness which are planted into the soil of the body. The first root of the disease to invade the body goes straight to the weakest organ. From that grow more root branches. It means that more organs are invaded by the sickness according to the Five Organs Relationship below. Above the soil grow branches and leaves—they are symptoms of the diseases.

So if a disease is left without treatment, its tree will continuously grow, and the patient will become sicker. The symptoms surface more and more.

What do we do? As preventive healthcare providers, we dig out the root to be sure the disease has no chance to grow more roots, invading more organs and growing more symptoms (leaves and branches). **As a patient, you should not stop your treatment when the symptoms go away because the root will keep growing, and new branches and leaves will continue to grow**. You might think that you're saving money by stopping treatments earlier. But you will actually spend much more money to remove the root, and the treatment will become much more complicated. You will then need a Chinese physician with higher skills, who will usually charge more, to take care of you.

Internal organs will be invaded by disease based on the relationship of the five elements. Heart disease affects lung and kidney health because they mutually restrain (see below picture). If organs locate on the diagonal line, the two organs mutually restrain, i.e. if one organ is unhealthy, it will cause dysfunction of the other two organs located on the other end of its diagonal line.

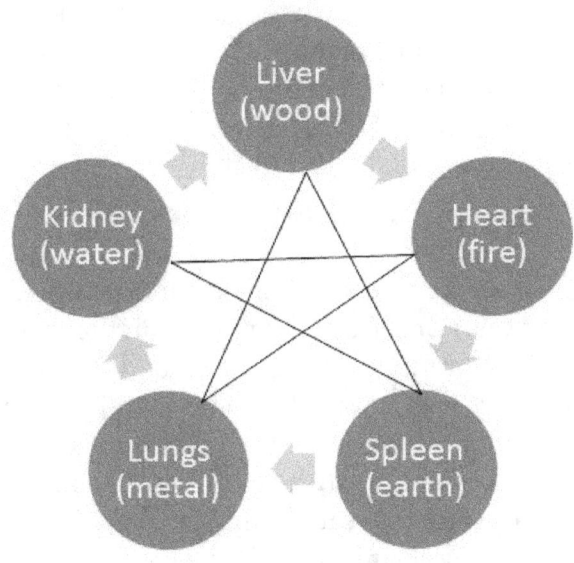

Fig 3 Five Elements

In the beginning, the effects are not obvious. But gradually, the body will send warning signs. Chinese medicine relies on those signs for diagnosis. The patient's body will begin to feel bad, and the person will start to get sick. Some recent Western medical machines can detect it. The infrared scanner can detect sickness earlier than other medical test equipment.

Different Disease Names in Western and Chinese Medical Fields

Due to the necessity of health insurance in the current health care system, Western disease names are widely used among patients and in the medical field. Even an acupuncturist at the last gate of the medical treatment chain ought to know them in order to communicate with patients. Additionally, it's important to know how patients were previously treated to see how their ailments could be addressed in a more productive way in the present situation.

Actually, the diseases known to Chinese medicine were well-identified, classified, and named thousands of years ago. The identifying names are fewer than those of Western medicine, and we follow the TCM diagnosis to treat. Even without knowledge of the Western medical label, we still can treat.

Some of Western medicine's tests can be helpful in our diagnosis and treatment results. But we never request invasive tests, most often because we are not the first-line health care provider for tough internal medical cases or serious injury cases in the Western medical system. Instead, we rely on the patient's body signs—they never lie. Of course, there will always be some tough cases where body signs and symptoms work against each other. In these cases, it can be a challenge to come up with the correct diagnosis. But a good Chinese physician who has read many cases and followed excellent Chinese medicine physicians or experienced more cases will rarely be confused.

Western medicine is different. Using the analogy of a tree, Chinese medicine treats the whole tree as a single disease. Western medicine lets a tree have many branches—each branch represents a disease and has its own name, and more names can be generated as new branches/leaves grow. And because new branches continue to grow, the names of diseases are ever-changing.

Only this difference, people think that Western medicine has more advanced researches and is more scientific than Chinese medicine. Therefore, we deeply hope that people can make judgments after they fully understand about Chinese medicine.

Chinese and Western Medicine Treat Diseases Differently

Through modern technology, Western medicine appears on the surface to be more dedicated in disease diagnosis and treatment. However, it's just that we have a very different treatment approach.

We've discussed how Chinese medicine views a disease. An excellent Chinese medicine physician treating a disease will dig out the root to avoid complications later. If you merely trim branches or cut the tree trunk down to the ground, more branches and leaves will grow because the root still remains.

When a patient gets an infection from bacteria, Western medicine uses drugs to kill the bacteria, but Chinese medicine treats the patient's constitution to turn his body into an environment unfit for the survival of bacteria.

Some people don't visit a doctor when needed, or they don't search for the person with the necessary expertise to treat their disease. As a result, the root cause grows deeper, and the branches keep growing. The disease affects more and more organs, and health grows worse as time passes. Those people sigh and say, "I'm getting older, and my health is getting worse." It may sound reasonable, but it's not true. Why is it that your next door neighbor who is the same age as you has never visited a doctor and hasn't taken any medicine, and his physical degradation is less than yours? You'd better search for the reasons!

The key to your health is in your hands. Only you have the key to open the door to your healthy life. There is no one—not even a doctor—who can do it for you. Only you can eat healthy, maintain a healthy lifestyle, and have a positive attitude. If you don't do these things and then go to a doctor expecting him to heal you, it won't happen. Once you are sick, all a doctor can do for you is make your sickness less severe. While the acupuncturists facilitate your body to do self-recovery.

I often hear patients talking about regret—that they acted "too late" and, as a result, will lose their lives or a damaged body part. There is no eraser for regret. What is lost is gone forever, and it is impossible to go back to the original! And who will bear the most pain because of your regret? Your family members, loved ones, and all of the people who care about you.

Health Standard

Besides standards set for diseases, in traditional Western medicine, there are no health standards.

Below is a healthy person's index set by Professor Ni, Hai Sha. By reading through these things, you can know if you are healthy or not.

1. Can sleep overnight without waking up.
2. Normal appetite: moderate intake.
3. The palms and the bottoms of the feet are warmer than the other parts of the body. The forehead is cooler than the palms. If the feet are covered when sleeping, the feet are cold.
4. Urination occurs five to seven times a day. The first urine in the morning is yellowish, and the later urines are light yellow.
5. There is one bowel movement daily. After menopause, it is better for women to have bowel movements twice a day. Stool is formed in a long strip (not as thin as a pencil, too short, or rounded) and is yellow-brown color. However, if more vegetables have been eaten, there could be a slight color to the stool. For example, if one ate a lot of carrots, the stool could have an orange tinge.
6. For a well-developed adult, upon waking up in the morning, the nipples or the penis are erect.

Besides the above-mentioned items, a healthy person should also be mentally healthy. He should be energetic, alert, in good shape, reasonably tolerant of the daily stress of life, happy, and appreciative of life. A healthy person should not only have a healthy physical body, but a mind and soul full of love and gratitude.

Body, mind, and soul all affect health and are affected by health.

An additional note:

1. Normal sweating means sweating in hot temperatures and during exercise. A person should not be easily sweating—that indicates a qi deficiency.
2. Normal menstruation means having a period every twenty-eight days with no dysmenorrhea or PMS.

What Blocks Qi and/or Blood Circulation?

There are many causes of blocked qi and/or blood circulation.

1. Wind, wetness, coldness, dryness, summer heat, and fire may cause arthritis and many other diseases that are not well known. It's wise to pay attention to them.

2. External injuries such as knife cuts, gunshot wounds, car accidents, falling, bruises, insect bites and other animal bites.

3. The qi stagnation can be caused by emotional constraints. Qi stagnation can cause phlegm and may even turn into blood stasis if prolonged, and then many unknown diseases can appear.

4. Internal bleeding can cause blood stasis. Due to the deviated organ function can cause phlegm or mucus or tumors or even cancer.

5. External coldness—coming from cold weather or even from the intake of cold foods or drinks—invades the abdomen, causing abdominal pain and diarrhea. There are both benign and severe diseases induced from external coldness. Please read Cold Foods Drinks Caused Problems Chart Rev 1[155].

    Since ancient times, the Chinese have had a saying— "Disease comes in from the mouth." Diet is essential to good health. Therefore the Zhou Dynasty (1046 BC—771 BC) set up four health departments: Medical Diet (in charge of food storage), Diseases Medicine (internal medicine), Ulcer Medicine (surgery), and Veterinarians[56].

    The incidence of some diseases is after a few decades. So, it does not mean that you can continue to accumulate onset etiologies.

    Such as teenage girls like to wear dresses that explored their umbilicus. Cold wind can enter from the umbilicus to the uterus, plus intake of cold drinks/foods in the summer, which caused their uterus to be too cold to impregnate and thus they become infertile. It's a most common infertility cause in the acupuncture clinics.

Some male patients played ball games in high school. Until 50 or 60 years old has heart pain or chest area pain mimic heart problem. By diagnosis, heart is normal. If you let the patient point where he feels pain, you can find the location has a soft tissue injury traced as ball hit.

There are tons clinical cases. We stop here after two examples. Later, in the Readers Discussion[137] or CHUEH Training Programs[198], we can see more of these kind cases.

6. When the accumulated etiology is beyond the body's ability to tolerate it, then the body becomes sick. Sometimes it is an intermittent disease, an overflow to give a warning. Other times, it is like a sudden burst of sickness or an acute emergency that requires hospitalization. It depends on what kind of protest the body gives to the patient.

    Western medicine often talks about the "silent killer." That concept does not exist in Chinese medicine. Our bodies give us warning signs long before we become ill. A good Chinese medicine physician can read them for you.

What Causes Pain?

There is a famous saying in Chinese medicine: "If it cannot get through, then there is pain." Where the qi and blood cannot pass through smoothly, pain is the result. This is the warning sign our body gives to us. If it's mild, a little massage can relieve the pain. If not, and the pain level increases or occurs more frequently, you may need to seek further help.

When dealing with pain, the worst case scenario is cancer. Cancer pain involves constant pain, localized heating, insomnia, and night sweats. Comprehensive Universal Energy Healing can help in most cases of pain. However, for cancer pain, one ought to get professional treatment. Universal Energy Healing should only be used as an auxiliary treatment.

Immunocompromised

Low immunity is related to physical, emotional, and spiritual problems. Stress and/or bad emotion are always the trigger.

The health of someone born with poor immunity is related to the parents, especially his mother's health. If the mother was in a bad mood during her pregnancy, taking medication during pregnancy, or smoking, drinking, or abusing drugs, or was abused, overdue herself, all could affect the child's immune system and even its vitality.

Please read: How A Mother's Health Can Affect a Kid's Health[168] and Emotional Disturbance During Pregnancy[169].

Acquired immune deficiency: Diet problems, bad mood, bad habits, smoking, alcohol, gambling, drug abuse, poor living conditions, poor hygiene, negative thinking, mental/economic/life stress, improper lifestyle, lack of sunshine, lack of exercise, excessive intake of drugs, chemical subtracted foods, working or living in an environment with toxins, excessive noise, harmful radiation…

People with high spirits usually have strong awareness, better moral cultivation, and know how to get longevity. But their strong responsibility makes them worry too much and work too diligently in an abnormal era where there are too many deviant behaviors and wrong doings.

The Causes for the Body's Internal Imbalances

The qi is constantly flowing, particularly the yang qi. It flows from the top to the bottom, and from the bottom to top. From the front outside of the body to behind the body and then back again to the front. The flow of the yang qi drives the body's internal balance. Thus, losing the normal free-flowing qi will cause an imbalance, and it will become possible to get sick.

Mood Swings

Huang Di Nei Jing • Su Wen • Chapter of Enumerating Pain Discussions:

The Yellow Emperor said, "I know that a lot of diseases are caused by qi. If angry, the qi goes up. If happy, the qi is lax. If sad, the qi vanishes. If afraid, the qi goes down. If cold, the qi congeals. If hot, the qi leaks out. If threatened, the qi flows in a disorderly fashion. If laboring too much, the qi is consumed. If thinking, the qi knots up. These nine kinds of qi are very different. What kinds of illnesses can be caused?

Qi Bo 岐伯 replied as follows:

1. Anger makes qi rebellious, and it goes upward. It can cause vomiting blood and diarrhea.

    NOTE: If there is severe anger, there is liver fire, which can cause one to vomit blood or stroke due to the fire traveling upward and the fire causing blood to flow out of the blood vessels. If the liver invades the spleen, it can cause diarrhea.

2. Happiness makes the qi harmonized, relaxed, and willing to attain. **Ying qi** and **wei qi** flow freely and benefit each other.

3. Sadness causes the Heart Meridian to flow rapidly and the lung lobes to expand and lift. This blocks the **upper energizer (upper jiao)**, and the ying qi and wei qi cannot disperse. The hot qi is trapped inside, causing the qi to vanish.

4. If afraid, the qi essence goes downward and retreats. The qi circulation cannot flow both upward and downward to connect together. Qi is blocked in the upper jiao. Because the upper jiao is blocked, if the qi of the lower jiao travels up, it is forced to return and causes the lower jiao to be distended.

5. If cold, the **zhou li** of the superficial skin and muscles closes to prevent coldness from invading the body. The qi cannot flow. Therefore, the qi congeals inside.

6. If hot, the zhou li is opened. Ying qi and wei qi flow smoothly causing qi to flow and the sweat to leak out.

7. If threatened, the heart palpitates, and the Shen (spirit) has nowhere to go. This causes anxiety, and the mind becomes uncertain, further causing disorientation of the qi flow.

8. Too much labor causes wheezing and sweating. Wheezing causes internal qi overflow. Sweating causes external qi (wei qi) overflow. With both the internal and external qi overflow, the qi is consumed.

9. If thinking, the mind is focused, and the shen is tied into something. Therefore, the rightness qi doesn't move freely as usual, and it causes qi knots.

Therefore, you know that emotions, doing too much labor, thinking too much, and extremes of cold or heat can disturb the direction, speed, strength, and the amount of qi flowing through the body. The abnormal qi flow can cause sickness.

Impact of the Cold and Hot Qi on the Human Body

Huang Di Nei Jing • Su Wen Chapter Thirty-Nine Enumerating Pain Discussions:

Qi Bo: Qi and blood in the meridians flow nonstop and circulate endlessly. If cold qi enters a meridian, it makes the flow slow down. Both the qi and blood circulation slow down and cannot flow smoothly. If cold invades outside of a meridian, it causes reduced blood flowing. If cold invades inside a meridian, the qi is blocked. As a result, there is acute pain.

If cold invades outside of the meridian, then the meridian becomes cold. If the meridian is cold, it makes the body contract without expanding. Contracting without expanding makes it shrink, and it pulls on the outside small collaterals.* Internal and external pulling is impetuous and causes acute pain. If heated, the pain stops.

If repeatedly invaded by cold, the pain injures the wei qi and becomes chronic.

> * *Think of it like a water supply system. If a segment of a main branch shrinks, and the flow through it doesn't reduce, what happens? Due to the strong pressure, the water flowing through should become faster. Its branches would also be affected by having a more rapid flow.*

If the cold qi stays inside the meridian, it fights with the hot yang qi and leads to the meridian being full. When the meridian is full, it causes pain that gets worse when pressure is applied. The cold qi stays, and the hot yang qi follows it to fight. This leads the qi and the blood to flow in a disorderly way. There is severe pain, and the area hurts when pressed.

If the cold qi stays between the stomach and intestines and below the diaphragm, the blood cannot disperse. The small collaterals pull and causes pain. When pressed, the stagnated qi and blood disperse. Therefore, when pressed, the pain stops.

If the cold resides at the deep hua tou jia ji (beside the spinal discs), you cannot reach it to press, and, therefore, pressing is of no benefit.

The Chong Meridian starts from Guanyuan (please refer to Appendix Five for its location) and follows Conception Vessel (Ren Meridian) through the abdomen upward. If there is cold inside the meridian, the qi in the meridian is blocked. If a meridian is blocked, its qi reflects it. Therefore, if you press on it, you can feel the qi jumping.

If cold qi stays in the back shu points (please refer to Appendix Five) located on the Bladder Meridian, then the meridian flows slowly and not smoothly. If a meridian flows in this way, the blood is deficient. If the blood is deficient, it causes pain. The back shu points connect to the heart, so there will be a pulling pain between the back and the heart. If you press on it, the hot yang qi will go there. Once that happens, the pain stops.

The Liver Meridian passes through the genital organ, up through the abdomen, and connects to the liver. If cold lodges in the Meridian, then the blood congeals and doesn't flow smoothly and the meridian spasms. Therefore, both sides of the front rib cage and lower abdomen will have a pulling pain.

If cold qi stays in the groin area, the cold qi flows up to the lower abdomen, and the blood flows slowly and not smoothly. Therefore, the abdominal pain pulls the groin area and causes pain.*

> * *There are connective tissues between the lower abdomen and groin area. The connective tissues shrink when cold invades.*

If the cold qi stays in the collateral blood between the small intestine and the diaphragm, the blood flows slowly and cannot enter the bigger meridian. If the blood sits there for a prolonged time without flowing, it forms an accumulation.

If cold stays in the five solid zang organs*, the qi in the zang organs rebels upward and leaks out. Yin qi (nutrients and oxygen) is exhausted, and yang qi (functional driving force) has not entered yet. There will suddenly be acute pain and then a coma. If qi (both yin and yang) returns, the person will be out of coma.

> * *The five zang organs are the kidneys, the liver, the heart, the spleen, and the lungs.*

If cold qi stays in the stomach and intestines, it causes the stomach and the qi of the intestines to move upward. Pain and vomiting are the result.

If cold qi resides in the small intestine, there will be pain there. If there is heat in the small intestine, it will cause internal heat injuries, heat up the bodily fluids, dry out the lips, and cause thirst. Stools will be hard and difficult to pass. It's painful due to the blocked small intestine.

Qi Bo said the five zang and six fu organs* that all has its healthy status showing places**.

> * *The six fu organs are the hollow organs—the urinary bladder, gallbladder, small intestine, stomach, large intestine, and Triple Energizer (San Jiao) of the three parts of the chest and abdominal cavities.*

> ** *The kidney's health can show on the face and most time under the eyes, in the hair, in the hearing, and in the energy. The liver's health can show in the eyes or around the eyes, in the eyesight, or in the tendons. The heart's*

health can show on the face, palms, four limbs, ankles, and in the body temperature. The spleen's health can show on the lips and eyelids or in the muscles. The lungs' health can show on the white part of the eyeball, the palms, and the skin.

According to the holographic theory that each organ's health also can show on the ear, palms, nails, fingers and bottom of the feet. There are so many ways to read a person's health without test equipment. Moreover, those signs can show far earlier than a machine can detect the health issues. That's why TCM can prevent sickness from reading those body signs. It's the most cost effective health care by preventing people from becoming sick.

Besides that, the emotion and mood also show an organ's health.

There are five colors to show healthy signs, the white is cold, yellow is heat, blue and black are painful. These are visual and could see them easily.

However, the colors that applying to health have more meanings than above stated. They will be covered gradually according to the book content. Here, we talk about cold, heat and pain relations.

Cold can cause pain, contraction of muscle/tendon/blood vessels and valves, phlegm, diarrhea, constipation, decrease in physical functions, and tumors. Please refer to Cold Foods Drinks Caused Problems Chart Rev 1[155]. If yang qi reaches the place where the cold qi is gathering, the symptoms of the illness will go away.

The evil heat (abnormal heat) can induce pain, push the blood out of the blood vessels, and cause dryness, thirstiness, yellow sputum, constipation, and mania. You need to soothe the evil heat and eliminate its source to avoid the illness.

Why Do People Get Sick, and How Can Sickness Be Avoided?

There are internal, external and non-internal, and non-external causes of illnesses. Now let's look at these factors and the circumstances that will cause people to get sick.

External causes. In general, when the righteousness qi is in deficiency, the wind, coldness, dampness, dryness, summer heat, and fire pathogens can invade the human body. These external pathogens can also be called external evils. They can cause both pain and sickness. So how can you increase the righteousness qi? Please find an acupuncturist or a physician to rid your body of its disease and pain. Meanwhile, practice Da Zhou Tian[152] (Chapter Five) every day and/or do meditation to help increase your righteousness qi.

Chinese medicine believes that if the body's defense qi is strong enough, no virus or bacteria following the wind, dampness, foods, drinks, or injury can harm the body. They either cannot enter the body or, after entering, they are killed. So they are not the primary root problems for health in TCM. The root problem is weak immunity from related organs or organisms.

Generally speaking, at the tight muscle and/or tendon area, the wei qi is weak. The muscle or tendon needs to be relaxed to avoid trouble later on. Wei qi is our body's defense to resist outside pathogens.

Internal causes: Negative emotions can make people sick. However, doing moral cultivation[170] can help you to avoid emotional diseases. Congenital diseases can be avoided through family planning. Before pregnancy, the future parents' constitution should be tonified.

During the pregnancy, tonify the fetus as well. Please read *"How A Mother's Health Can Affect Kid's Health?"*[168]. As a healthcare provider, I deeply hope that a pregnant woman and the future child's health can catch your attention. If a pregnant woman is mentally or physically abused, it will often cause future mental and physical troubles for the future child. The child also has a lot of trouble. The influence could be a whole life tragedy thing. Who swallows the most pain? The pregnant mother!

Non-internal and non-external causes means that the bodily and/or mental injury was caused by something such as a car accident, being bitten by a toxic insect or animal, intake toxins or loved ones suddenly passed away, Preventing unexpected injuries and accidents can address non-internal/external causes. It also can be addressed by doing good deeds and having good intentions or through moral cultivation to let things go easily.

The Causes of Degeneration

According to the theory of use and disuse, the causes of degeneration are as follows:

1. Being lazy and getting no exercise causes the qi and the blood circulation to decline. The toxins inside the meridians cannot be carried away, and the nutritious elements cannot be carried in. This leads to organ and tissue degeneration.

2. Taking drugs to help your body function, ingesting healthy food to aid in the body's digestive functions, or using health accessories and/or equipment* to replace active movement with passive exercises makes the yang qi decline. Bodily movements are what generates yang qi. The human being is an animal, and animals are supposed to be active.

   If use any kind of supplemental enzyme, the body will eventually stop producing that enzyme. It goes from being secreted in low doses to not being created at all. In TCM, we strengthen the spleen to let it push enzymes from the pancreas or related organs.

   Using health aid accessories/equipment means without them, no exercises or those are passive to activate the body function such as using infrared ring, all of their functions have fewer benefits than actively exercising.

   All of the above can cause the body's natural function to decline. Taking insulin reduces the pancreas' secretion of insulin and causes the pancreas to shrink because there is no longer a need to gradually secrete insulin.

3. The attitude is not right. Some people always depend on others. They have lost the ability and confidence to do things on their own.

The human body is like a house or a car that needs regular repairs and maintenance. Not following a health regimen can cause a yang deficiency and/or an injury to the yin. This may be because of internal emotions, external pathogens, or other internal causes. Without timely treatment, organs and tissues may not get adequate nutrition, and they will atrophy. Fortunately, if it's not too bad, it is reversible.

This is much like a house falling into disrepair. Some things are easy to fix, some are difficult, and some cannot be repaired at all. It depends on the damage that has been done.

The Causes of Aging

Some older people are more energetic and look better as they age. Some become senile and doddering as time passes. Age is not the real reason for the physical and mental degeneration, but the following things are responsible.

1. There is no health care and no exercise.
2. There is not a healthy diet, living habits, and lifestyle.
3. The person is overworked and has consumed too much yang qi.
4. The person has the wrong mindset.
5. There is abuse, and the person does not know how to end it.

Investment Revenue Exercise

Get a pen and a piece of paper ready. Play one of your favorite songs, one that is peaceful and calm. Read the following steps, and then do them. Repeat it daily.

1. Take a deep breath three to five times and enter the meditation state.
2. Imagine a scene that shows your longevity, such as the happy life you want to have and having many generations of family living nearby.

3. Think about the outlook on life and the physical appearance that you would like have when you are older.

4. Think about the maximum age you would like to reach. How do you want your life to be then? Do you want to be happy? Do you want your life to be meaningful? Or would you rather lie in bed with lost mobility and no self-esteem?

5. In your life, what are the five things that you feel are the most important? You can summarize them or break them down into the following five areas—your health, career and business, your relationship with your family members and friends, money and time freedom, such as how much money you want to have in your bank while you retired. Where do you want to spend your retirement? How many hours do you want to work per week or per year? What level of philanthropy do you want to achieve?

   Donate regularly or set up a non-profit organization to support what you want to accomplish. Set up a foundation to give funds so that your community has a place to borrow money for their business and/or family emergencies.

6. Right after your meditation, immediately write down your responses to numbers two to six, and mark them according to their priority.

7. Using the priorities you came up with in number six, list your goal for three years, for five years, and for ten years.

8. Subdivide each goal into small steps.

9. Looking at your answers to number seven and eight above, consider what can do each month to move toward your goals. If it seems that there are too many things to do, put your focus on the three most important things. Review your priorities every three to six months, and reorder them as necessary.

10. Follow your plan to reach your goals. If you need private consultation or would like to join the group class, please reserve our The Dream Builder Coach Program[171].

CHAPTER FIVE

How to Get The Universal Energy to Improve Health

● ● ● ● ● ● ● ● ● ● ● ● ● ● ● ● ● ●

"There is the rightness qi existing in the universe in various forms!"

Wen, Tian Xiang Zhen Qi Ge

The Differences of the Qi from Qi Gong and the Universal Energy

Qi from the qigong is derived from the qigong practitioners' long-term practice of accumulating qi. When the practitioner uses his qi to do a treatment, that consumes his accumulated qi.

People are born with the ability to use the cosmic energy. Even if you don't use Comprehensive Universal Energy Healing for a long time or you lose the ability to use it, if you practice at least five minutes of qigong—Da Zhou Tian[152] or put your palms facing each other, like holding an invisible ball between two hands and manipulating them as in playing tai chi (or translated as tai qi qigong) or as you wished way to play with your hands—the universal energy can be restored on your hands.

Practicing the Da Zhou Tian[152] has the added benefit of opening the whole body's acupuncture points, improving qi and blood circulation, boosting immunity, and encouraging a stronger universal energy and power. If during a meeting or class time, you feel tired or have mild discomfort, play with your hands under the table or while sitting on a flight and use it to recover the universal energy on your hands. It is a convenient way to help yourself.

Universal energy is inexhaustible. If it is used to treat patients, it does not consume the healer's energy. Instead, the universal energy travels through the healer into the client's body to do the healing job. Both the healer and the client can gain the benefits of improved health at the same time.

The Power of the Universal Energy

The universal energy is boundless. Its positive energy is strong enough to balance negative energy to maintain order in the universe. It enables all life to survive. This book series will help you to understand it better. Using it can sometimes heal health problems and get the desired results more quickly than with formal medical treatments.

For example, in ten minutes, it adjusted a slightly thoracic vertebrae to back to normal position. Within forty minutes of a hip replacement, it eliminated the pain from inflammation, a lumbar disc narrowing, and a pinched nerve caused by a Governor (Du) Meridian qi deficiency. The patient felt comfortable after one adjustment, but since he was an elderly with a lot coldness in his body and a long history of illness, a one-time adjustment was not enough. He had to get more adjustments and use other therapies like moxibustion with acupuncture treatment along with an herbal prescription and /or self-hypnosis to treat the root problems and avoid having trouble later.

It took only three minutes to relieve a right shoulder pain in one patient for six years. When the pain did return, the pain level was reduced. A few years ago, this same person fell onto a brick floor from a two-story high ladder. Later, he practiced the Da Zhou Tian[152] and did the universal energy healing daily by himself. The pains in his whole body improved every day.

Another person had a cold for a week without having time to visit a doctor. She had productive coughing and continuous watery running nose. But after using Comprehensive Universal Energy Healing for around five minutes, her runny nose stopped. In fewer than an additional five minutes, her cough stopped as well. Her testimonial is posted at Cold Flu[150].

There are numerous other cases that have had surprising results— so many that we cannot list them all. You can read some of them in Chapter Eleven, and please keep visiting the reader's discussion[137] to polish your knowledge and your healing skills.

Unfortunately, up until now, the main switch for the positive energy of the universe has yet to be discovered. By pushing this switch, we would be able to resolve all human catastrophe. But since there is no switch available to us, the existence of a variety of medical therapies continues to be of much value.

Everyone ought to make an effort to utilize spiritual and moral efforts to repair themselves and their bodies. There is no proxy for this. For people who do not exercises and who drink icy water, causing cold body constitution, they should stop drinking cold water, exercise, and take fu zi[*1], rou gui[*2], or raw ginger to expel coldness in the body and change their body constitution to avoid sickness. For chronic injury or sickness, there could be a blood stasis that requires the intake of herbs and/or acupuncture with moxibution treatments to rid them of the blood stasis. Using only the Comprehensive Universal Energy Healing to do adjustments is not enough to totally solve those problems.

*1   Fu zi is *Aconitum carmichaelii Debx*. But it should be used only under an herbalist's prescription to avoid too much heat added into the body. Extra heat can push the blood out of blood vessels, causing internal bleeding and possibly other health issues.

*2   Rou gui is *Cinnamomum loureiroi Nees* with a thicker skin. Supermarket sold has less treatment value. The medical grade rou gui only can intake in the cold weather, In the summer, it is easily to cause nose bleeding if intake more dosage due to the hot weather. Therefore, it's better under an acupuncturist's prescription.

Energy and Emotional Relationships

Please refer to **Raise Up Your Energy Frequency to Avoid Sickness**[160] and buy David R. Hawkins M.D. Ph.D's book of Power vs. Force to check your emotion and frequency score. If you want to raise your score, you can adopt the emotion and mind setting at the score of 500 or above.

A zealous person always feels gratitude, happiness and has a high frequency. If a person is easily angered, complaining, or has negative emotions or sickness, there is qi blocked in his/her body. When using universal energy healing to do an adjustment, his/her reaction level will be proportional to the severity of the blockage. We will mention it in more detail in Chapter Eight. If the client has poor qi/blood circulation or meridian blockage, the adjustment time should be extended. There will then be a stronger turning better reaction during adjustment.

The turning better reaction is a natural body reaction during the healing process. We will discuss it throughly in Chapter Eight.

How to Make Hands Have the Universal Energy?

Practicing the qigong of the Da Zhou Tian[152] can open the acupuncture points of the body and allow you to accept universal energy. **If you practice the Da Zhou Tian every day, your ability to accept universal energy will be gradually increased.** When you practice the Da Zhou Tian[152], do every movement five times, including kai gong (at the beginning to induce qi flowing) and shou gong (at the end to dismiss the qi). This can usually be completed in five minutes. If the body is cold or there is phlegm in the lungs or excessive blockage, it will take longer practice to feel the energy in the hands. This kind of person can do more chest expanding with the kai gong movement. It will also be difficult to feel warmth in the hands in the case of the brain being too hectic and restless. Please take the time to take a couple of deep breaths or do more kai gong movements in a slow speed with deep breathing until the brain calms, and then do the Da Zhou Tian[152].

If using universal energy healing often to help people improve their health or do self-healing, the hands will have stronger universal energy. In the Acknowledgements, it was mentioned that a good-hearted person always helps people, and his/her hands' energy is relatively stronger. If one practices the Da Zhou Tian[152], the effect will be even stronger. It increases the effectiveness of adjustment and can therefore help more health issues.

Da Zhou Tian

Prepare: Stand with your two feet apart and parallel at about the same width of your shoulders. Close your palms, and hold your arms straight forward, parallel to the floor.

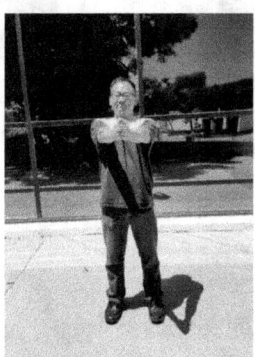

Pic 61 Arms straight forward and parallel to floor

Kai gong (to induce more qi flowing at the beginning of the qigong): Try to match your breathing with each movement. Inhale, and slowly open arms horizontally as far as they can go. Exhale, and slowly move the arms back toward each other horizontally and close the palms. Repeat the two movements until you can feel the heat between the two palms when closing the palms*. Do this three more times. Now, the qi is able to flow freely in the body. Not all people can *feel* the qi flowing, so it's okay if that's the case.

NOTE: When exhaling, if you use your nose instead of your mouth, you can keep the qi circling inside your body. The qi will flow inside your body without leaking out of your nose.

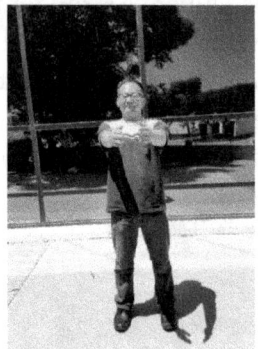
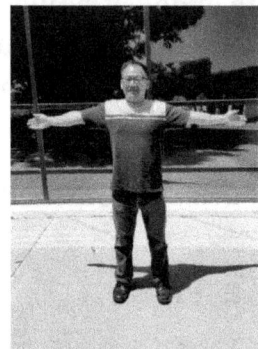

Pic 62 Inhale & Slowly Open Arms   Pic 63 Until Arms are Fully Opened

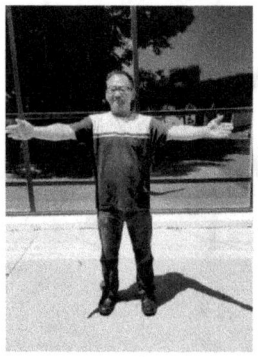
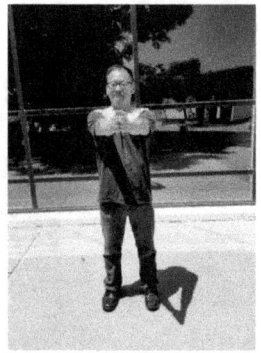

Pic 64 Exhale & Slowly Close Arms   Pic 65 Until Arms Closed Together

   *   Some people do not feel warm but feel a tingling in their hands or arms. It means the qi is flowing. In Western medicine, the heart beating pushes the blood flow. In Chinese medicine, besides the heart beating, the meridian's qi also moves the blood. The qi is the main drive for the flow of blood in TCM (Traditional Chinese Medicine) Theory. Some people might feel cold air coming from fingertips or the body—this is also good news as it means the body function is recovering and expelling extra coldness out of the body.

When the qi is weak, it pushes less blood. When the qi is stronger, not only can the person feel it flowing better but can also feel more blood flowing. When blood flows freely, the blood vessels must expand to allow for the increased flow. During the expansion of the blood vessels, the outside nerves are affected, thus generating the tingling sensation. The sensation disappears when the local blood vessel is fully expanded. Therefore, the person feels the tingling sensation until the whole blood vessel is expanded.

Meridians usually run parallel to the blood vessels and nerves. However, a meridian is not the same as a nerve because some branches of a meridian do not have a nerve branch following their route.

After kai gong, touch the tip of your tongue to your upper gum to connect the Conception and Governor Vessels (Ren and Du meridians). In the beginning stages, you will do this to guide the qi flow to follow the hand movement. However, after practicing several times, when the hands move, the qi will flow without you having to guide it. Your qi flowing will be controlled by your subconscious.

When exhaling, when both hands move to the proximity of the umbilicus, raise your anus up and hold your abdomen inward to avoid the qi being dispersed. Doing so constrains the qi to flow in the middle line of the body (within the Conception Vessel or called Ren meridian).

a. **Inhale:** Qi from Huiyin CV 1* (Ren 1) goes upward → Governor Vessel (Du Meridian) (along the spinal cord) →GV 20** (DU 20).

   * CV 1 is the Huiyin, located at the midpoint of the two lower orifices.

   ** GV20 is the Baihui located at the crossing point of the two ear apexes upper connection line and the line along the nose to the top of the head.

   Exhale: Qi from GV 20 (DU 20) goes downward →Conception Vessel (Ren Meridian, centerline of the front body) →CV1 (Ren 1).

b. **Inhale:** Qi from CV 1 (Ren 1) goes outward and upward →Groin Area** goes upward→ SI 9/10 (the connection line of the upper arm and posterior of the body).

   * Groin Area is the front folding line between the body and the upper leg.

** SI 9/10 are on the connection line of the upper arm and posterior of the body truck.

Exhale: From SI 9/10 → Lateral of the Arm (the yang side, also known as the darker side of the arm) →PC 8.

* PC 8 is the Laogong located at the point of the third fingertip when counting the thumb as the first finger and the pinky as the fifth. When making a fist, it is the middle finger touching a point in the palm.

c. **Inhale:** From PC 8 →Arm Yin Side (the white side of the arm) → CV 17* (Ren 17).

* CV 17 is the Tanzhong located at the midpoint of the two nipples or the midpoint of the space between the fourth and fifth rib for older ladies.

Exhale: From CV 17 (Ren 17), goes downward → Conception Vessel (Ren Meridian) → CV 1 (Ren 1).

d. **Inhale:** Qi from CV 1 goes upward→ Conception Vessel (Ren Meridian)→ Zhong Ge*.

* Zhong Ge is the diaphragm. It is meeting line between the yin part of the lower part of the body and the yang part of the upper part of the body and is the transverse line of the lower ribs.

Exhale: From Zhong Ge → Lateral Side of Body → Yang Qiao Meridian loacted on the lateral side of the legs →KI 1*.

* KI 1 is the Yongquan located at the depression point when the foot is in plantar flexion.

e. **Inhale:** Qi from KI 1 goes upward→ Yin Qiao Meridian, located on the medial side of the legs →CV 4 (Ren 4).

* CV 4 is the Guanyuan, located on the Conception Vessel (Ren Meridian) between the umbilicus and the horizontal ramus of the pelvic bone and 3/5 of the distance below the umbilicus.

Exhale: Qi from CV 4 goes downward → CV 1. This distance is very short. In order to get better function, do this as slowly as possible.

Shou gong 收功 (at the end of the qigong to dismiss the qi. Otherwise, the qi will move to unwanted rout.): Move the palms upward (you can also raise the body up as well) until reaching the maximum and inhale (using only the nostrils). Then, press the palms downward (lowering body to its normal position) and exhale (again, use only the nostrils). Repeat two or four or six times.

For a demo, please watch the Da Zhou Tian[152].

Please note, fully extend your arms while practicing the Da Zhou Tian[152] so that you can get the maximum qi flowing inside your body and get the most benefit, no matter whether it's for your own health improvement or for increasing the effectiveness of your Comprehensive Universal Energy Healing power.

Attention:

1. Avoid doing Da Zhou Tian if the weather is hot, you have high blood pressure, you have blood vessel blockage (your tongue's body will have a purplish tinge— darker purple means severe blockage), you've been drinking wine, or you're just in an angry mood[152]. Blood vessels could burst in your head, and you could have a stroke.

2. Do not practice the Da Zhou Tian[152] before going to bed to avoid your energy being boosted up so much that you cannot fall asleep.

3. People who have undergone surgery should not practice the Da Zhou Tian[152] to avoid tearing the wound.

4. Before doing any exercise, please discuss it with your physician to avoid any accidents.

5. Some people have phlegm in the lungs, and their arms cannot open up to 180 degrees. You do not need to force yourself to open that far. Only open your arms as much as you can and as much as is comfortable. If keep practicing, the angle of the arms opening will grow larger.

   While I worked on a cruise ship, a guest came to my health seminar, and his arms could open horizontally less than sixty degrees. I asked him to practice opening and closing his arms in that fashion, repeating twenty to thirty times in each session. On the third day, he came to another of my seminars and was thrilled to tell me that he could open his arms one hundred and eighty degrees.

I had a patient whose lung capacity was only 1000 cc. She began to open and close her arms horizontally once or twice a day for ten to fifteen minutes. Two weeks later, her lung capacity increased to 1500 cc. It's a small movement, but it has great effectiveness in improving weak lungs.

For people who frequently catch colds or the flu, who cough and feel uncomfortable in the chest, who have bad skin or dry skin, who smoke or have had lung injuries before, or whose lung capacity has been impaired in some way, practicing the opening and closing of the arms twenty to thirty times per day can improve lung function, enhance immunity and lung capacity, and improve the appearance of the skin. It also benefits those whose lung qi could not descend, causing constipation, or those whose heads sweat when eating hot food or drink or has heat or sweating on head.

6. Some people have a motor mind and cannot calm down. It's better to do a few deep breathing exercises first and then do the Da Zhou Tian[152]. Focusing on slowing down the breathing and opening and closing the arms slowly helps to calm the brain.

7. Any organ that is not functioning well can cause a cough. We cannot blame the cough solely on the lungs. Please refer to the *Huang Di Nei Jing • Su Wen • Cough Theory*. We will teach you how to diagnose your cough and how to do adjustments for a cough in a future book.

8. After practicing the Da Zhou Tian[152], you should be able to feel the qi and the blood flowing smoothly and comfortably through your body. The Conception and Governor vessels (Ren snd Du meridians) are now open, activating the thymus gland, kidneys, and bone marrow—the organ responsible for primary immunity—as well as the spleen and other organs of the secondary immune system. Thus, the whole body's immunity is increased.

How Can People Who Cannot Stand Firmly Gain Universal Energy in their Hands?

People who cannot stand firmly can sit to practice the Da Zhou Tian[152] They can move the hands to induce the qi to flow and get the same effect.

How Can Bedridden People Get Universal Energy in their Hands?

In the sports arena, it has been widely demonstrated that doing exercises in the imagination can have the same results as doing exercises on the playground or in the field.

Therefore, bedridden people can practice the Da Zhou Tian[152] in their imagination. If the hands and the arms are mobile, they can move as much as possible to the extent their health will allow. This will help to generate the yang qi. Yang qi is the force that will improve the body functions, enhance immunity, and aid in recovery. And as I've mentioned before, people are animals, and animals keep moving to stay alive!"

How to Do Healing After Getting the Universal Energy?

If possible, invite your client to practice the Da Zhou Tian[152] with you. By doing so, he will have a stronger qi flowing inside his body. The first benefit is if the client has a motor mind (his brain is too busy), this allows him to calm down. The other benefit is that it increases sensitivity and receiving power.

If the site does not allow you to do the Da Zhou Tian[152], you can let your client follow your instruction to do deep breathing until his brain can calm down. Let your client give you a signal by lifting a hand or a finger when he is calmed. You can then let him stop to do deep breathing. Meanwhile, pay attention to the elapsed time.

Later, you can soothe the motor minded person's liver, strengthen his spleen, or strengthen his kidneys as needed. The length of the adjustment time should be proportional to the time it took him to calm down.

Be cautioned that there are other factors involved, such as body constitution and how long the health problem existed. For a cold or a weak constitution, the adjustment time should be longer. For chronic diseases, the adjustment time should be proportional to the length of the disease. As you practice more Comprehensive Universal Energy Healing and gain more experience, you will gradually know how to control the adjustment time.

If you visit readers discussion[137] to ask a question(s) or post your experience, you are doing good deeds which can help speed up your learning. We would also like you to share your adjustment experience(s) on the Da Zhou Tian[152]. By doing so, you can increase your frequency.

We encourage you to practice the Da Zhou Tian[152] (only five minutes a day) or do meditation every day. Anytime you can, use your hands to help yourself or others without practicing the Da Zhou Tian[152] before the adjustment.

For the symbol of the adjustment points, please refer to Appendix Five for Important Acupuncture Points and Organs.

Usually, you can put one hand (either your left or right) on top of the head at **Baihui U3**. Put the other hand on the forehead between the eyebrows. Your hands can be placed directly on the client's body, or you can keep them a few inches away for the adjustment. Keeping some distance transmits more energy to the client. The energy power is actually proportional to the distance.

However, if the client cannot feel the heat from your hands, you'd better put them on his body first until he is able to feel the heat of your hands. Then gradually move your hands away.

However, when the client's body is too cold that can make your hands also be colded to lower your adjustment effectiveness. If this is the case, you can use your thumb to do acupress at geshu BL 17 (Appendix Five, back shu point, 1.5 cun laterla to T7.) on the client's back. BL 17 can activate whole body blood flow. Until the client's body warmed up, then you can keep a distance to make adjustments.

The best way to make adjustments is to keep hands a couple of inches away from the client's body without touching the client.

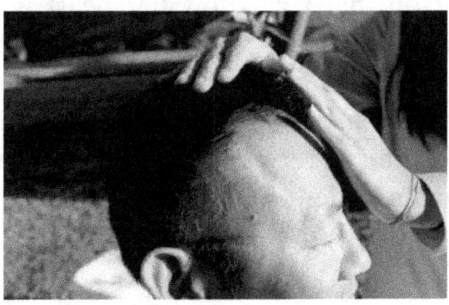

Pic 66 Baihui U3 & U1/U2 area to make people calm down.

The client will tell you in a short time (usually within two or three minutes) that he feels calm or cozy or comfortable. Next, you can combine the universal energy with the universal codes to do healing. Please read the next section for how to apply.

For adjusting different health issues, please read Chapter Ten How to Handle the Emergency Situation and Chapter Eleven Some Commonly Seen Health Issues in Healing. Please pay close attention to our future new book announcement[172].

The Benefits of Practicing Universal Codes

This book asks you to combine love, gratitude, sharing, and collaboration—the four universal codes—and Comprehensive Universal Energy Healing and practice them in your daily life. Do your best to practice them for at least twenty-one days to allow them become a part of your daily life or a part of your character.

In combining the four universal codes with Comprehensive Universal Energy Healing, and in reading this book, you will be able to heal other people or be healed yourself. Follow the book's methods to practice, and you have many chances to experience how effective they can be in improving your health and life.

The four universal codes are the keys to open the universe's prosperity, happiness, and good luck for you. Each code unlocks a different treasure for you. You can use them individually or combine all to treat people.

Such as a person that you know her heart was broken by her husband who has a girlfriend and wants to divorce. During the healing process, you try to find chances to let her feel gratitude also feel how lucky that it's not her fault and she can be released earlier. Using the lucky feeling to replace be abandoned and betrayed. The gratitude is the main code to be practices. If add, add love to love herself.

For a depression and hopeless person, you can emphasize love from his family, friends, even the God or the universe to let him find the strength to move life forward.

For a regular person, you can let your client experience all of the four codes.

• Love

This story happened in the simplicity of a countryside. The local residents trusted people and were friendly to others.

One day, as John played in the front yard, he saw three elderly people nearby. They looked tired. John walked up to them and asked, "Would you like to come to our home to rest for a little bit?"

One of them replied, "That would be good. Thank you. But, you'd better go back to ask your parents' permission."

John ran home and talked to his parents. His parents welcomed the guests, so John ran out and invited them in.

Another of the three said, "We cannot all go in together." And then he pointed to his companions and introduced them to John. "This happy man is Success, this better dressed fellow is Fortunate, and my name is Love. Please go back and ask your parents which of us they'd like to invite in?"

John went back to talk to his parents again.

His father said, "Invite Success in. I need to be successful."

John asked, "Can we invite Fortunate? I like his dress and would like to hear his fortunate story so I can learn how I might be able to dress so handsomely."

Then his Mom said, "We are a friendly village full of love, trust, and friendship. They travel around, so why not invite Love in to let us learn more about outside people. Later, when you grow up and want to go outside for your future, we can know about where you choose to go, and both your father and I will feel comfortable with your choice." All of them agreed with her idea.

John went out to invite Love in. Shortly after, Success and Fortunate followed. John and his parents didn't understand and said to Love, "You told us that only one of you could come in. Why did they then follow?"

Love laughed happily and replied, "It's our mission to share our stories with people. Usually, people only ask Success or Fortunate. So they only can have one in to share the skills to get what they want. However, when people invite me in, Success and Fortunate come in as well to witness people who possess and give love to others, to hear about the kind of success and the fortunate stories that were created from a loving mind."

It's normal and necessary for everyone to accept and give love. Without love, there is nothing that can go right.

Everyone has to love himself first.—his holiness, purity, and health. To do self-healing and to maintain a healthy, productive, and youthful vitality is an expression of self-love.

Using your hands to do Comprehensive Universal Energy Healing for your loved ones is a form of noble love. Helping someone you do not know represents great love because giving love to family members, friends, and relatives is a lot easier than giving love to a stranger.

The noble performance of purity, kindness, mercy, bravery, wisdom, and courage to help others overcome illness is pure love. This kind love does not ask for feedback and is not greedy in giving.

• Gratitude

Two retired classmates decided to travel around the world together on foot. When they were college students, one was a class leader, and the other was his assistant class leader. They were good partners.

The class leader, William, was a smart person with innovative ideas and ambitions. The assistant class leader, Henry, appreciated and respected William's smart ideas and ambitions. They collaborated very well and managed to perform a lot of miracles together in their college life.

When encountering difficulties in their travels, Henry complained. After Henry's complaints, William always pulled out a piece of paper to write them down, but he'd end up throwing it into the trash can before he fell asleep.

When there was joy that was created from Henry, William wrote it down and kept it until the next city when he could post it with their pictures on his blog and social media on the Internet.

Near the end of their travels, Henry asked William why his complaints had been thrown away, yet William had posted good things online.

William replied Henry, "I feel so grateful that you can accompany me on my dream. I wrote unhappy things to when I noticed your disappointment with me. If I was right, I kept my decision to myself and ignored your complaint. If I was wrong, I modified my plan and got your agreement. And then, I cleared it from my memory.

When you have a better idea, I let everyone know it. Don't you think that after we go back when we hold classmate reunion, people will ask questions according to my post? Do you want to them ask happy things or unhappy things?

When I get older and be alone at home, I only want all of the happy memories company with me to support my breathing for each day.

Moreover, you were always curious about how my business was so successful. It's one of my secrets of how did I treat my subordinates that I learned after graduation. I am never greedy to show my gratitude to the people who helps me or make my day."

If we give gratitude to our parents, caregivers, and anyone who has helped or benefited us, it reminds us to always think about the source of our favors. And it also lets the receiver of the gratitude feel comfort.

If we are grateful when we look at what we have, we will feel contentment and remain in an abundance mentality, rather than feeling dissatisfaction and embracing insatiable greed, stinginess, and dissatisfaction. All of these harm our spirit and moral cultivation.

Whenever I drive on the highway, I always pray. "The Super Power! I give my gratitude to You! Please give Your love to everyone on the road!" The result is always a smooth drive to my destination. Inevitably, I feel even more gratitude for the day in all sorts of hidden things and moments.

My spiritual friends often mention that gratitude leads them to good fortune. They have better interpersonal relationships with the people who surround them, and their lives becomes more enjoyable.

After reading this book, you will also practice gratitude. You will gradually notice more and more people, things, and moments worthy of your gratitude. And there will always be happiness in your mind. Your health and fortune will grow to be better and better.

• Sharing

When I mention sharing, it reminds me of holding the "new product launching workshops" among conservative company engineers in Taiwan about forty years ago. In the beginning, there were only one or two engineers who came back from the US who wanted to share their newly designed test equipment.

The speaker shared the function of the equipment, the design ideas he had, the problems he encountered in his design, his solutions to those problems and how he implemented them. Then there were discussion sessions where recommendations could be collected from colleagues.

I never thought that two to three months later, engineers would be clamoring to participate. In each workshop, there were two to three new designs launched. Technical discussions between engineers increased enthusiastically.

In my private life, when I shared my culinary dishes with my friends and neighbors, I received more people's tasty foods on our dining table. When I shared the fruits that grew in my back yard, I got more varieties of organic food shared back with me.

When I shared my treatment experiences and encountered treatment problems, I gained different views and research findings that could help me better solve my problems.

It's common in school and in the workplace to see people bring food to let friends enjoy delicious foods and taste new things, learning new things available in the market. Besides the fun of sharing, you also have the experience of being the provider and from the provider to become the beneficiaries. There is a famous saying that says, "To be a provider is happier than a receiver!"

• Collaboration

We read in elementary school that a father told his kids that a single chopstick is easily broken, but a bundle of chopsticks is not. In telling this story, the father educated his children on the benefit of teamwork.

The saying "Many hands make light work" also clarifies the benefits of collaboration. In today's era of high tech, we need many different professionals involved in order to achieve our goals.

The benefits of human collaborations are often just the sum of a simple addition problem. In the case of Comprehensive Universal Energy Healing, however, the collaboration benefits are totaled using multiplication rather than addition. This deeply matches the necessity in today's era of cooperating for scientific innovation. More important is the understanding between the people taking care of each other that they are mutually interdependent.

How to Make Your Adjustment More Effective

- ## Mindset

  - ➢ Mindset that a Reader Should Have
    - o Treat this book as a health maintenance book rather than a medical book to treat diseases! It must go through careful clinical trials before it can be used as a medical reference book. I am seeking ways to let it be included within the medical research scope in order to benefit the public.
    - o This book can be used as an auxiliary therapy for any severe diseases and to heal mild discomforts.

      In today's busy life, you can use it for your own health maintenance purposes. When you go to bed, put your hands on your liver, spleen, or any other part of your body that is weak, and do self-healing. While you are at a meeting or watching TV, you can put your hands on any site that needs healing.
    - o If you keep doing more healings, your healing power will continue to increase. It doesn't matter if you heal yourself or others. I always heal myself before I sleep—I put my hands on my organs to strengthen them. During a workshop or any time I have to wait, I do self- healing.

  - ➢ The Healer and the Client's Mindset and the Basic Understanding

    All of the healing experiences and testimonials listed in the book are for reference only. The healing effectiveness is related to the healer's mindset, spirit, healing time used, as well as the client's mindset, spirit, severity and duration of disease, and healing environment. During the healing process, there's no need to be rushed. If there is a worry in your mind, the healing effectiveness will decrease because the worry will generate negative energy to block the qi from flowing smoothly.

During the healing process, the healer or the client having thoughts about immediate success and quick recovery could possibly induce the reverse result. However, if the client imagines the happiness after recovery and gives gratitude for the universal unconditional favor, abundant love, and the healer spending time to do the healing, it will positively benefit the healing effectiveness.

The healer and the client must be quiet during the healing process. It helps the qi and the blood to circulate freely in both bodies and benefits healing. However, during break time, if the client gives feedback to the healer about his feelings or any improvement, it will help the healer to improve later results. If needed, during the adjustment, you also can communicate with each other calmly and gently.

If you have any question, please go to the book website Readers' Discussion[137]Q & A[153] to ask questions according to the chapter content and get input from others.

The Comprehensive Universal Energy Healing and abundant love are coming from kindness and all kinds of noble characters. Therefore, using the same kind mindset to access the website of this book's readers' discussion[137] and related content to ask or answer a question(s) is pertinent and can accumulate your good deed rewards.

In this chapter, you will learn that any intention, thoughts, mind setting, and behavior induces the universe's feedback, and that is directly related to your health and fortune.

Your healing results are better if you are out of the wind. If indoor, and facing a fan or air conditioner which is blowing strongly and making it very cold, this is not benefiting the healing. A quiet place is better than a noisy or attention-disturbing environment. If, right before doing Comprehensive

Universal Energy Healing, the healer drank a cold drink or ate cold foods or washed hands with cold water, the client will feel that coldness coming from the healer but not the healing power. The healer should rub hands or do Da Zhou Tian[152] to warm them up, and then do energy healing.

> ## The Mindset a Healer Should Have

It's better first to start doing your Comprehensive Universal Energy Healing on yourself or on someone who trusts you. Then apply it to others. It's also a wise idea that, after accumulating sufficient knowledge and experience for specific health issues, you start by doing healing for those familiar issues only. In doing so, you will not delay people from visiting a health professional on time if needed, and you will avoid later guilt for possibly causing irreversible consequences. It also helps you to avoid situations where a patient's serious illness could change quickly, and you don't know how to handle it.

The healing effectiveness is not decided only by how long or how many times the healer did the Comprehensive Universal Energy Healing. If a healer is willing to accept the challenge, when he encounters different situations, he is always looking for more effective healing methods. This is much better than the healer who follows only one healing method without caring whether the healing results are good or bad.

It's better for the healer to be open-minded and humble and never to promise a healing result to the client. There are never any promises where medical treatments are concerned. There are too many factors involved, especially when there is no way for you to control the client's thinking, lifestyle, diet habits, and environmental influences.

It's important for you to ask your client when and how the uncomfortable situation commenced. If the client's pain was from an injury, there might be bone fractures, dislocation, sprains, or cerebral concussion. All of those need professional diagnosis and treatment. If there is a severe, sharp pain in the right lower abdomen, it could be appendicitis, and the client may need to go to the emergency room immediately.

Please do not feel discomfort in telling your client to seek a medical professional's help. When you have accumulated enough knowledge and experiences, you will have a better idea about the necessary healing time for each healing, the healing frequency, and the break time between two healings, as well as the possible total healing period. At that point, you will have more chances to reduce your client's medical costs by staying with you.

> ### The Mindset that a Client Should Have

It's important for the client who accept Comprehensive Universal Energy Healing and believe that it does positive things for health without harm. The discomfort felt during the healing process is a temporary transitional reaction and a necessary process for getting better. We call it a "turning better reaction." Relax your brain, body, and mind. Give gratitude for the chance at healing in order to let the universal energy flow freely in your body. Doing so helps you become better sooner. Chapter Eight will talk more about the "turning better reactions." You can read Chapter Eight before you accept the healing.

On the other hand, pain may be caused by your improper posture or accessories. Maybe the height of your pillow does not match the length of your neck, and that is causing your neck pain. These things should be corrected to prevent pain.

In some situations, you may need to change your diet, keeping away from cold foods and drinks to avoid the coldness causing stomachache, abdominal pain, and diarrhea. Please read Cold Foods & Cold Drinks Caused Health Problems[154] or get a quick glance at Cold Foods Drinks Caused Problems Chart Rev 1[155].

If your lifestyle is not healthy, you will need to make a change. In order to have better energy and immunity, don't overwork yourself and go to bed early before 10:00 p.m. to avoid dreams and nightmares or insomnia that may wake you up in the night.

Do moral self-cultivation to avoid evil thoughts, cultivate kindness to earn happiness, and practice Da Zhou Tian[152] every day to balance yin and yang and stay away from sicknesses.

How to Combine Universal Energy and Universal Codes

When adjusting the client who has a health issue, ask her what her religion is. Then ask her to give gratitude to her God. If she has no religion, ask her to give gratitude to whoever is most deserving, such as parents or spouse, or to the universe for supplying everything she needs to support her life.

When the client gives gratitude, both you and the client can feel the increase in the energy flowing in the client. In the majority of cases, it increases at least twofold.

Next, tell your client, "Imagine that one whom you gave gratitude gives you a lot of love in return. The love becomes golden with heat and light and starts flowing quickly from your head into your body, fulfilling your body. It starts to overflow, flowing out of your body and filling this room (or this space, or this garden—it depends on where you are)." You can ask immediately, "Do you want to share it?"

In general, most people will nod their heads. Immediately, you and your clients will feel the heat increase several times. If you are curious, you can double check with your client for the increased heat (energy). For two more years, I adjusted numerous people, and there was only one man who did not have increased energy. It may have been due to the fact that he was an MD and had an intention against it.

When doing Comprehensive Universal Energy Healing, if the client thinks about love and expresses gratitude to the source of love, the universal energy in the body will grow instantly. If he is willing to share with others, the power of the universal energy will increase exponentially. If there are more healers or crossing hands/arms to do self-healing, the universal energy has a synergistic effect that is significant and much more powerful than doing by one person without collaboration.

By now, you should see that there are without a doubt universal codes that regulate us and are directly related to our health. You might have never noticed it before. But please, from here on, please pay attention to your intentions and your behaviors—what you do and what you say.

For the person, who does not want to share at first, you'd better adjust his heart to make him happier and more willing to share later. Usually, this person has heart problems or had his heart hurt by someone.

When more than two healers collaborate to do universal energy healing, its strength and effectiveness is the synergy of adding two healer's energies together. For example, one healer may have three parts of energy, and the other healer has five. But when they work together, their overall energy is more than ten parts energy when doing Comprehensive Universal Energy Healing.

The universal energy flows in the two healers and in the client. Soon after, the client will feel the two healer's energy as the same, and if you invite the client to join you to do healing by putting his hands on himself, his hands will very quickly have the same temperature as yours. I always invite the client to join in to speed up the healing or give him the ability to adjust his root problems at home.

Investment Revenue Exercise

Practice the Da Zhou Tian[152] every day. It's better to practice it in the morning so you can have one whole day to feel energetic. In the beginning, if you cannot have a full energetic day, you should spend five minutes practicing the Da Zhou Tian[152] again when you feel tired to recover your energy.

Once you have enough energy on your hands at any given time, you no longer need to practice the Da Zhou Tian[152] before doing the healing. When you have enough energy, it means that when your palms are a few inches away from your skin, you can feel the heat. When you get to this point, you can put one hand directly on the top of your head (U3) and the other hand on your heart to improve blood circulation and increase oxygen capacity. Then your energy will be back. However, if you keep practice the Da Zhou Tian[152] every day, your health improved and you have stronger healing power in your hands.

Try to find ten people as your practice targets and then fill in the following table. At this time, regardless of whether they have health problems or not, you can apply Comprehensive Universal Energy Healing to them. It is important to ask for consent to apply healing.

Put one hand on the Baihui and the other hand on the forehead. Until your target person can feel the heat of your hand and feel the qi traveling, ask his feelings. When there is a positive feeling such as calm, then follow the steps on how to combine the universal energy and universal codes together to practice until he is willing to share and nods his head. After you finish with each person, make notes in the table below.

Note:

If your client has headache, put one hand on Baihui (U3, DU 20) and the other hand at the painful area to relieve the pain. This only addresses the symptom instead of solving the root problem.

If the target feels heat and pain in head, wave your hands around the head and move them downward to assist in cooling. This also only helps the symptom instead of solving the root problem.

No	Name	Time Used	Client's Reaction
1			
2			
3			
4			
5			
6			
7			
8			
9			
10			

CHAPTER SIX

Healing Points
● ● ● ● ● ● ● ● ● ● ● ● ● ● ● ● ● ● ●

"Diligence lets study be proficient, amusement causes it to be uncultivated. If only following instead of thinking, the profession accomplished will be..."

Gu Wen Guan Zhi • Jin Xue Jie, Yu Han

Universal Abundance

The universal abundance is inexhaustible. More exciting is the high diversity and numerous alternative resources so that there is no worry about a shortage.

After the gasoline crisis in the world that brought with it a high cost of living for everyone, we later discovered a new technology to get gasoline from shale. There is also a Japanese invention using water to replace gasoline as fuel. It has not only dropped the cost, but has also carried with it new benefits.

With farm land in short supply, Israeli people are hanging boxes in which to plant foods. Fewer insects damage the plants, and they are able to export foods as well.

There are not really any limitations in life. Too often, our thinking is self-limited and we worry too much about negative considerations and fear of failure. Not thinking of innovation and breakthroughs have generated unnecessary competition, fighting, theft, robbery, fear, cheating, greed, and ahost of other selfish and unethical behavior.

If everyone could only live based on what Confucius said—"Do unto others, do not impose on others"—we would all be born with the natural abundance. If we focused on steadfastly finding the proper way to develop our talents, doing our best to take responsibility, and only accepting a fair share without doing damage in the process, then everyone's life would be abundant.

Every generation's lifetime talents have been already written in the genes to pass on. That's why hypnosis and self-learning with practice can wake up the talent and get extra achievement.

In addition, there are twelve-strands in DNA that document everyone's personality, personality traits, talents, and life mission. They also link us to and communicate with higher dimensional space. There are two strands that can help to repair the other DNA strands[203]. They can be easily covered by greed, selfishness, jealousy, anger, ignorance, and other negative emotions and unethical behaviors. However, they can also be lifted and/or improved through the right education or medication[204] and be transformed into a noble soul which can enjoy the abundant resources of the universe[207, 208].

If you give gratitude, open your loving hands to share the Comprehensive Universal Energy Healing, and collaborate with others to make adjustments and improve others' health conditions, you'll be surprised to see the door to your life's treasure cave gradually opening. If you give gratitude daily and take advantage of more chances to open your loving hands, it can help you avoid many of the puzzling routes within the treasure cave and reach the treasures more directly. Besides that, you will also discover that in your life, there are infinite blessings of love, praise, and priceless treasures waiting for you!

You can hardly imagine the universe's abundance. The universe's divine love fills the world with streams of helping. Listen to the small voice of your great self. All difficulties have solutions.

Focus on positive thinking. Take action, and solve the problem instead of falling into frustration. If you read the biographies of great people, high achievers, and great inventors, they will validate the fact that thinking positively brings great rewards.

More importantly, even when a resource is contaminated, there are other resources substituting it such as the alternative energies. Plus Israel is a shortage of land and water country, but they adopt agriculture skills, to export goods and flowers.

The key is that do you have the courage to break through the difficulties for the public interest, to solve the problem.

Modern medicine is an example. People trust the medical profession and blindly hand their health over. Because medicine is big business and today's society's health care system complex, medical care is not cheap. It's even worse when the patient spends a lot of money but cannot regain his health. All kinds of treatments flourish—and they're full of both good and bad.

So universal divine love gives self-healing back to the earth. You must practice self-hypnosis, hypnosis, qigong, meditation, music healing[205], moral love, gratitude, sharing, and collaboration. A person should be the most sensitive to his own body's needs to avoid a small discomfort turning into a serious illness and bearing unnecessary suffering.

Waking up between 1:00 - 3:00 AM treats the liver, and reduces the risk of liver diseases including liver cancer.

Or, when one just falls down, apply Comprehensive Energy Healing on the injury spots to avoid qi stagnation or blood stasis later, there will be no pain left later.

The Universal Abundance Relies on Everyone's Maintenance

Modern society has twisted the important values, making it all about money, social rank, and fame rather than personal contribution to the community, the universe and its net worth of abilities (potential resources and abilities minus debts).

There exist huge biases: over-decorated without helping poverty, but not laugh prostitution, without thinking, but simply imitates advertising. Such as despite one's neck length to buy counter pillow and causes neck pain to spend more money, overeating meat causes wastage of natural resources and creates a diabetic patient, polluting the earth and destroying the ecological balance of the environment by too much material shopping only for own interests.

People do things purely for profit without caring about anyone's health, such as using chemicals instead of natural food, attempting to sell or cover up the products that aren't supposed to be sold because they damage the health. Despise the person who damaged their health due to contributing too much to others, there are people who hurt the others without sense; the killing power of the language to put people down such as against people who are not in our group, label people to limit their freedom such as for their intelligence or ADHD who are too active, bipolar kids who are too sensitive or artistic to put them on drugs or refuse them to enter a regular classroom, indigo kids to put too much focus or stress on them.

If you use diet to cut down sweets or meats or you use acupuncture to calm ADHD down, to develop indigo and bipolar's artistic or literature ability, letting them express could be a better way to treat them.

Please watch the YouTube video: The Indigo Evolution full-length documentary Indigo Children[205] to find how the educators faced problems for indigo. It's the same for education fund shortage for the others as labeled as ADHD. If the Comprehensive Universal Energy Healing can be broadly applied to cut down medical costs to increase the education fund, numerous kids and their family, plus their school teachers, will get a huge benefit. It's more meaningful to correctly use the society's limited resources.

There are too many consciences that need to be awakened, too many morals and spirits that need to be improved*. It's now the time to renew the universal codes to purify our hearts, improve our health, and reduce human disasters such as chemicals added foods that have caused so many severe diseases.

---

* There are those who use material items as a way to measure the value of a person. It's not uncommon for someone to purchase a nice dress or jewelry for an event, just to return it for a full refund once it's over.

Others will make a complaint, even if the service has a positive result, in order to not pay or cut down service fee or claim lawsuit to get benefit.

We read a lot of stories about millionaires who started from scratch. We're also familiar with the stories of those who splurge excessively and plunge from wealth into debt. We know the consequences of only withdrawing from our bank account without depositing. It's our obligation to use our love and our hearts to manage the universal abundant resources! How do we fulfill these obligations? By carrying out the universal codes and practicing them always!

Therefore, we should not only make adjustments on the physical body, we should also adjust psychologically. Let us start with simple and easy codes already mentioned in the book—love, gratitude, sharing, and cooperation. We should use these codes to modify our behaviors and what we say. In this way, we increase our on-hand tools—positive emotions like love and positive words by gratitude words[208]—and can strive to obtain different universal resources for our use.

The universe has seemingly infinite resources, and if one resource becomes polluted or depleted, there will be another to substitute. But think about the discovery of a new resource and the time it takes to become be widely available—it can take a long time. And it may not be available for everyone to enjoy at the start. It may not be affordable.

Garbage from the United States used to be dumped in poor countries. China used to dump garbage where poor people lived, etc. People today, for their own convenience, drink bottled water, producing tons of plastic waste. We are purposely and knowingly producing too much waste, and we overeat meat without thinking about the animals' cries before they are killed. Where is our humanity?

Have you ever thought about the price we pay for our inhumanity? How can not caring for others—humans, animals, and the environment—escape universal condemnation? The answer is that there is no lucky person who can be waived from universal retribution, even though when you look it seems to be silent.

When you express gratitude or share, you can reap positive rewards. In contrast, there can also be a negative reward through accidents or disasters. However, karma often delays the negative in favor of giving chances to partake of the divine love of the universe to allow people can correct their mistakes.

Psychological Adjustment Point

Please go through the Investment Revenue Exercise at the end of this chapter.

The Main Adjustment Points on the Body

In Appendix Four, Basic Traditional Chinese Medicine Theory, we mention that the body has more than a thousand points which communicate with the universe. They are the switches for the body's numerous physical functions. They are both the diagnostic points and the treatment points. Naturally, some points have more extensive features than the others. In addition, all of the acupuncture points are connected directly or indirectly. When the body has no blockage, they are interlinked. If blocked, they may not be well connected.

Our body always gives us signs before sickness. The related acupuncture point(s) also show tenderness. The more severe the problem, the more tenderness, you will experience. Remember, there is no silent killer in Chinese medicine.

A patient could not sleep well from one to three clock in the mornings for a while. Later, when more symptoms came out—unhappiness, night sweats, general pain, and then pain with warmth in the liver area—he was diagnosed with liver cancer. Why was he not treated when there was a sleeping problem? It would have avoided a series discomforts and maybe even have caught it before it turned into cancer.

We separate the healing points into the front and the back of the body to facilitate memory and application. The important acupuncture points are summarized in Appendix Five, Locations for Important Acupuncture Points and Organs, with pictures for your reference at any time.

- ## The Front of the Body

There are many schools using energy to heal diseases. Traditional Chinese medicine uses acupuncture points. Other schools, like yoga and Reiki, use the chakra. It is also possible to use organs to do healing because organs serve as the pump on the meridian's pathway. They have the function to soothe the whole meridian's qi and blood flowing.

According to your preferences and experience, you are free to choose which approach to use. Because I am of the Chinese medicine origin, I thought it best to write this book based on the Traditional Chinese medicine. But I equally respect the contributions of the other schools to the public health.

- ## Yoga and Reiki's Chakras

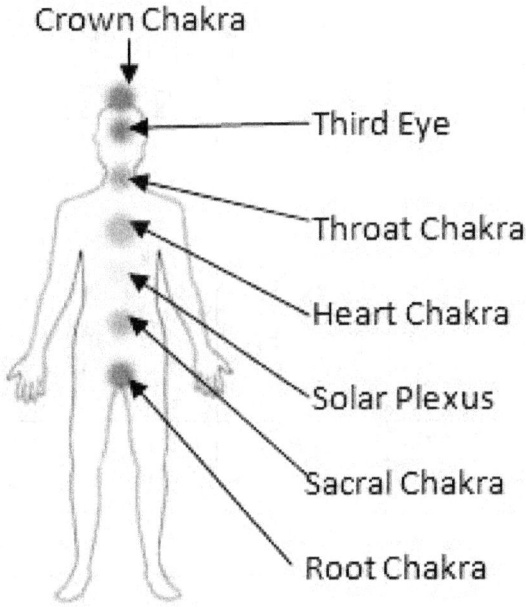

Fig 4 Chakras Chart[206]

Chakras Locations and Functions

Chakra	Color[23]	Acupuncture Points[21] (Front)	Function[23]
Crown Chakra	purple	GV[20]	Self-improvement; pausing for universal wisdom and harmonious fusion with the universe; spiritual connection to the divine universe without transgressing the ethical boundaries.
Third Eye	Indigo	Yingtang	Connects with the pituitary and pineal gland, brain and nervous system, eyes, ears, and nose. Has the ability to integrate the brain to think rationally and sensibly, intellectually and truthfully. Further development of vision rather than fantasy and the ability of insight into the truth and self-awareness.
Throat Chakra	Blue	CV[22]	Has the ability to express the internal voice to the outside. Based on good critical thinking skills, leadership, or creativity, it bravely speaks out of the inner feelings.
Heart Chakra	Green	CV[17]	It's the whole body system's axis and emotional confluence point. It maintains a close relationship with self and the others. People with a healthy heart chakra are happy, are approachable, are good at sharing, have good interpersonal relationships, are forgiving, loving, and merciful, and carry out their dreams.
Solar Plexus	Yellow	CV[14]	The central power of the energy field, the spirit of wisdom and the strength to act, can grasp and handle a moral crisis, practice self-restraint.
Sacral Chakra	Orange	CV[6]	Ability to desire intimacy, willing to take risks to create, can turn failures around into successes.
Root Chakra	Red	CV[2]	Pursuing and reproduction for future generations provides a sense of security.

Chakra Locations and Adjustment Table

Chakra	Back Point[21]	Physical Dysfunction
Crown Chakra	Baihui GV[20]	Mental disorders and body pain.
Third Eye	Fengfu GV[16]	Brain and head-related problems including brain, eyes, ear, nose, head diseases.
Throat Chakra	Dazhui GV[14]	Endocrine problems for reproduction, growth, metabolism, digestive and personality problems.
Heart Chakra	Lingtai GV[10]	Heart problems and lost love feeling.
Solar Plexus	Jizhong GV[6]	Digestive problems including diabetes, fatigue, low self-esteem and confidence.
Sacral Chakra	Yaoyangguan GV[3]	Reproductive and water retention problems, cold emotions.
Root Chakra	Yaoshu GV[2]	Mental: Personality bias is to be dominant or weak without feeling satisfaction their daily life, fear or abuse without emotional ease. Physical: Reproductive problems and problems related to lower abdomen and lower limbs.

"Chakras (chakra) means the wheel, which is the energy of the rotating disc, or rotary, coupling with the body of the spine and central nervous system in human skin at the periphery of the top three to four inches. Chakras neurally network with direct access to the body. They rotate clockwise, and the spiral galaxy rotates in the same direction. Each chakra has its own unique vibration frequency, respectively, with one of the colorful rainbows."[24]

If you do not know how to use your hands and start to make an adjustment, use the above table as a reference. In addition, you can put one hand in front of the Conception (Ren) Meridian position and the other hand behind in the Governor (Du) Meridian corresponding points. Allowing the qi to go back and forth horizontally through the body is better because it means that there is no blockage between your hands and the covered area.

• Acupuncture Points and Organ Locations

Codes are in parentheses (this series book code, acupuncture point code).

Please refer to Appendix Five, Locations for Important Acupuncture Points and Organs.

There are important points on the Conception (Ren) Meridians: Zhongji (CV 3 or Ren 3), Guanyuan (CV 4 or Ren 4), Qihai (CV 6 or Ren 6), Shenque (CV 8 or Ren 8), Zhongwan (CV 12 or Ren 12), Juque (CV 14 or Ren 14), Tanzhong (CV 17 or Ren 17), Tiantu (CV 22 or Ren 22); Points on the Governor (DU) Vessel: Shenting (U2, GV 24 or DU 24), Yintang (U1), Baihui (U3, GV 20 or DU 20).

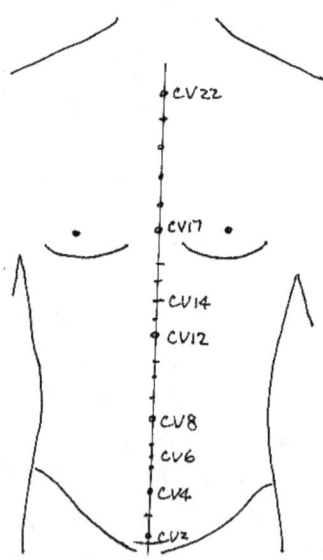

Fig 5 Important Points on the Conception Vessel

The Front Mu points in the front of the body: Zhongfu中府 (LU 1), Tanzhong膻中(CV 17 or Ren 17), Juque巨闕(CV 14 or Ren 14), Tianshu天樞(ST 25), Shimen石門(CV 5 or Ren 5), Guanyuan關元(CV 4 or Ren 4), Zhangmen章門(LR13), Qimen 期門(LR 14), Jingmen京門(GB 25), Zhongwan中脘(CV 12 or Ren 12), Riyue日月(GB 24), Zhongji中極(CV 3 or Ren 3).

Eight confluence points: Zhangmen (LR 13), Zhongwan (CV 12 or Ren 12), Yanglingquan (GB34), Juegu or Xuangzhong (GB 39), Geshu (BL 17), Da Zhu (BL 11), Taiyuan (LU 9), Tanzhong (CV 17 or Ren 17).

• Diagram of Organ Locations

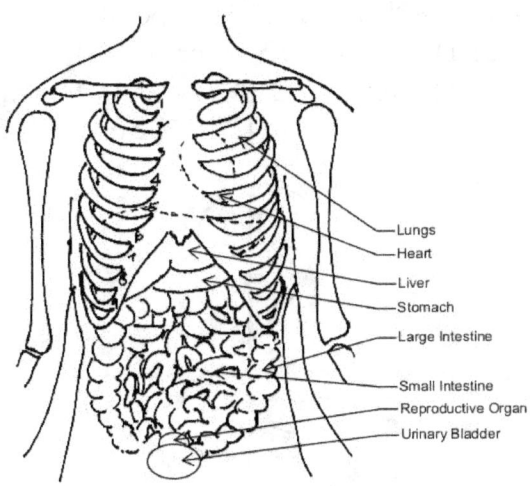

Fig 6 Front View of Body Organs

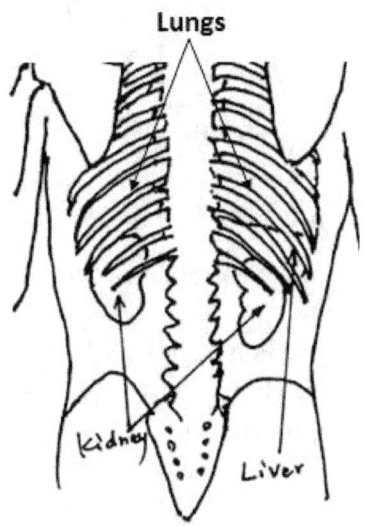

Fig 7 Back View of Body Organs

• The Back of the Body

The most important points are located on the Governor Vessel (Du Meridian).

- **Acupoint and Organs Location:** codes in brackets (this series book code, acupuncture point code)

  Governor Vessel (Du Meridian). points: Baihui (U3, GV 20 or DU 20), Dazhui (U4, GV 14 or DU 14), Shen Dao (U5, GV 11 or DU 11), Zhiyang (GV 9 or DU 9), Mingmen (U6, GV 4 or DU 4), Yaoshu (waist) (U7, GV 2 or DU 2).

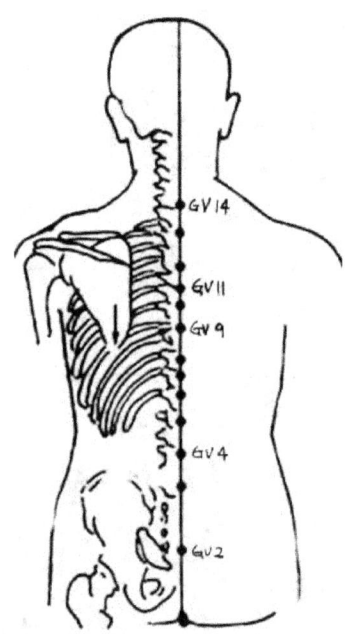

Fig 8 Important Points on the Governor Vessel

Back Shu Points: Feishu (BL 13), Xinshu (BL 15), Geshu (BL 17), Ganshu (liver) (BL 18), Pishu (spleen) (BL 20), Sanjiaoshu (triple energizer) (BL 22), Shenshu (kidney) (BL 23).

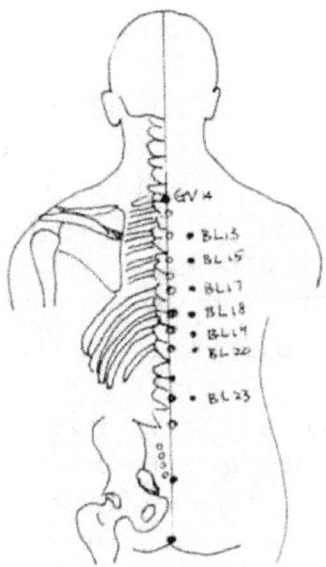

Fig 9 Back Shu Points

• Lateral of the Body

Dabao (SP 21)

The Dabao SP 21 locates at the mid-axillary line in the sixth intercostal space. It can treat problems within the chest. If the internal organs are not harmonized, there will be tenderness when pressing on it. It can balance the internal organs but can also treat whole body aches and pains. If combined with ST 36, it can treat weakness of the four limbs.

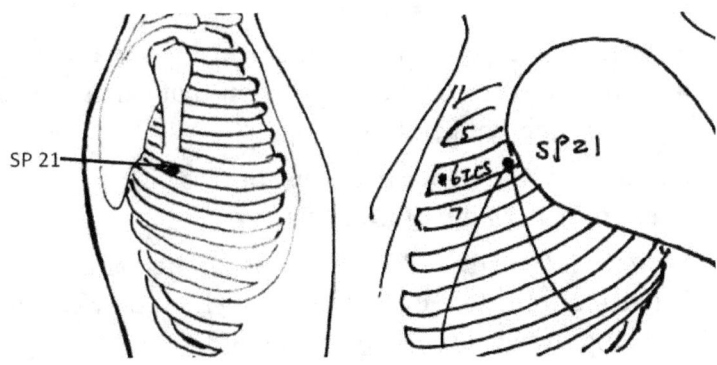

Fig 10 Dabao SP 21

Investment Revenue Exercise

Currently, the body's most important adjusting points are the points located in the Governor (GV or Du) Vessel, the Conception (Ren) Vessel, and organ locations. You'd better do your best to remember them all. An easy way is by learning one point each day and then reviewing them daily. Eventually, you will know all of them. If you can find a partner to study with you, that can benefit you both.

Try to look at the diagrams in this chapter, Appendix Five - Locations for Important Acupuncture Points and Organs, and the table below (at the end of the chapter) and memorize them. Print the pictures and post them around your house so that you're always studying them. When applying Comprehensive Universal Energy Healing to your family member(s), you can bring the pages as a reference. Do not be nervous—repeated practice will make you perfect. Learning in a relaxed manner is more effective. But do not be lazy in your practice because you never know when you might be needed to use your healing. In case of emergencies, you will be glad when you have a trick to help people and maybe even save lives!

Psychological Adjusting Points

This book emphasizes love, gratitude, sharing, and collaboration. Let's think a little deeper about them and ask some vital questions:

1. Love
   - Besides making love on a bed and using gifts to show love, is there any other kind of expression that exists to show love between different genders?
   - In addition to the love between couples or men and women, does any other kind of love exist?
   - How would you describe the love of parents for their children? What about the love of brotherhood? Love between employer and employee? Love between friends?

- Of all the kinds of love mentioned above, what kind love do you have a shortage of or do you feel you're not good at? Do you want to keep it that way? Or do you want to make a change? If you said yes to change, what action do you want to take? Can you set a goal for it and plan for your steps?

- Does love only exist between people? Can we expand this love to other things in the world or the universe?

- Do you love your pet or any other animal(s) in your home? If yes, how do you describe that kind of love? What attitudes and behaviors do you use toward to them?

- Do you agree that any living animal has the same right as humans to access natural resources and live with dignity?

- Have you ever noticed the love and sentiment between animals is sometimes nobler than between people? Have you ever noticed the animals' frustration and sadness when they are facing humans' ruthless abuse and slaughter? What can you do for them?

- Do you love nature? Do you pay attention to and study the interdependence and balance among all species in nature? Please watch "How do wolves change the river ecosystem?[183]".

- Are you a defender of this balance, or are you here to provide a better balance? Or are you just a balance spoiler?

- What can you do to help nature? Do you recycle? Do you make an attempt to reduce waste? Are there other things you can do?

2. Gratitude

- Regarding the people, things, and life around you, do you have more complaints or more gratitude?

- If you feel you have more gratitude, do you feel gratitude at specific moments or at many times in each day?

- Are you willing to go to this book's website reader discussion[137] to share your gratitude for and your harvests from every chapter with friends and readers who have the same mindset as you to make the world a better place for everyone to live?

- If you have more complaints, are you willing to write them down to exchange and discuss them?

- After seeing things from the other side's perspective, do you still complain? If so, we recommend that you put effort to communicate with the party or find a trustworthy friend or a professional or member of the clergy with who you can discuss your concerns. You can also go to the book's website reader discussion[137] to express your concerns and get other readers' opinions and thoughts. If your efforts to resolve your complaints failed, do you plan to take action to leave the person?

- Body health affects the health of the heart and the spirit health. If after you did Comprehensive Universal Energy Healing, your body still does not feel comfortable, we recommend that you seek Traditional Chinese Medicine treatment or another medical professionals' help for your health.

3. Sharing

Different groups of people or individuals may have ideas and viewpoints to share. Consider filling in the following table. Feel free to lengthen the form if necessary.

Group (or Individual) Name	Members of the Group	The Thing(s) that You want to Share
What would you like to share?		

What you would like the others to share with you?		

4. Collaboration

Do you have the opportunity to work with others? You can always find a few people do Comprehensive Universal Energy Healing with you. (If too many people are involved, it will be too crowded. Two to three people working as a team is more common. Five people can work as well by standing or sitting to the front, back, left, and right of the person to be adjusted.).

Even if you are using the CHUEH to do self-healing, you can cross your hands or arms to get the synergy effect without a second person to join you.

5.

The name of the person who works with you	What health issues do you want to improve?	Your goal to achieve	Expected date to achieve the goal	How often do you want to work with the person?

Notes

Investment Return Practice Table

Adjustment Point	Adjustment Point Location	Function (What Item Can be Adjusted)
U1		
U2		
U3		
U4		
U5		
U6		
U7		
BL 13		
BL 15		
BL 17		
BL 18		
BL 20		
BL 22		
BL 23		
SP 21		
CV 22		
CV 17		
CV 14		
CV 12		
CV 8		
CV 6		
CV 4		
CV 3		

Memorizing all of the above points will help you a lot in the rest of your life.

Take it slow—you can remember three to four new points a day. And review the previously learned one daily until it becomes part of your daily life knowledge. It will be just like driving a car. You can stop driving for a week or a month, but when you sit back in the driver's seat, you always know how to operate the car.

CHAPTER SEVEN
Hands Position for Healing
•••••••••••••••••••••

"The heart is the monarch of all the organs;...
Therefore, sadness, grief, and worry make the heart
change. When the heart changes, all of the organs
are shaking."

Huang Di Nei Jing• Ling Shu•Chapter 28 Oral Asking

The whole body receives universal energy when making adjustments. Then, through both hands, you transmit the universal energy to the client.

As stated in Chapter Two, The Root of Health and Wealth, the root of health in life is the smooth flow of the qi. When the energy can flow freely in our bodies without blockage, almost no sickness exists. Health problems can come from the mind, spirit, or body. They mutually influence each other.

Theoretically, no matter where you put the hands, the universal energy can go through them and transmit to the client's entire body. But if the client has health issues, his qi and blood circulation are blocked. This can also block the universal energy from flowing freely inside the body. If the blockage is severe, you should move your hands around to help release it because that is necessary in order to obtain the expected result quickly.

As we mentioned before, the universe is abundant. Therefore, there are numerous ways to make adjustments. The correct one depends on the clients' needs, the site conditions, the number of people involved in the adjustment, and the environmental constraints (the patient is lying down, cannot stand or turn the body, or prefer sto sit for the adjustment).

Each client will have different adjustment needs, according to his own health situation. This is different from Western medicine which generally uses a unified treatment protocol for each disease rather than taking the individual into account.

As an example, two patients have a cough. The first patient's cough is caused by a kidney blockage, and therefore we should adjust the kidneys. The second patient's cough is due to a liver problem, so we must instead adjust the liver to stop the coughing. In Chinese medicine, this is called the same disease with different treatments.

If one patient has problems with his heartbeat, and the other person feels tired, we will do the same for both of them and adjusting the heart. These are different diseases but are treated in the same way. Adjusting the heart for tiredness helps the blood circulation and supplies more oxygen and nutrients to the brain.

There are several methods you can use to place your hands. You can apply them separately or together. There is no specified order in most cases. Usually, we let the client feel comfortable and calm down first. The same words apply—be relaxed enough to learn constantly but without being lazy. Communicate constantly with the client to understand their feelings and thoughts. Please refer to Appendix Five Locations for Important Acupuncture Points and Organs.

Put Hands on the Acupuncture Points Mentioned in the Last Chapter

As you face the front of the person to be adjusted, put your hands mainly on the chakras or affected organs or discomfort locations. If you are in the back to do the adjustment, the hands are mainly put on the U1 and U3 or U1 and U8 position and on the organs or discomfort locations, depending on the client's needs.

Yoga or Reiki healers can put hands only on chakras to make adjustments.

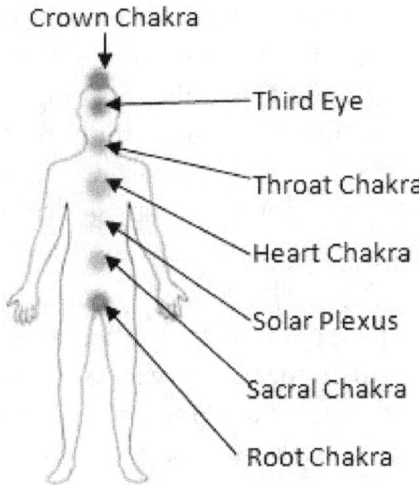

Fig 11 Chakras

Generally, put hands on the U1, U3 first. To be more effective, cover U1, U2/U3 together or U1/U2 together and U3 first to calm the client down. Depending on the health issues, this will usually have better results due to it activates the hypothymus and pineal glands. If the client has a motor mind and you cannot calm him down, you can teach him to do Da Zhou Tian[152]. Or alternatively, let him close his eyes and take three to seven deep breaths until the brain calms down. Follow this by combining the universal codes as stated in Chapter Five to adjust U1 and U3. Then let the client adopt an attitude of gratitude to accept the adjustment.

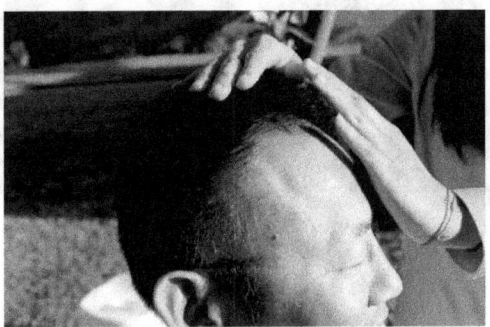

Pic 67 The adjustment that covers U1, U2 and U3 in the same time

According to the client's needs, adjust the heart between U1 to U8 and move the hands. The hands can stay hands at each location for ten minutes, extending or shortening the time depending upon the severity of the sickness. Generally speaking, if the problem occurs continuously for six months or intermittently for more than three years, it is considered chronic. For chronic diseases, the adjustment time needs to be longer. You must also get rid of the root problem of the chronic disease. If it is an acute condition, after the symptoms have gone, things are usually okay.

If the time interval is not long after an adjustment, and the occurrence repeatedly appears, it's necessary to consider removing the root cause. If the onset of symptoms is seasonable or has been occurring for years, it is also necessary to address the root cause of the disease.

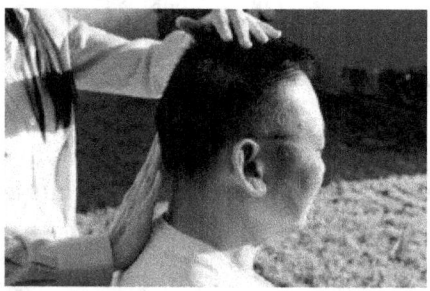

Pic 68 Bai-Hui and Back of Neck

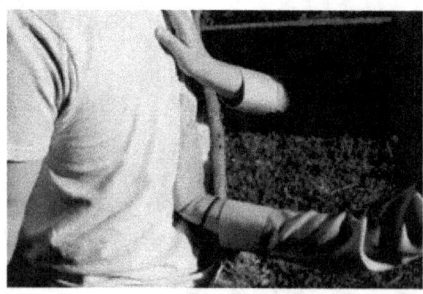

Pic 69 Upper Spine

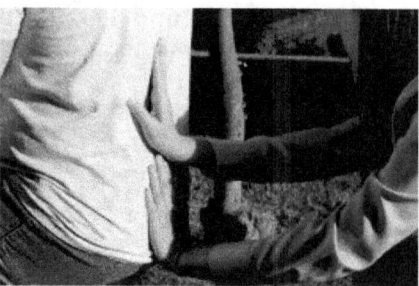

Pic 70 Lower Spine

Putting your hands on the spine can adjust organ, muscle, and tendon problems located at the level of the hands. The discs that the hands cover can benefit as well.

Remember that if you are adjusting a different gender or a stranger, especially if the area to be adjusted is a sensitive or private area, you'd better not put your hands directly on the body. You can keep a distance of two or three inches or more to avoid misunderstanding by a third party or the client's discomfort while you are doing the adjustment. Psychological discomfort can cause the client's qi to stagnate and waste your adjustment time.

If the area is in a sensitive area—for example, a male adjusting a female's heart—it's better to ask permission and put hands on the back of the female's heart first. When the client feels the heat from your hands or you feel that the client's energy is flowing, then you can move the hand from the back of your client to the front heart location with some distance to make adjustments instead of directly touching her chest. Because the cosmic energy has radiation and a reflective function, you can make adjustments from a distance. Cosmic energy can penetrate clothing made of materials with soft textures.

If your energy is strong enough, you can emit enough energy from one corner of a room to adjust a person at the diagonal corner of the room.

Hands Put on the Location of Discomfort

Put one hand on the U3 and the other hand on the painful or uncomfortable location. Both hands can also be in the same location of discomfort, just keep one hand in the front and one hand in the back. In the ideal adjustment case, you will feel the qi move from the front to the back and from the back to the front. That means the blockage is no longer present. The pain and discomfort are totally gone.

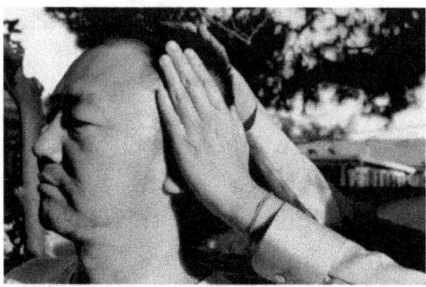

Pic 71 Adjust the left side migraine

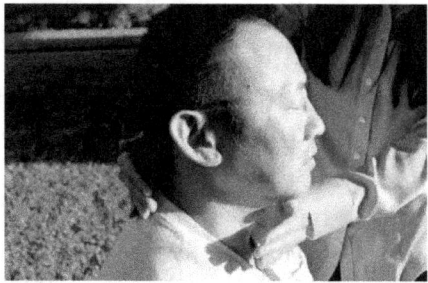

Pic 72 Put hands on the throat to adjust
the throat discomfort or dysphagia

Put Hands on the Organ that has Deviated Function(s)

You can put your hands on the location of a painful or poorly functioning organ to make adjustments. You can also put hands in front of and behind the same organ to do the adjustment. Prolonged emotion affects the heart. The heart is the monarch of all organs, so putting your hands on U3 and the heart area, or U2/U3 and U5 locations will alleviate the high stress of modern life , and both the liver and heart will benefit.

Where tumor, cancer, or bleeding are concerned, if the qi can penetrate the back and front of the problem area, it means the local blockage is well-adjusted. If it is your desire to adjust your client to rid him of the root problem, please refer to Chapter Four to determine whether he reaches the health standards or not. If not, refer to Chapter

Eleven for the pain, stress, and insomnia adjustment. For any other diseases, future books will teach you how to do those adjustments.

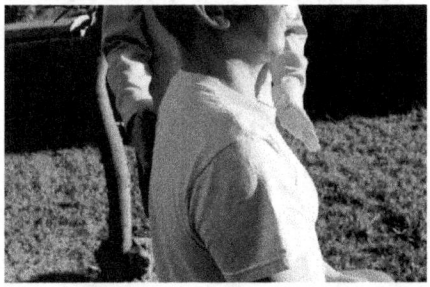

Pic 73 Put hands in the front and back
of the Heart and also cover T5

Adjust According to the Mother and Son Relationship

In the diagram below, the clockwise direction represents the mother and child relationship. That is the mother's organ is always helping the son organ to be stronger. Therefore, if the son organ is weak, Traditional Chinese Medicine tonifies the mother organ to let it generate a strong son.

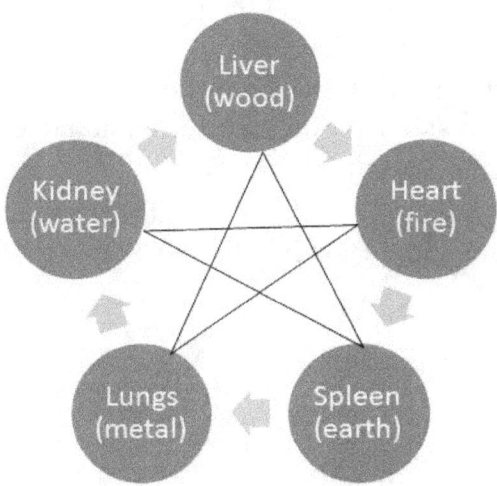

Fig 12 Mutual Generating and Invading for the Five Elements

For example, if the heart is sick, put your hands on the heart and liver positions to treat the mother (liver) and son (heart) together. Or if the kidney has problems, put your hands on the lung and kidney to tonify the mother (lung) and the son (kidney) together.

Address the Invading Relationship to Avoid Sickness

Organs are mutual invading if they locate on a diagonal line.

If the spleen is sick, you should put hands on the kidney and liver area to prevent the sickness from moving to the liver or kidneys. If your spleen problem has already induced a kidney problem, it is good to adjust the heart as well as the spleen and kidney.

Moving Hands

Aside from moving your hands from area of discomfort or pain to another, some additional guidelines are listed below:

1. When your hands are too cold, rub them together to warm them up first. If the client's body is cold, and the client cannot feel the heat in your hands, it's better to press your hands to the client's body until the client can feel their warmth and then move your hands away with some distance.

    When touching the client's body, be careful not to place hands in sensitive areas, and always ask permission to put hands on the client before beginning.

2. Keeping the hands at a distance from the body actually transmits more cosmic energy to the client. Greater distance transmits more energy.

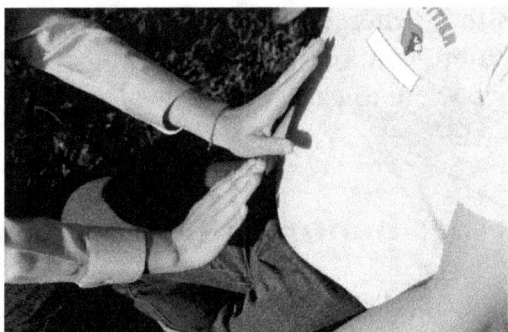

Pic 74 Keep distance from the body to
transmit more cosmic energy

3. When adjusting the area of discomfort or pain or poor organ function, if the lower part of the hands closer to the ground feels warmer than the upper part, it means that the lower part of the body has a blockage. Swing your hands gently downward a couple of times to get the stagnation flowing downward. The accumulated heat will disappear, and the patient will feel more comfortable.

   This movement can help phlegm in the lungs to move downward. The client will feel there is more room in his chest will breathe easier and deeper. It also can expel liver toxins and move them to the large intestine.

4. After the adjustment is finished and before concluding the session, move your hands slowly downward a few times to soothe the client's qi flow in the adjusted area. If you have adjusted many areas, from the top to the bottom, scan all parts that have been adjusted, area by area. If you've adjusted the legs, for example, then soothe the qi from the kidney to the knee or ankle or foot, depending on where you made the adjustment.

Methods for Stimulating Energy Flow

For severely blocked locations with severe coldness, blood stasis, tumor, or cancer cells, after resting the hands on the area for a while to warm it up, and once your hands feel warmer, move your hands away from the site and come back again to press energy on the target area. It gathers more energy to hit and break the nodule, and the client will feel more comfortable. But do not do it too often. You should wait for a while to gather more heat under your hands and then do it again.

How to Further Improve Effectiveness?

In Chapter Five, we talked about how to combine cosmic energy and the universal codes to enhance health. We also mentioned about how collaboration can have a synergistic effectiveness. You can watch the quantum physics cartoon of the Dr. Quantum's Double Slit Experiment[182] to get a better understanding of this concept.

It will strengthen the adjustment effect if four people mutually adjust each other. Instead of pairing by two persons as a team, a group of four work better. Let three people adjust one person and take turns. The person being adjusted should join in and do self-healing.

If only two people mutually adjust, it is always better to let the person to be adjusted put his hands on his body to collaborate in the adjustment—even if the person to be adjusted has never practiced any qigong or Da Zhou Tian[152] or adjusted any one. Even if he has no heat in his hands or the hands are cold, all hands will have the same temperature later because of transference of energy. It will have the effect of two persons adjusting one person.

No matter how many healers are doing the adjustment for the client, it is always better to invite him to join in and do self-healing in order to speed up the effectiveness. But if the client refuses to join, we are always tolerant of his enjoyment of the adjustment, and we respect his decision.

If you are doing self-healing, and the liver is invading the spleen, for example, so that it cannot properly absorb nutrients under stress, it is better to cross your arms to put them on the liver and spleen area instead of putting left and right hands separately on the liver and spleen area. When you cross the arms, the energy from both hands have that synergy effect.

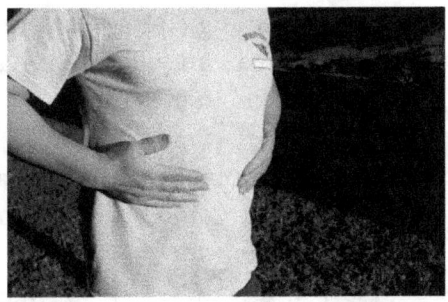

Pic 75 Hands on Liver & Spleen, No Crossing

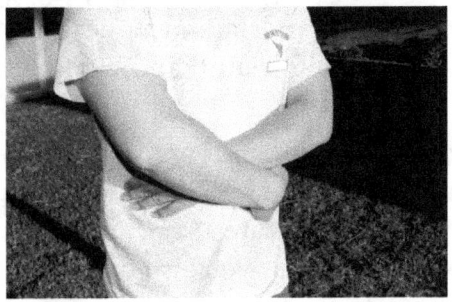

Pic 76 Crossing Hands on Liver & Spleen

Putting left and right hands separately on the liver and spleen area has less effect than crossing the arms to put them on those areas.

Investment Revenue Exercise

Medical science is a practice- and result-oriented science. If you are able to get plenty of experience adjusting the others and being adjusted yourself, you will learn better and much faster. You will have more chances to exchange experiences with others. You will have a chance to read and think. You will be able to modify or correct your diagnostic, analytical, and adjustment skills and theories. This will help you improve faster.

Because there is a huge difference from one person to another, you, as a client being adjusted, should be patient and reply your healer's questions to help him provide better services to you and others.

1. After you get the cosmic healing energy in your hands, put your left hand on your spleen area and your right hand on your liver area. Your arms are not crossing. When you get the sensation of the energy flow, remember what it feels like. Then move your right hand to your spleen area and your left hand to your liver area. Now, your arms are crossing. When you feel the energy flowing, compare the sensation to what you felt when your arms were not crossed. Do you feel there is a stronger energy flowing when you cross your arms?

   Review again: In order to get the healing energy, you can do Da Zhou Tian[152]. If your hands are already warm enough, you do not need to do Da Zhou Tian[152] and can make the adjustment directly.

   Keep in mind that if your hands are warmer, your client will feel more comfortable, and the result will usually come sooner and quicker. Even if your hands are already warm, there is no harm in doing Da Zhou Tian[152], and you also can invite your client to do it with you for better results.

   When you stand behind a person helping him doing the adjustment, when he feels the energy flowing, let him put his hands in front of his body in the relative position of your hands. Then let him relate to you the energy changes.

2. When you are being adjusted, you can personally experience the difference with and without placing your own hands to collaborate in making the adjustments. The difference in feeling will be obvious, especially when the healer's energy is very strong.

3. Find one or more persons to adjust you and really feel the relation of the healing results to the number of healers involved. At the beginning, pay attention to the energy differences in each person's hands. After a period of time, see if all hands have the same energy.

4. Enjoy the happiness of learning new knowledge and maintain a sense of joy as your experience grows.

   Too often, I see practitioners do not change treatment methods and stick with what was learned. It leads many treatable diseases become none treatable or requiring treatment for a long time without getting off treatments. I have solved the patient's problem, just add a little bit more thought or try a different angle to solve the problem. Learn to be flexible in practicing and use your brain to conquer your client's problem. You will be the hero of your client to make him better.

My acupuncturist friends or classmates used to ask me: "Your treatment is so powerful, but, I cannot notice it from any medical book that I had read or from school instructors who taught us."

If diseases can follow medical textbooks or published medical books to be treated well, there does not need so many healthcare practitioners and research funds, but a lot diseases are still being labeled as a "death" situations or patients keep forever sick. It's not right and against the universal divine love.

However, "the greatest way is the simplest way". There does exist a switch that sets in our DNA to turn diseases and disasters away. It's the "ethic".

Ethic was emphasized in the traditional Chinese history. Now, due to my great editor, Lori, I did more research and found from scientist proof in a series videos collected in CHUEH Video 1[203].

High ethic can open a two key DNA strands to repair the rest of the DNA stands. Meanwhile, they allows us to commune with the high dimensional spaces to acquire wisdom and abundances. You can jump to Part 4 to watch it.

It explained why we can ask our great self to heal ourselves. When our ethic has no blockage, our great self can directly communicate with us.

The learning opportunities are endless. If you grasp them, your life will not be boring, and your ambition will not be worn out by bland days.

5. The reason I teach you to experience different feelings is to train and raise your sensitivity. It will be a great help in your life. Many people are always busy and never have the feeling of being alive in the moment. If this is your case, practice Comprehensive

Universal Energy Healing more, and you will be surprised to find that a lot of fun is accompanying you.

This also trains you to not fall in the case that suddenly, you are sent to an ER room due to you not sensing the early warning signs of your health. Clinically, we can see a lot of these kind cases.

CHAPTER EIGHT

Turning Better Reactions and the Needed Mindset During Healing

When will and thought are harmonized, then the spirit is focused and straight, the soul lingers, regret and anger cannot generate, internal organs will not be affected by pathogens.

Huang Di Nei Jing • Ling Shu • Chapter Forty-Seventh Root of the Organ

In any treatment, with poor health turning into a better health situation, there will be changes in the body. The changes are not necessarily pleasant. It's like fixing a house—a wall has a leaky water pipe, the water seepage caused moldy walls, plumbers have to knock out the wall to get to the pipe, and maybe some pipes need to be cut. The waste heap might be uncomfortable, and it may also cause inconvenience. But it's a necessary thing.

The body needs to go through the transferring process. In the health care field, we call this process the "turning better reaction." I ask you to read the following carefully so that when you encounter this when doing an adjustment, you will not feel panic or worry about a loss.

Commonly Seen "Turning Better Reaction"

Blockage in the body is a very common thing. When there is any blockage, the amount of qi or blood or lymph flowing through the blocked channel will be smaller. The meridian qi stagnation is caused by emotional issues, wind, coldness, or dampness or whatever. It can gradually lead the stagnation to be phlegm or blood stasis or a nerve conduction problems such as numbness or pain or other discomfort sensation to warn us to take an early action to remove the blockage and avoid costly sickness. And until the blockage becomes severe, it will have symptoms.

Phlegm can cause conditions such as autism, epilepsy seizures, cancer, COPD, emphysema, pneumonia, tumor, cysts, dizziness, over weight, hyperlipidemia, lymph node tuberculosis, bone tuberculosis, pineal gland swollen, chronic fatigue syndrome, Meniere's disease, and so on.

There is visible and invisible phlegm in the body which can cause diseases that are unsolved to western medicine but could be well treated by good Chinese medicine physicians more than a couple of thousand years ago.

Blood stasis can cause pain, lymphatic nodule, tumors, cerebro-vascular accident sequel, stroke sequel, pulmonary heart disease, bleeding, purpura, and so on.

When cosmic energy enters into the body, it will increase the amount of qi flowing through the body. Thus, when it goes through the blocked area, it can generate different levels of discomfort. It's like a high-pressure jet of water passing through a section of blocked and narrowed pipe. The flow will either open the stagnation or burst the pipe if the pipe wall is not thick or strong enough.

During the flowing of the high pressure water, the pipe wall bears a higher pressure than usual. In a person, this will generate all sorts of uncomfortable sensations to warn the person in order to avoid that unwanted bursting of the water pipe. We will teach you later how to handle that discomfort.

In general, the strength and frequency of the "turning better reaction" will decrease except when the blockage is severe. Then the bad sensation can become stronger. That means this area needs special care. You can either put a hand there to help unblock it or seek professional help.

For a severely blocked area, if the increased meridian flow can't unblock it, the discomfort in the spot will be proportional to the increased pressure acting on it.

In my acupuncture practice, I add a needle to the area of discomfort to solve the problem immediately. I always joke to my patients that their body is smart to ask for needles from me so that it can recover sooner. The total treatment time can be reduced and the root problems be taken care of. You can read about that in Appendix Six Author's Cases Sharing.

As the adjustment progresses and meridian flow is unblocked, the turning better reaction will disappear. This does not mean that the turning better reaction will not appear again.

Whether it was a healer or maybe a client who had emotional stress or lack of rest or didn't practice the Da Zhou Tian[152] or meditation when doing the adjustment or getting adjusted, coming out of the turning better reaction—or having it become severe after it had already disappeared or reduced—is normal.

Note:

1. When doing the adjustment, the client's body blockage will not go to the healer's body. During the adjustment, the cosmic energy goes through the healer and transmits to the client's body. Therefore, any body discomfort in the healer or the client's body is induced by their own body's blockage. Both the healer and the client's body blockage will be reduced as more adjustment is done. However, if the time between two adjustments is too long, the effect achieved by the adjustment could be reduced or totally lost, or the blockage could get worse.

Sometimes the time between two adjustments is not long, but the uncomfortable sensation grows worse. This is not the fault of either the healer or the client. One reason this may happen is that the client's natural situation is getting worse.

2. Please recall that when qi and blood cannot pass through, it induces the pain. A patient had traffic accident decades ago. Each week, when she visited her acupuncturist, due to the acupuncture treatment it can increase qi flowing that can pass through the blocked spot, that makes her feel pain reducing.

   After treatment, without the external force (needles or cosmic energy) help, patient's flowing qi decreased, cannot pass through the blocked spot, the pain returned. Usually, the pain level reduced, it means the treatment works. I will give an interesting case below.

   However, due to real stagnated qi by the car accident the problem had not been solved. The patient experienced worse pain episode than before.

   Think of a section of pipe that is blocked, if the blockage is not totally opened up, then the dirt in the flow passing through that section will easily stop at the blocked spot to make the blockage becomes worse.

   In human's body, the dirt is the cells metabolism waste.

3. Another reason is that due to our body's natural tendency to protect itself in order to maintain daily mobility and viability, our alertness to the discomfort is reduced. After adjustment, the body experiences some repair and recovery. The painful sensations are awake and alert. Thus, we feel worse.

4. If a patient has five pain spots. The number one painful spot catches the patient's attention. When the worst pain solved, then the fourth painful spot catches patient's attention. It's so common in the clinical practice. The patient usually doubt that the 4th painful spot is the new pain generated. Actually, it is already existed for a while. The same as the fourth painful spot solved, the third painful spot comes out to catch patient's attention. Until

all of the five spots be solved, then, there is no more pain feeling for the patient.

5. Besides the hidden pain situation stated above, there are also hidden internal health issues due to the healing digging to the root problem, it can induce an old symptom that did not well treat comes out.

   It likes a swimming pool had some stones in it, you could not see them when the water is dirty, when you drain the water, the dirty water level going down, you can see the stone that is not supposed to be in the pool comes out.

6. I had a case that induced worse situation after treatment that is worth to share with you:

   A female friend had severe blockage all over the body. She came to ask curing her legs curve. According to diagnoses of her tongue, pulse and visual observation, I improved her sleeping problem and balanced her body to feel more pleasant than before.

   Then, I started to cure her legs and got over miles of her expectation. She told me that in China, practitioners gave up her case already.

   After another treatment, due to needing her help for some of my personal stuff, I let her stay with me overnight.

   The next day, she told me that she woke up at midnight and had severe heart pain with weakness in her heart. The weakness prevented her to get up and woke me up. I asked where was the pain. She pointed at the GB 23 zhejin location. She was worrying about that she has severe heart problems. I told her no worry. I gave her some needles to increase her heart Qi flow to avoid the heart pain and weakness sensation in order to eat breakfast.

   Later, I checked out the most painful spots on her upper body along the foot showing gallbladder meridian. The spots were checked on the previous day without pain. Those spots pain was caused by the previous day curing her leg and hip, removed a lot toxins in her legs' gallbladder meridian. That increased flow in her upper body's same meridian and caused the new pain.

The worst spot is at GB23 that connects to the heart directly. Its blockage can cause heart problems.

This is a situation that I always can solve; a decades, chronic disease in limited treatments. It induced me not so rely on herbal treatments. No matter Eastern or Western medicine practitioners are trained to use herbs or drugs to treat internal organ function problems. However, it is the case that the internal organ problems are caused by soft tissue problems instead of the organ's function problem.

7. For example, there is a plastic container set on the table, the container body was squeezed by surrounding stuff to be deformed. The lid cannot fit in the container. So, if kept changing the container instead of taking away the pressure on the container body, it does nerve work and gives a solution. Due to this it can be seen and easily understood. But, for the internal medical problems, it cannot be seen, even hardly to be found by MRI or CT scan until it becomes very severe.

More cases can read at Heart Pain Cases 210 and Decades Stomach Problems 211.

8. Deeply, this book shares some of my clinical experiences to treat what the other MDs and/or acupuncturists failed to treat and let you have another angle to view diseases.

If you think that an organ due to its soft tissue is abnormally pulled by the other soft tissues, how can it function right even under its normal original organ function?

Patients with heart problems have either hyper or hypo pain sensation. After the heart problem gets better, the painful sensations disappear. For example, a patient with heart disease does not feel pain from needling. After the heart problem is resolved, he can feel the pain from the needle pinching his blood vessel.

After the body repairs itself, the numb sensation will go away, and the body will gradually become more sensitive. For a hypersensitive person, the feeling will become normal to be not so hypersensitive. But he will sense the survival threaten situations such as feeling pain before a severe blockage causes a worse sickness.

9. A severely sick person's body blockage is more severe. In this situation, the reaction from both the healer and the client will be stronger. As stated before, it's due to encountering a stronger blockage, there is more reflected the qi flow back and more pressure induced at the blockage spot.

10. If the healer has no body blockage or the blockage is mild, there will be no uncomfortable sensation.

How to Handle Commonly Seen Situations

1. When a water pipe is blocked, the front end wall of the pipe bears higher pressure than is proportional to the severity of the clotting. In humans, because the yang qi travels around the body from the top to bottom, left to right, front to back, outside to inside, and inside to outside, when the yang qi hits a blockage and can't penetrate it, it will be reflected back. This will make the local temperature higher than the other areas.

   If this happens, wave your hands downward several times to guide the qi and encourage the loosening toxins to move downward until the extra heat dissipates. It will also make the client feel more comfortable. If there was phlegm in the lungs, the client will feel increased lung capacity and be able to breathe in more air. Be careful, though, not to over-wave or wave too fast and lose useful healing heat on the hands.

2. During the adjustment, the healing induces the qi to start flowing. The sick site may feel sensations of soreness, numbness, swelling, pain, coldness, heat, or tingling, This is a normal phenomenon. The internal body energy balancing produces the sensation. The following are some of the more common "turning better reactions."

   - **Soreness**—The lactic acid freed from muscles or tendon fibers causes this sensation. It will disappear as long as they flow out and away from the site. It occurs most in overused areas of the body—for example, when you stand too long or walk or run too much, your legs will be sore, and typists often feel soreness in their shoulders.

If you are always on your feet, please read Raise Your Legs 90 Degrees Up Against the Wall[175] to avoid wearing your knee cartilage out and stomach diseases.

- **Heaviness**—Accumulated metabolic waste (toxins) freed from muscle or tendon fibers causes the heavy sensation because the toxins are particles and carry weight. As the toxins are carried away by flowing qi, the heavy sensation will be gradually reduced, and you will feel lighter. Meanwhile, the local tight tissues gradually recover their original elasticity and softness.

- **Numbness**—Accumulated metabolic waste freed from muscle or tendon fibers press on the blood vessels and nerves, producing numbness. The numbness will dissipate as those toxins flow away, and normal sensation will come back. The client will feel lighter even during the adjustment.

- **Distended**—This sensation is caused by mild qi stagnation due to local qi suddenly gathering more than usual in one place.

- **Pain**—This sensation is induced when qi and blood attempt to pass through a severely congested site but cannot do so easily. The more severe the pain, the more severe the local blockage. The pain usually subsides by itself as long as the toxins are carried away. If not, moving a hand or two hands to the site will help reduce the pain sooner.

- **Coldness**—It's the yang qi pushing the internal coldness out of the body. After the coldness is gone, the body feels warmer and more comfortable.

If the coldness is strong, ask the client to seek professional medical service or ingest raw ginger or other warm herbs and practice the Da Zhou Tian[152] to help expel the coldness in the body.

- **Heat (Warmth)**—If a local site feels warm, it's due to the yang qi hitting a site of severe blockage, such as blood stasis, a cancer site, or a nodule. There will be a warm sensation, and you might even see the skin in the area turning pink or red. The warmer the area is, the more blockage at the site. Both the color and heat will disappear if doing an adjustment long enough. If not, the client should seek medical service.

- **Tingling**—In Chinese medicine, qi pushes blood flow in addition to the force of the heart pumping the blood. When qi is weak, it pushes less blood. Due to the universal energy entering the body, more qi flows, and that, in turn, causes more blood to flow.

  When the blood flow rapidly increases, the blood vessels rapidly expand. The increased blood pressing on the blood vessels causes the nerves in the blood vessel walls to produce the tingling sensation. This tingling sensation disappears quickly but transmits along the blood vessels in the direction of the flow until it reaches the end of the vessel.

- **Mild electric shock**—Qi is composed of electrolyte particles. Therefore, it flows like a current. Usually, people do not feel it. However, once the strong cosmic energy enters the body, the qi flow becomes suddenly strong and induces a sensation similar to a mild electric shock.

- **Muscle tremor**— These are caused by extra water or fluid inside the muscle. The cosmic energy pushes the qi to flow. This, in turn, induces water waving, which generates the muscle tremors.

- **Body rocking or doing circular movement**—Some people entering a deeper state of meditation can have this kind of movement, and it can sometimes become more pronounced. In order to avoid the client losing his balance and falling if he is standing or sitting to accept the adjustment, you can wake him up by lightly tapping on his shoulder.

  Meanwhile, tell the client not to focus on his body movement. You want to avoid it becoming more severe because agitated movement can reduce the effectiveness of the adjustment. Tell him to imagine that he is as stable as a mountain. Continue to do the adjustment.

- **Yawning**—This indicates the body's shortage of oxygen to support qi and blood flow. Yawning can quickly get more oxygen to the body and is a necessary reaction for the body to do repairs.

- **Falling asleep**—This happens when a client is overworked and fatigued or does not get good sleep at night. Sleeping can facilitate the body's internal self-regulation and repair. If the client is sitting or standing for the adjustment and has a tendency to fall down, you can simply pat his shoulder to wake him up. Otherwise, just let him sleep and do the needed body repairs.

- **Feeling dizzy or feeling dizzy and sleepy**—Teng, Wen Gong (at Mencius's time) mentioned that if a medicine cannot cause the turning better reaction of a dark dizziness sensation, it cannot help a client recover. In some people, when they are getting the right treatment and when the body is doing self-repair, there is a special brainwave produced that can induce a dizzy or sleepy sensation. It's normal.

When a "turning better reaction" comes out, even if the healer or the client feels uncomfortable, the healer can usually continue with the adjustment. The symptom will most likely be reduced. If it isn't, move one hand to the U3 (Baihui or GV 20 or DU 20) and the other hand to the location of discomfort and apply the universal codes, as well, to reduce the symptoms faster. When there is accumulating heat on the hands, gently wave them downward several times, and the discomfort will gradually disappear.

If the uncomfortable sensation persists or is severe, you'd better investigate more possibilities by asking the client to see if there is any history of illness related to the site or the discomfort. If you do not know how to handle it, recommend that the client seek the help of a medical professional.

Besides learning the "turning better reactions," you'd better read Chapter Nine and Ten before adjusting people whom you are not familiar with to avoid regret later.

Preparation for the CHUEH and the Needed Attitude

Find a clean, quiet, calm, and comfortable environment to make adjustments.

Preparation for jobs and the proper attitude are very important. The healer and the client should release their bodies of any loads such as bags, purses, or anything in the hands. If you know the time of the adjustment ahead of time, it's better to wear loose clothes, wear as little jewelry as possible. Do not wear accessories on the body, and to remove or loosen anything that is tight to not block the qi from flowing.

If possible, the client should wear no makeup in order for the healer to observe the facial color changes and practice such observations during the adjustment.

Close your eyes, arms falling naturally, and put your hands on your thighs. Take a deep breath three to five times, and then breathe evenly. Sit quietly for five to fifteen minutes. If the site is appropriate, the client and healer(s) can practice the Da Zhou Tian[152] together. Please refer to Chapter Five to learn the contraindications for the Da Zhou Tian[152]. Then relax your mind, be calm and quiet, and remain in a state of gratitude and happiness, ready to embrace the opportunity for Comprehensive Universal Energy Healing.

If you're going to be outdoors, be sure it's not cold, windy, raining, or in the hot sunshine. If you're indoors, check to be sure the air conditioning is not too cold and the location is not too crowded.

Ask your client details about the health issues that he is most concerned about and thinks which need to be improved.

What is the health issue he is most concerned about? Where is the location of the health issue? What is the sensation in that location now? If the issue has been intermittent, what is the frequency? How long does it last, and how often does it happen? How severe is it? When does the client feel better or worse? What makes the client feel better? Has he had any treatment before? What did the medical professional tell him? What was the treatment result? What is the ideal situation that the client would like to reach? How would he like to collaborate with you?

Then start to make the adjustments.

We will introduce the adjustment methods in Chapter Ten, Chapter Eleven, and in later books in the series which will focus on specific health issues.

If you want to do a good job, you'd better learn Chapter Nine, Ten, and Eleven well. Learning how to make good adjustments to make the client feel better is important, but if you want the ability to help unknown people in any situation, you'd better first learn when it is necessary refer a client elsewhere and when he needs an ER service.

If referring your client elsewhere, it is best to let the client visit his family doctor instead of referring him to a medical professional where he may spend money without getting any result and come back to complain to you. However, it is always good for you to have trusted professional medical referral information on hand so that when the client really feels helpless, you can help.

For beginners, do not rush to seek meritorious efficacy. The adjustment effectiveness is related to many factors.

The healer: Knowledge, skills, attitude, moral cultivation, emotion, mindset, patience, washing hands with cold water or not, having just eaten cold foods or drank icy water?

The client: The severity of the sickness, duration of the health issue, client's body constitution, diet, lifestyle, exercise, emotion, job/family/environmental influences, mindset, attitude, follows instruction or not, beliefs, thoughts, moral cultivation, personality.

The environment: Indoor or outdoor, weather, pollution level, noise, lighting, temperature, crowded area, wind, air conditioning, fan, odors, fresh air or lack of it.

Except for some accident and emergency cases, most ailments come and go quickly. However, things like heart disease and stroke have developed for a while even when the onset was acute. The client is not supposed to expect immediate effectiveness. It's better not touch the kind of client who asks for a one-time adjustment to solve his health issue. He would be adjusted and treated once and subsequently conclude that it did not work. It would be a mistake in judgment on your part and an improper conclusion on his.

The body needs time to recover, especially in the chronic cases. It likes a learning curve, only repeated study (treatments) and within a short time to boost another study (treatment) to make the knowledge (health) staying constant in memory (the body).

Even if a pain is long-term, accumulated result of an acute injury, once surgery is done, the pain or illness appears to be removed. It looks fast. However, most of the side effects can still be seen years or even decades later. The body needs time to repair and rid itself of the root cause.

Being adjusted often is the fastest way to eliminate the root cause. Climbing the mountain from the valley of the current situation directly to the peak of healthy status is the shortest distance. The total cost to you in terms of time and money is the least. If the interval between two adjustments is too long, new symptoms will surface as your health deteriorates. It then becomes like climbing a mountain with jagged rocks and varied peaks. It takes extra time and money. But the client has only himself to blame.

For example, if you drink often, the alcohol poisoning is stored in the liver and will gradually cause the tendons to lose their softness. If you sprain a part of your body and get adjusted, the pain will go away because the qi and the blood flow will be soothed. It does not mean, however, that it will not hurt afterwards.

Later, due to coldness invading the body or drink more alcohol, the original painful area will have pain because the tendon has shrunk again. Therefore, in cases of not feeling pain, it's better to do more adjustments so the energy can flow from left to right and from back to the front. Additionally, it is necessary to treat the root problem causing the tendon tightness. Usually, the liver controls the tendons. Abstaining from alcohol is the solution. Doing deep breathing for fifteen minutes and meditation will help your body gradually lose its desire for alcohol.

This series will better acquaint you with many diseases' sources, pathogens, etiologies, and prognoses so that your adjustment results will be improved.

As long as the mindset is correct, universal energy returns with a love of positive energy. So far, universal healing energy is the only treatment that has the advantage of no side effects, no required medical devices, no equipment limitations, no medicines*, inexhaustible sources, no discrimination between poor and rich people, environmentally friendly, and beneficial to both the healer and the client. It comes from the equity of universal love. Everyone, from birth to death, has only twenty-four hours a day. You can use this time to color your life and create your own life transcript.

* For severe blood deficiency clients, tonifying herbs are still needed.

There is no need to complain, to hate, to regret. Nonstop learning and creating, continued hope, and patience will one day bring the good life to you.

Here to share with you: You Can[184].

The correct mindset to do adjustment is nothingness—a mind full of gratitude and enjoyment. If familiar with the possible situations, doing the adjustment will cause no worry, no fear and no rush, and you will make the adjustments with ease.

Evil cannot conquer rightness. Keep this concept in mind, and have the faith to deal with life and people. Do not have narrow vision, but instead be bright and sharp. In this way, through your lifetime, you will reap the benefits of it. These benefits can be both visible and invisible.

The visible benefits could be getting promoted, making money, having a good spouse or a child. The invisible benefits include having good fortune and avoiding bad luck—perhaps encountering a disaster that through good fortune you're able to avoid or bear. If you've accumulated enough good deeds, the extra credits that are left over after your life ends can be carried over to your descendants.

Whenever possible, do the best you can to do good deeds without caring about the returns. Universal love is unlimited in abundance. You will experience its power from practicing Comprehensive Universal Energy Healing. As you grow older, you will learn that karma is real. If your good deeds have not been rewarded, it is not yet the right time. There is nothing that will erase your fair reward, so do not be preoccupied or tempted to reduce your frequency. Keep your generous and charitable spirit, and upgrade your frequency. The rich rewards will be beyond your imagination!

Investment Revenue Exercise

Please find a comfortable place that is safe and quiet with no interference and no wind. Let go of all your chores and distractions.

Close your eyes and take a deep breath three to five times. Keep taking deep breaths, as necessary, until your brain is empty. Then meditate quietly. When you meditate, ask yourself these questions:

1. In your memories up to now, do you have joyful things that are worthy of your gratitude?

2. Can you think of anything that seemed to be a disaster at the time but had a blessing hidden inside that is worthy of your gratitude?

3. Think about your love of nature. What pleasures do you have in nature that are worthy of your gratitude?

4. Think about your family, friends, and coworkers who are friendly to you. Has anyone helped you? Who has cultivated you and is worthy of your gratitude?

5. If these are too many things, and you cannot think about them all at one time, you can meditate every day and think about one item per day. After giving your gratitude, think about what has changed in your mind. Find the party and let him know your gratitude. Pay attention to his reactions.

6. If a person gives you a favor and receives gratitude from you, how much joy will you convey to him? You may want to meditate every

day and find something to be thankful for on that particular day. The next day, share with those for whom you feel grateful.

I wish that you every day be immersed in bliss!

CHAPTER NINE
Time for Referral
•••••••••••••••••••••••••

Saint does not treat already sick. But treat before sick. He does not manage disorder but manages before disorder. It is what speaking of. When disease already formed, then treat with herbs, or already disordered, then manage it. It likes digging will when thirst or build casts and the awl while fighting. It is too late!

Huang Di Nei Jing • Su Wen • Chapter 2 The Great Theory for Turning the Divine Essence at the Four Seasons

We mentioned in Chapter Four how a Chinese medical physician views diseases. It's better to take care of the root problem as soon as possible. If the adjustment is not effective, for the benefit of the client, it's better to refer out as soon as possible to avoid delaying the needed treatment.

When the Client's Condition is Hardly Improving

Sometimes you will run into the following situations:

1. You did a long time adjustment for the patient, but there has been no improvement.

2. After adjustment, the client's situation was improved, but the effectiveness was not maintained for long. Extend the adjustment time length or increase the adjusting frequency to shorten the

time between adjustments. If you cannot match the client's needs, it's time to refer him elsewhere. Please read How often should I get treated?[158].

3. In certain situations, you don't know how to handle the adjustment or professional knowledge that you do not have is needed in order to help the client get better (i.e. The client's life is in danger, his sickness is severe, he has sharp pain, severe bleeding, diarrhea, stroke or infection.

All of the above situations are when you should refer out. Let the client find a Chinese medical physician (an acupuncturist) or other medical professional to get treatment.

When Encountering Situations You Do Not Know How to Handle

There are some things you can do if you are not a well-trained or experienced medical professional and encounter situations you do not know how to handle.

1. You can either follow the aforementioned "When the Client's Condition is Hardly Improving" or refer to Chapter Ten How to Handle the Emergency Situation.

2. To enhance your own medical knowledge, you can buy our company's series of books or go to each chapter's Readers Discussion[137] to enhance your healing experience. Read medical books or seek a medical authority for advice.

Investment Revenue Exercise

1. In the United States, dial the 911 emergency number to call an ambulance. If you are outside the United States, please find your local medical emergency phone number. In Taiwan, call 119. In China, call 112. For other countries, please check out the emergency numbers all over the world at Appendix Nine # 214.

2. Think about times when you would need to call an ambulance? If there is a severely sick patient at home, ask your doctor or nurse under what circumstances you should dial an emergency number or call an ambulance.

3. In life-threatening situations, people are often incoherent and panicked. The following are some things often asked in emergency calls. You can memorize the answers or print this out and keep it by the telephone.

   • For the severely ill patient, there are situations when you need to call an ambulance. It's better to consult his doctor about this before the emergency occurs so that you know what to do.

   • The client's injury or condition should be reported.

   • Keep the patient's name, gender, approximate age, and address at his current location so that you can locate it quickly if needed. Provide your telephone number for further contact.

   • Explain what happened to prompt your emergency call.

   • What kind of emergency treatment has the client had in the past? What treatment is he currently undergoing?

   • The ambulance should transport the patient to the nearest hospital or a hospital designated by you.

Please do not hang up the phone before the person on the other end does.

CHAPTER TEN

How to Handle Emergency Situations

• • • • • • • • • • • • • • • • • • •

As we look ahead into the next century, leaders will be those who empower others.[4]

Bill Gates[212]

There are many emergency situations—seeing a fire, witnessing an armed robbery, suicide. They should all be called in. But this chapter is limited to emergency situations you could encounter during Universal Energy Healing adjustments.

If you have a first aid certificate, follow your professional approach to handle an emergency. Nonprofessionals can refer to this chapter as a guide.

Situations that Require Immediately Calling 911

If any of the following situations occur in the workplace, you should immediately notify the supervisor or department secretary and call the emergency number for an ambulance. If you are doing the universal energy healing adjustment in someone's home, you should ask the family members to call immediately for an ambulance. If it happens in your own home, you should call the emergency number to request an ambulance.

1. The patient rolls his eyes suddenly.
2. The patient is suddenly blind or restless.

3. The patient cannot move, loses sensation, or lapses into a coma.

4. A client that you are familiar with suddenly cannot recognize you.

5. White foam comes out of your client's mouth (unless you are already aware of a previous history of epilepsy).

6. The patient suddenly becomes incontinent and urinates.

7. The patient has a stroke.

   For severe stroke patients, there are open and closed syndromes in TCM (Traditional Chinese Medicine).

   Open syndrome: faint breathing, extremely cold in the extremities, profuse sweating, mouth open but eyes closed, hands open, urine flowing, pulse extremely thin and weak.

   Closed syndrome: lockjaw, red face, rough breathing, excessive phlegm, hands clasped, pulse is slippery and wiry or deep and slow.

8. Heart attack, angina

9. Shortness of breath, cold sweats

10. Coma

11. Continuous bleeding or severe bleeding

12. Sharp pain or severe injury

Be Ready to Answer the Following Questions in the Emergency Call:

- Patient's name, gender, estimated age, address, landmark (if any), telephone number

- What happened?

- Before the ambulance comes, ask what you should do and not do.

- If it's necessary to send the patient to a hospital, ask what you should get ready to bring with him?

- If you are in a public area and there are others in need of emergency care, report how many people were injured and explain their injuries? What are the symptoms?

Wait until the other side has finished speaking, and then hang up the phone.

What Should and Shouldn't You Do List before the Ambulance Comes?

1. Absolutely do not move the patient! It is likely to make the situation worse and can cause irreparable damage.

   If someone falls and is unconscious, you should call the emergency number. If you cannot determine that the patient is without fracture or dislocation, it's better not move him. If a nonprofessional person used improper methods to move the injured person, it could lead to paralysis. Even if well-intentioned, you could get have to deal with a lawsuit from the family members.

2. If at home and the patient needs to go to the hospital, help him prepare the necessary documents and items—medical cards, medical-related information such as medications, recent test reports, ID, hospitalization fee, door keys, and hospitalization necessities such as clothing and toiletries. It would be helpful to have all of these things prepared and in a bag in case a trip to the emergency room if necessary.

3. While waiting for the ambulance before it arrives, keep the following in mind:

   - If the patient had a stroke and is in a coma, does not recognize anyone, starts foaming at the mouth, or has sudden incontinence, put one hand at the top of head U3 and the other hand at the other position on the head.

   - If the patient has rolling eyes, and it is caused by a high fever, put one hand on the neck Dazhui (U4, GV 14) and wave downward quickly to assist in heat dissipation. Otherwise, do as stated above.

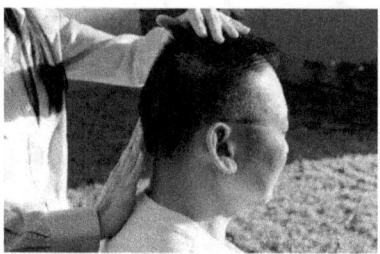

Pic 77 Baihui and Dazhui (Vertical)

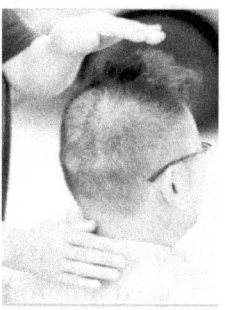

Pic 78 Baihui and Dazhui (Horizontal)

Put one hand on the Baihui and the other hand on the Dazhui (can put hand horizontally) and wave hands downward to disperse heat.

- If encountering a heart attack or cardiac arrest, put one hand on the head Baihui (U3, GV 20) and one hand on the heart.
- If suddenly blind, put one hand on the head Baihui (U3, GV 20) and one hand at the back of the head just above the skull. Or put one hand to cover the eyes and other hand put at the back of the head just above the skull.

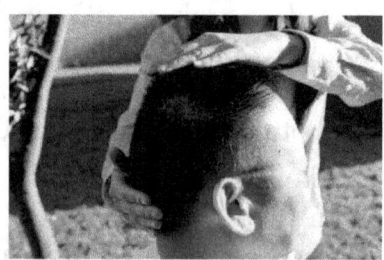

Pic 79 Baihui U3, above the skull

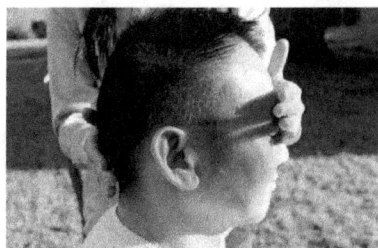

Pic 80 Eyes and above the skull

- If the patient is restless, have him do deep breathing to calm his body and mind. If the patient can sit down, put one hand on Bauhui (U3, GV 20) and one hand above the back skull, or one hand on the eyes and one hand above the back skull.

- If sudden incontinence and out flowing pi or pu, one hand on the Baihui (U3, GV 20) and one hand on the umbilicus or at Mingmen. The kidneys control pi and pu. Mingmen locates on the back between the two kidneys. The umbilicus is on the front of the body and at the opposite side of the Mingmen.

- If short of breath and having cold sweats, put one hand on the Baihui (U3, GV 20) and one hand on the heart and left lungs, or one hand on Tang zhong and one hand on T3/T5.

- If the patient cannot move because of the pain, put one hand on Baihui (U3, GV 20) and one hand at the painful place. Otherwise, if it's too far away to cover the Baihui and the painful place, you can put both hands at the hurt place. If the pain is in the chest or abdomen, then put one hand on the painful area and the other on the relative height of the spine. If the pain is on an upper limb, you can put one hand on the wrist, elbow, or shoulder to determine which one is closest to the pain location. If it is in the lower extremities, put one hand on the knee or hip and thigh connection joint or ankle to see which one is closest to the pain location. Please refer to Chapter Eleven for pictures.

- If bleeding, put one hand at Baihui (U3, GV 20) and one hand at the bleeding area to help stop the bleeding. If the head and bleeding area are far away from each other, put both hands on the bleeding area. The yang qi can stop the blood flow to the outside and keep it flowing in its normal route.

A Common Emergency Situation on Flights

A male patient with heart disease drank wine at a high altitude, resulting in a heart attack and shortness of breath. Even with the oxygen mask, he still had difficulty breathing, his body temperature dropped, and he broke into a cold sweated and had a pale face.

This was an emergency experience in 2012 on a flight over the Pacific Ocean. A male premed* passenger went to help first. Because of the lack of medical facilities and supplies, the pre-made could do nothing besides monitor the patient's blood pressure and heart rate.

* Premed means an official medical certified first aid professional.

So I squatted down to put my index finger to the patient's right ST 36 to do acupressure. Soon after, the patient pulled off his oxygen mask and his symptoms gradually subsided.

Because the flight attendants told me that this was the most common emergency case in airplanes, I included it here for your reference. Maybe someday you will use it to save a life.

1. Use the index finger or thumb to do acupressure on Zusanli (ST 36)—downward direction toward the inside of the leg to do circular massage, and then turn down. If you face the patient's left ST 36, you do the acupressure clockwise. If face the patient's, right ST 36, you do counterclockwise acupressure. When the alcohol in the patient descends downward from the stomach, and he is breathing smoothly, he will voluntarily remove the oxygen mask.

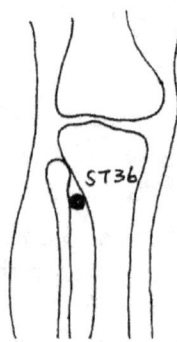

Fig 13 ST 36 on the Right Leg

2. Do acupressure at BL 15.

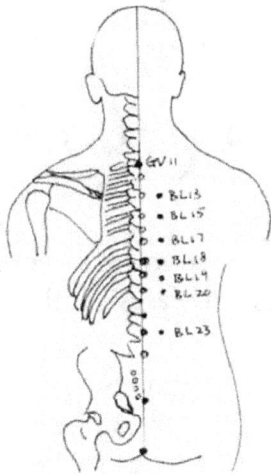

Fig 14 Back Shu Points

Xinshu (heart) BL 15 is below the fifth vertebra spinous process (T5) at the midpoint of the spine and the shoulder blade's medial edge. Or, by the intersection of the lower edge of the scapula and the spine, go up two vertebrae, and it is the fifth vertebra lower process for the majority of people.

3. At the Zangmen (LR13), do acupressure to soothe the patient's qi and make it flow smoothly. After wine enters the stomach, it goes to the liver and disturbs the qi's normal flowing route.

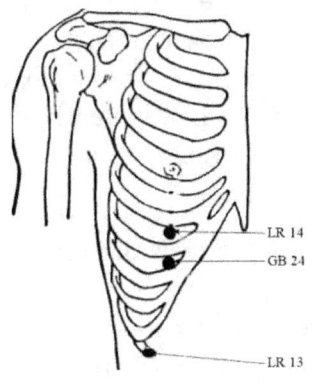

Fig 15 LR13

Zangmen (LR 13) locates at both lateral sides of the abdomen at the inferior end of the eleventh rib end.

The above acupressure took less than ten minutes.

Using the Comprehensive Universal Energy Healing

Because you do not have practical experience, you can follow these steps to help in emergency cases in the absence of professional medical staff on the plane:

Use the index finger or thumb to do acupressure on Zusanli (ST 36) in a downward direction toward the inside of the leg, doing circular massage, and then turn down. If you face the patient's left ST 36, you do acupressure counterclockwise. If face the patient's right ST 36, you do counterclockwise acupressure. When the patient's alcohol descends downward from the stomach, and he is breathing smoothly, he will remove the oxygen mask.

- Put one hand at the head Baihui (U3, GV 20) and one hand at the heart location. Or put one hand in the front of the heart and one on the back of the heart to make the heart function more normally again.

Or do acupressure at the Xinshu BL15.

- Put one hand on the head Baihui (U3, GV 20) and one hand on the patient's right side liver location. Or one hand in the front and another hand on the back of the liver location to soothe the alcohol in his liver. When you feel your hands inferior (lower) part is warm, wave your hands gently downward to guide the wine into the large intestine.

Or do acupressure at LR 13.

- Ask the patient where he feels discomfort. Put one hand at the Baihui (U3, GV 20) and one hand at the uncomfortable place until the patient feels comfortable. Or put your hands on the location of discomfort with one hand in the front and one hand in the back of the body until you can feel the heat traveling between your two hands. Ask the patient to follow the Chapter Five How to Get the Universal Energy to Improve Health to improve his health. Also ask the patient to always practice gratitude, sharing, collaboration, and other good spiritual codes.

- Please keep in mind that this is for emergency cases. You have no obligation to adjust irrelevant discomfort such as knee pain or elbow pain,

  If a patient has suffered a heart attack as in the above situation, but it is not caused by drinking, you do not need to massage the ST 36 and LR 13, but still follow the rest of the above steps.

Investment Revenue Exercise

1. If there are people with heart disease who live or travel with you, you should print this page and keep it within reach. When you have time, memorize it in case of emergency.
2. Know when your client needs ER care and you need to notify the client's family members for an ER care.
3. Understand the local ER laws and have the local ER phone number and address readily available.
4. Accidents happen, so be prepared for the unexpected. Brainstorm how you might make an emergency stretcher out of rope, clothing, sheets, and long sticks in case of emergency.

   You can also go to universalenergyhealing.us for instructions to make an emergency stretcher.

Attention:

If there are professional medical personnel on site, let the professionals take charge of the emergency case.

CHAPTER ELEVEN

Some Commonly Seen Health Issues in Healing
●●●●●●●●●●●●●●●●●●●●●●●●●●●●●●

Yin and yang are the way of the universe, the discipline of all things, the source of changes, the origin of life and death, the house of gods and spirits, and treating diseases should seek its root.

Huang Di Nei Jing • Su Wen • Chapter Five The Big
Theory of the Yin and Yang

This chapter's contents are from my clinical experience, but please use everything contained herein for reference only. This is not a formal medical textbook.

As a reader, if you can go to the book's Readers Discussion[137] to share your adjustment experience and/or ask questions, you will help more people get benefits from the Comprehensive Universal Energy Healing!

Besides the healer following the instructions in this book to put hands on clients, the client also can follow the healer's instruction to put his own hands on his body to do a collaborative adjustment, especially in locations that are hard to reach for the healer, to speed up the adjustment results. As the healer is adjusting the legs, the client can put his hands on U3 (GV20 or DU20) and the heart, to help the whole body circulation, or the kidney, to help the lower body's circulation.

It's better for the client to follow the healer's instruction except for when the healer asks the client's opinion for where to put hands. In any collaboration, if there is a commander and a follower, things run smoother. Usually, the healer is in charge, so it's best that the healer acting as the commander.

If there is more than one healer, they can take turns being in charge of the adjustment. That way everyone can have the experience of being in command. Being a commander can speed up the Comprehensive Universal Energy Healing learning process. It's a valuable experience to be in charge of healing and makes for quicker and more complete learning.

If there are any differences in opinion, they can be discussed after the adjustment. The client's feedback is invaluable in helping the healer improve later adjustments.

Please refer to the Chapter Two case summary table for the location of hands for various adjustments and the approximate time used. But please don't feel you must adhere to the exact time. Everyone's health situation is different, so the adjustment time needed will vary for each individual.

The following paragraphs recommend where to place your hands to use Comprehensive Universal Energy Healing (CHUEH) for pain syndromes. During the healing process, if both the healer and the client give gratitude and collaborate, it can bring a faster result.

Pain

This chapter covers only mild pain situations. The best advice I can give you is that if the client is in severe pain, it's better to let him visit a doctor or emergency room. If you're one to jump around in books, please be sure to read Chapter Ten to avoid not recognizing the danger signs.

For patients who have very high pain tolerance, mild pain indicates something that is already a severe case. Take, for example, a chief nursing officer when she felt pain and visited a doctor. The doctor showed her an x-ray showing that her discs were already all gone. Another male patient had never felt pain in his back until on one day he could not bend at all. His x-ray showed that some of his lower back vertebrae had already fused together. Both of these people were too busy to pay attention to their body's warning signs.

Lower right abdominal pain could be appendicitis and require a visit to the ER. For common visceral pain, you could go to a Chinese medicine physician or an MD who adopts natural ways to treat to take care of you.

If the pain is mild, and you can use Comprehensive Universal Energy Healing, put one hand on the head Baihui (U3, GV 20 or DU 20) and one hand on the area of visceral pain.

If it is a pain caused by coldness due to cold wind, cold food, or cold drinks, stop ingesting the cold food or drink immediately and, protect yourself from cold temperatures and wind. Please read Cold Foods & Cold Drinks That Cause Health Problems[186] or briefly look the chart of Cold Foods & Drinks That Cause Problems Chart Rev 1[187]. You can ingest ginger soup or cinnamon tea with honey at as hot taste as you can tolerate until your body warms up.

Please buy the cinnamon at a Chinese herbal store that carries a better quality cinnamon with a thicker skin. Grate fresh spice for the tea. Due to its herbal grade, you cannot overdo the dosage. The regular dosage if taken long term depends on your body coldness. You can start with one to three grams per day. When your body starts getting warmer, you either decrease the dosage or stop taking it altogether. The three grams per day can be used in the winter. Use one gram per day or none at all in the summer to avoid becoming too hot and getting nosebleeds. In the fall and spring, you can vary the dosage depending on the weather.

I'd recommend using ginger soup instead of cinnamon honey tea in the summer. Ginger is a lot safer to use even though it has a slower effectiveness.

In general, Northern Chinese medicine schools adapters used to use stronger herbs to treat yang. Yet, the southern Chinese medicine schools adapters are used to tonify yin. The long term treatment results have huge differences.

If the pain is chronic, there might be blood stasis or an organ problem. You should suggest a visit an acupuncturist to help with the blood stasis if it's severe or chronic, and you can also adjust the related organ(s).

For muscle pain, you need to adjust the spleen or the spleen and kidney in combination. The spleen controls the muscles and the four limbs. If the kidney yang is deficient, it can lead to a spleen yang deficiency.

In case of stress, dining outside often, or taking drugs or ingesting chemicals of any kind, you should adjust the liver or do a liver detox exercise that we will cover in our next book.

If the client has an aversion to cold, the lungs will have to be adjusted because they control the skin pores that prevent coldness from invading the body. If there is phlegm in the lungs, expel the phlegm using CHUEH. If the phlegm is sticky due to smoking—either in the present or in the past—you should refer your client to an acupuncturist for help in expelling the phlegm. Otherwise, getting old, a flu could induce a severe pneumonia.

If the coldness is from ingesting cold foods or drinks, tell the client to stop the behavior immediately. If it's the summer or he is in any hot environment, instruct him to drink water slowly, as close to body temperature as possible.

Water that enters the stomach should be vaporized by the stomach heat in order to quench thirst. Cold water does not vaporize quickly. Its low temperature slows down the process until the stomach is full of cold water. Then you are full and cannot drink anymore, so the thirst remains, and the coldness has caused physical damage which accumulates as time passes.

If there is a string-tight type of muscular pain, it's better to use acupuncture to quickly loosen the muscle and alleviate the pain.

A string-tight muscle is a long strip of muscle bundles that is harder than the nearby muscles. If you press on it, the client will feel soreness or pain. It's shaped like a rope and can feel as hard as a string or cable, hence its label. Similarly, there are string-tight tendons.

The string-tight type muscle and tendon treatments have not been covered by medical schools. We include it as an acupuncturist continuing education class.

Some people do self-massage or visit a masseuse or a massage therapist, but they may not know to use a strong blood circulation activating massage oil. That can leave skin injuries or, more serious, cause muscle fiber injuries. The muscle layers are hard and without elasticity. It's difficult to separate them even with regular acupuncture or a skilled massage therapist. The adhesive muscle fibers can best be treated with herbs or skillful tui-na* or massage therapists.

> * Tui-na is similar to massage but focuses more on acupuncture points and meridians. Plus there are more skills from ancient Chinese medicine only. However, Acupuncture schools do not teach the deep skills in general. They can follow private masters to learn.

The liver controls the tendons. If there is tendon pain or tightness or hardness, the client should drink less wine or no wine, reduce stress, and keep away from processed foods and stop dining outside to avoid taking in food additives and poisons which cause toxins to accumulate in the liver.

If going to bed too late, he should change his lifestyle and go to bed before 11:00 p.m. The gallbladder's detoxification time is from 11:00 p.m. to 1:00 a.m. From 1:00 a.m. to 3:00 a.m. is the liver's detoxification time. If you miss the detoxification period for a long time, poor organ detoxification can allow toxins to accumulate in the organ and cause health problems due to blockage of proper organ functions.

If have liver problems, such as hepatitis, liver cirrhosis, or fatty liver, you can look for qualified Chinese medicine treatments. There are many well-documented successful cases of treatment.

Arthritis involves tendon and muscle problems. The liver, spleen, and kidneys should be adjusted. Clients with rheumatoid arthritis should turn to Chinese medicine treatments.

The auxiliary adjustment for the arthritis is to put one hand to cover the Shendao 神道 (U5,GV 11 or DU 11)/Zhiynag 至陽 (U6, GV 9 or DU 9). The other hand is put at the head Baihui 百會 (U3, GV 20 or DU 20).

Later, put one hand on the Mingmen (U7, GV 4 or DU 4) and the other hand on the arthritis spot. Then move hands to put on both kidneys.

At the end, adjust the liver and spleen.

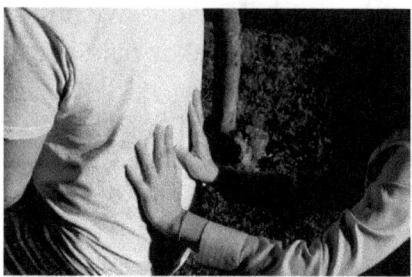

Pic 81 Left hand: spleen/kidney, right hand: liver/kidney.
One stone for two birds

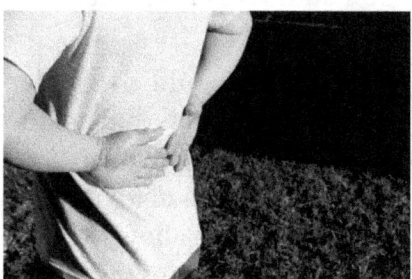

Pic 82 Put two hands on the back in both kidneys' locations

You can adjust two kidneys by yourself. Put your hands behind the kidney with dorsal side, or put your palms beside the umbilicus on the front to cover the kidneys, or cross your arms to adjust both kidneys. It doesn't matter in the second two examples whether it's the palm or dorsal side of the hands—they all have the same adjustment effect.

For the coldness pathogen invading the body and inducing arthritis or muscle and tendon pain, adjust the lungs. The lungs control the skin and the pores on the skin. If the pores can't close well, the outside coldness will enter to cause pain.

If often have back pain, nocturia, or dark circles under the eyes, there is a kidney yang deficiency, and you should adjust the client's kidney. In addition, adjust the kidney's mother, the lungs.

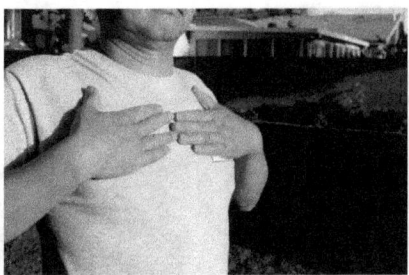

Pic 83 Put Hands on Lungs

When adjusting the lungs, if the pinky finger of the hand feels more heat, gently wave your hands down two or three times to guide the heat downward. The client will usually feel more comfortable and be able breathe deeper and easier.

If the heat cannot be reduced, there might be sticky phlegm or a foreign substance in the lungs, and it's better to seek medical help without delay to determine the cause and get proper treatment.

There are strong herbs that expel sticky phlegm with a foreign substance by vomiting out and acupuncture skill to expel sticky phlegm. There are also qigong exercises to help you expel phlegm, but slower than visit a professional.

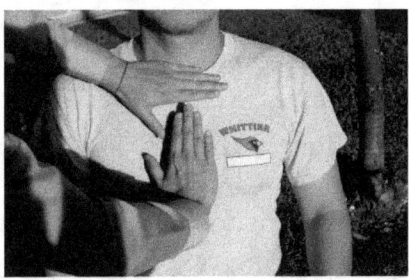

Pic 84 Adjust the esophagus or respiratory problems.

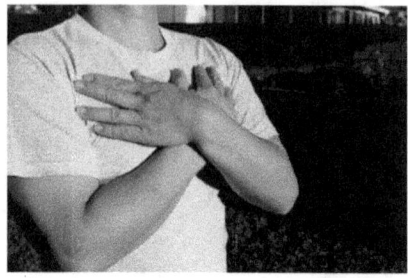
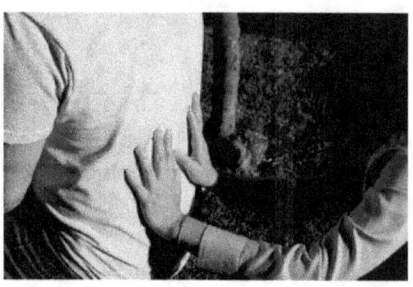

Pic 85 Adjust the heart and lungs   Pic 86 Adjust the kidneys

Adjust the calf, knee, ankle problems

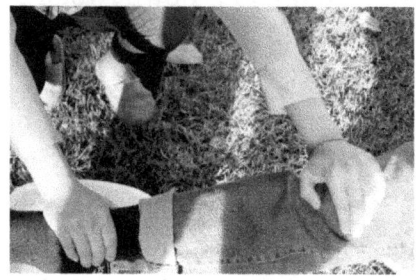

Pic 87 One hand on the knees, one hand around the ankle

If there is bone pain or bone injury, adjust the kidney and the local bone pain area. The kidneys control the bone. For bone pain, bone injury, or osteoporosis, your client can also find good Chinese medicine treatments.

For a bone dislocation in the US, look for a chiropractor for treatment. If in Taiwan or China, look for a Chinese medicine physician or a bone adjustment doctor's help. There is a very powerful herbal formula that helps to increase bone density. It's very sad that many powerful herbs and herbal formulas safely used for more than million years have been prohibited in the US. For example, the inner skin of the chicken gizzard is an excellent herb to open up the appetite. It has other functions as well.

If have osteoporosis, you should avoid dairy products and excessive animal protein intake. In order to expel extra animal protein, calcium is often used to carry them out of the body. Therefore, the countries that drink more milk have more and severe osteoporosis cases[188, 189, 190]. Also stop drinking carbonated[191] drinks. They are a strong acid and cause bones to lose calcium.

If you want to maintain more calcium and mineral in the bone, instead of taking calcium pills that cause kidney stones, eat onions, wheat, and asparagus to increase calcium absorption. Prevent bone mineral destruction by eating nuts and whole grains[192].

Protrusion of the vertebral bone (spinal bone), spinal bone displacement, disc displacement, disc stenosis, pinched nerve, and humpback are all due to a Governor (Du) Meridian qi deficiency. Muscles or tendons are tight because they have shrunken in length and had become accustomed to those situations.

Auxiliary adjustment can put one hand to cover the Shendao 神道 (U5,GV 11 or DU 11)/Zhiynag 至陽 (U6, GV 9 or DU 9). Another hand is put at the head Baihui (U3, GV 20 or DU 20). Or put one hand to cover the Shendao神道 (U5,GV 11 or DU 11)/Zhiynag 至陽(U6, GV 9 or DU 9) and another hand on the Mingmen (U7, GV 4 or DU 4). Then one hand at Mingmen (U7, GV 4 or DU 4) and the other hand at the problem area. Later, put hands on both kidneys.

Because the muscles and tendons are stiff or tight, it is wise to also adjust the liver and spleen. For disc displacement, disc stenosis, and pinched nerve, before the end of the adjustment, put hands on the stiff muscles located between the spine and the side of the trunk. This will relax these muscles on both sides to avoid the pulling from that will cause bone and disc problems again. Because the muscles and tendons tighten up, the wei qi becomes weak and coldness invades. If it's severe and beyond the help of CHUEH, acupuncture and moxibustion can be used. If it's more severe, acupuncture and moxibustion plus my external herbal treatment can be used for treatment. That can accelerate the result and solve the root problem.

Another alternative is sitting in the sauna. Always bring a bottle of water to compensate for water loss. The coldness will allow the sweat to flow out.

If you have high blood pressure, it's best not use a sauna or steam room. If your high blood pressure is mild, you can have someone accompany you for safety, staying no longer than ten minutes. Also pay attention to your body heat to avoid its temperature a further increase in the room.

Please also avoid leaving a sauna or steam room and immediately entering a cold environment. Big temperature changes can cause unexpected health issues for patients with high blood pressure and blood clotting, patients with clots in the head, and the elderly or qi/blood deficient patients. It could cause a coma, a stroke, or cause you to pass out and fall.

If the body of your tongue has purple color, it means that you have blood stasis in your body. If it is located at the head[213] from a palm reflexology chart and has a purple color, you'd better not enter the sauna or steam room. Instead, you can visit an acupuncturist. TCM can clean the blood and treat the organs to avoid blood clotting. Western medicine can only thin the blood.

The purple color is due to red blood cells stacked together and carry less oxygen that turn the artery to be purple color like a vein's color.

A sauna is best for letting the coldness get out the body through sweating. Because it's in a dry air, sweating is easier.

Be alert to signs of any discomfort. If you feel uncomfortable, leave the sauna immediately, but do not enter a cold room right away—the heat will push more blood to the head, and the coldness will shrink the blood vessels, causing a stroke.

Ankylosing spondylitis treated well with acupuncture. There needs to be some clinical trials for the efficacy of using CHUEH to make adjustments.

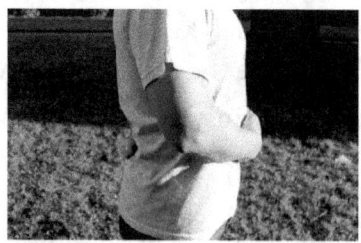

Pic 88 Self adjusts the Mingmen and umbilicus.
Put hand in the front and back at the same height.

For the slight misalignment or displacement of the spine and disc narrowing or back stiffness or tightness, you can try to hang on the monkey bars for a couple of minutes to correct the spine. But be cautioned to hang only three to five inches above the ground and avoid jumping down and impacting the bad spine. If it is too high, you can use a stool or stepladder under the feet.

Please be patient. The problem was not created in one day. It will take time to correct it.

Another way to correct the spine is to copy the ballet dancers when you sit down by extending your legs 180 degrees out. It does take time, however, to correct your spine. Some people sit in this way every day for a year and can go without surgery.

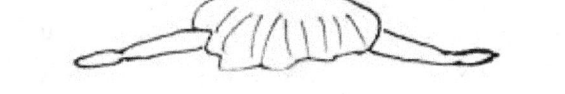

Fig 16 Use a ballet dancer sitting posture to correct spine misalignment

Of course, you can find a good chiropractor to correct your spine and an acupuncturist to loosen the muscles and tendons. This will get you a quicker result.

Once the spine is corrected, you will find that all organ functions get better. You will have a healthier body.

For any pain, you can put one hand at the top of head Baihui (U3, GV 20 or DU 20) and the other hand at the painful area. Or put both hands on the spine at the same level of the painful spot or the problem organ(s).

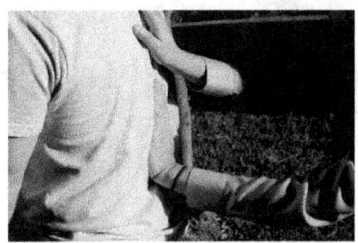

Pic 89 Hands on the Upper Spine

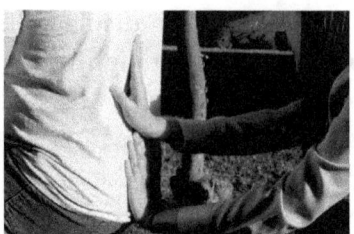

Pic 90 Hands on the Lower Spine

Back pain causes, consequences, and treatment methods are listed in the Back Pain Chart[197]. Please refer to the end of this chapter.

For discomfort of the knees, ankles, elbows, and wrists, you can put hands around them to adjust, or a healer can put one hand on the head Baihui 百會 (U3, GV 20 or DU 20) and the other hand on the heart. *Huang Di Nei Jing • Su Wen • The Chapter Seventy-Fourth-The Must True and Great Theory* "All kinds of pain, itching, and skin ulcers belong to the heart problem…" So for pain, itching, or skin ulcer problems, you can adjust the heart.

If there are knee problems, then put hands around the knee.

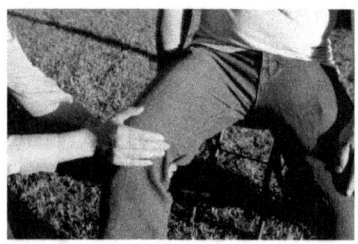

Pic 91 Hand around the knee

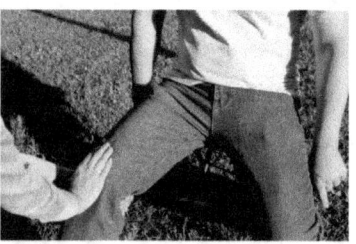

pic 92 Hands on the knee

Adjust calf or knee or ankle problem

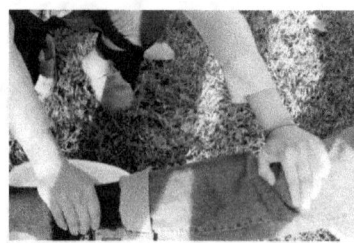

Pic 93 One hand on the knee,
one hand around the ankle

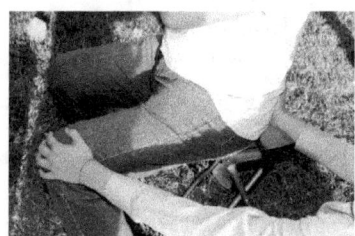

Pic 94 Adjusting knee, hip, and thigh problems

If swelling is causing pain, put one hand on the head Baihui 百會 (U3, GV 20 or DU 20) and one hand at the edema site.

If there is swelling in the thigh, then put the other hand on the same side of the kidney.

If the swelling is in the lower leg, put one hand around the ankle and the other at the back of the knee. If both ankles are equally swelling, put hands on heart to treat the root problem.

After the swelling is reduced, if the swelling is in the upper body—the head, face, upper limb or upper trunk—put hands at the front and back of the body in the lung position and then in the spleen position until the heat penetrates between the front and back of the body. You and the client should be able to feel the adjustment if it is well done. If you cannot be sure if the heat has penetrated, you can verify it with the client. If the client can feel it, you can soothe the qi* in that area and then move hands to adjust the next spot. If feet are cold that need to cover during sleep, the kidney also needs to be adjusted.

> * Soothing the qi means to move hands from the top to bottom of the adjusted area two to three times to make sure qi is flowing smoothly.

If the client also has nocturia* or a cold body constitution, put hands on both kidneys to adjust. If there is an aversion to cold, adjust the kidneys and lungs.

> * Nocturia is waking up in the night to pass urine. It is common in the elderly who have a kidney yang deficiency or a young person without a kidney deficiency but who drinks too much water before going to bed.

If the edema is in the lower extremities, put hands on the spleen and kidney, respective to the location. If one hand is behind the back, and your hand is big enough, you can cover both the spleen and kidney.

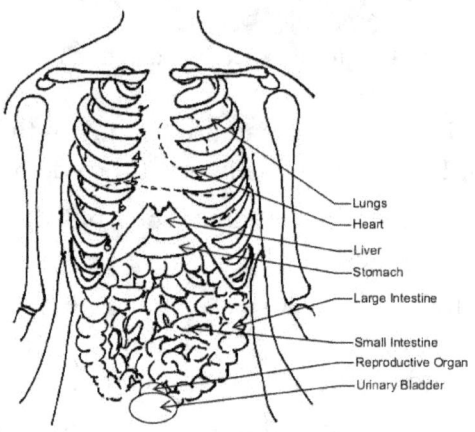

Fig 17 Body Organ Front View

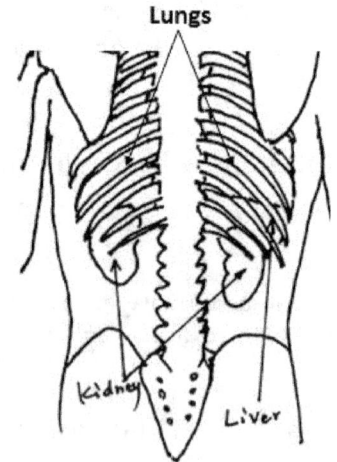

Fig 18 Body Organs Back View

For whole body pain, sit at the side of the client. Put one hand at Zhiyang 至陽 (U6, GV 9 or DU 9) and one hand at the Qihai 氣海 (CV 6 or Ren 6, below the navel).[215]

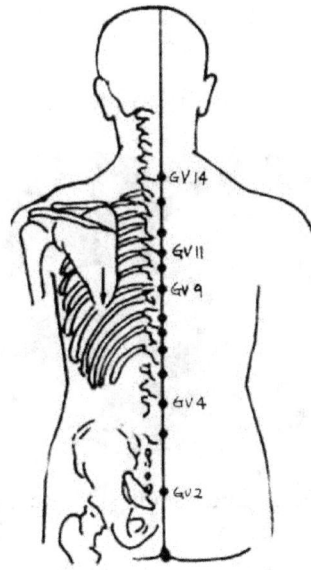

Fig 19 Zhiyang 至陽 (GV 9 or DU 9) is located at the lower edge of the seventh thoracic vertebral process, or intersection point, of the connection of the bilateral of the scapula's lower edge crossing with the spine.

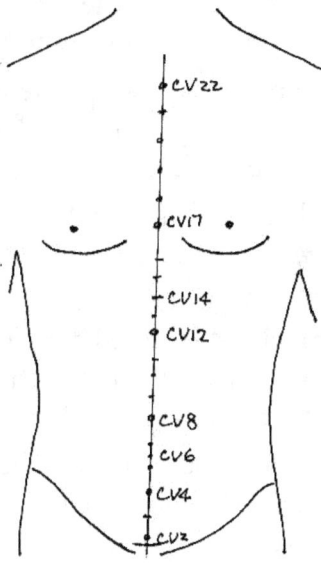

Fig 21 Qihai 氣海 (Ren 6) is located in the abdominal midline, 1.5 cun* below the umbilicus

*   Cun is a measurement unit in TCM acupuncture. Please refer to the Appendix Two Glossary *Cun* 寸.

For headache, put hands on the painful places.

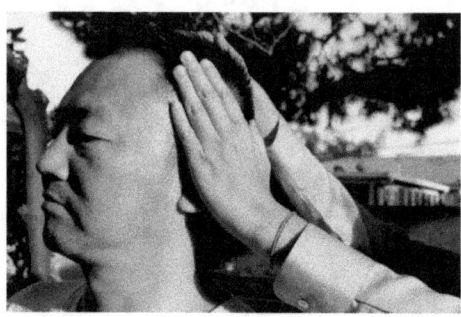

Pic 95 Baihui and painful side of a migraine

When adjusting the stroke patient's head, if the healer feels heat under his hands, and the heat is not reduced after waving the hands, he should consider there could blood stasis or a tumor or an abnormal nodule and refer the patient to an acupuncturist who will use herbs to clear the blood stasis. Otherwise, the blockage will block either brain or emotions or body functions depending upon its location.

Chinese medicine can not only solve the blood stasis, but also treat the root problem(s) causing it. It's a fact based on 250 million years of the wisdom of Chinese medicine.

If the inside of the head feels hot and painful, you can cool the heat at Dazhui 大椎 (U4, GV 14 or DU 14) and expel the phlegm in the lungs.

Acupuncture treatment used to needle this GV 14 to immediately reduce a high fever. Meanwhile, add points to treat the cause and root problems to boost up the immunity.

The neck serves as our body's cooler due to all of the yang meridians goes up to the head that brings a lot yang (warm) Qi to the head.

If there is phlegm in the lungs or neck is too tight, the ascending yang qi goes to the head and cannot descend down, it's one of the reasons that causes the head to hurt. And that causes head sweating when intake hot foods/drinks or in a hot environment.

You can also wave your hands downward after applying CHUEH at Dazhui and expel the phlegm in the lungs. Or loosen the neck if needed.

If the heat does not reduce after waving your hands, there might be severe problems inside the lungs. It could be sticky phlegm or foreign particles in the lungs. Ask the client to get a medical professional's help as soon as possible to avoid severe health issues later.

Heat in the head can be caused by a tumor or blood stasis in the head or phlegm in lungs. The head yang cannot descend past the phlegm in the lungs, and the extra yang stays in the head to cause heat. If you ingest too many cold foods or drinks into the body, either the stomach heat rises up to the head or the coldness invades the body, especially the head,

If you have had a stroke for a long time, you also need to adjust the four limbs. For a new stroke, concentrate on adjusting the head to expel the blood stasis is helpful except the bleed area has too much blood dried out that needs herbs to help.

If there is dead blood in the head, the heat under the palm(s) cannot be reduced by waiving hands. You need ask your client to visit a health professional to remove the dead blood.

Adjusting shoulder problems

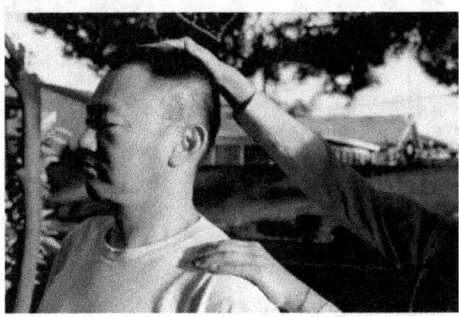

Pic 96 Baihui and shoulder

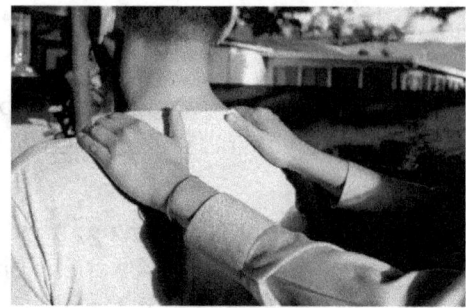

Pic 97 Both Shoulders

Adjusting upper limb problems

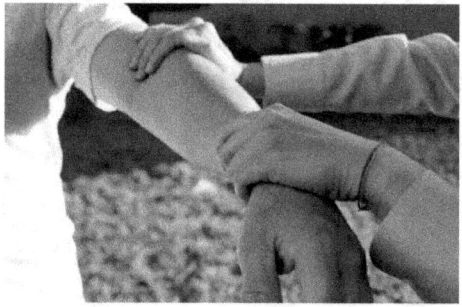

Pic 98 Adjusting elbow, wrist, forearm problems

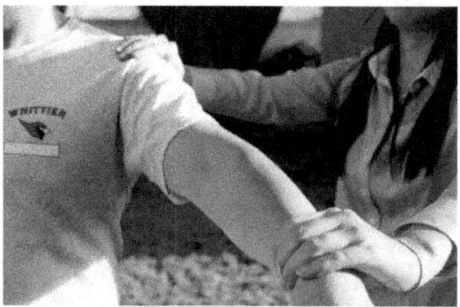

Pic 99 Adjusting discomfort between shoulder and wrist

Adjusting abdominal problems

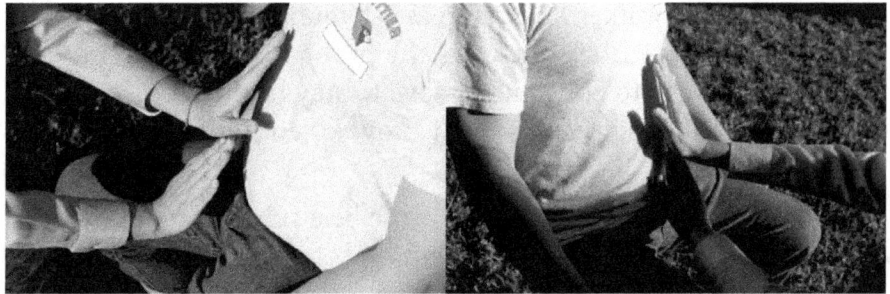

Pic 100 & Pic 101 Adjusting abdominal problems

If a person easily falls down, falls often, or falls for unknown reasons, he can look for an acupuncturist's help. There are a couple of possible causes.

1. Most likely the back of the neck muscle is tight. That blocks the qi and blood from flowing up to the head, causing a poor flow of qi and blood to the cerebellum. That causes a loss of balance. Please read Poor Balance[196].

2. Deficiency in both qi and blood are causes of falling down. When you suddenly stand up, blood cannot flow quickly enough to the head to supply enough oxygen. Dizziness is the result. Besides standing up slowly, look for a good acupuncturist to solve the root problem of qi and blood deficiency to avoid falls in the future. Falls can cause numerous other health issues including but not limited to bone fractures and coma.

   Iron intake is not the total solution for anemia due to iron shortage is not the single cause of anemia. The spleen cannot absorb iron is a main reason. For a pregnant woman needs extra iron to supply a fetus needs, small red beans (chi Xiao duo 赤小豆 is sold in Chinese Supermarket) soup is good to supply irons. That's nature and can help to leach out the extra water in the body.

3. If there is water sitting above the diaphragm, when the body moves or on a boat or in a car, that disturbed water leveling can cause dizziness.

4. Translocation hypertension, a drug's side effects, high blood viscosity, or internal medical problems can cause dizziness.

Relying on a walker or cane to assist you in walking or avoiding walking altogether does not solve the problem. Human beings are animals that need to constantly move to stay healthy. Once we lose mobility and flexibility, plus don't move often, more health issues will emerge.

Traditional Chinese Medicine is the best solution to take care of the root causes of dizziness and falling.

If a client has fallen and is unconscious, call an emergency number immediately. Do not move the person to avoid injuring them further. Nonprofessional emergency personnel using improper methods to move the fallen person can cause paralysis.

Even if it's well-intentioned help, there was a case, that the helper got a lawsuit from the family members due to the victim could avoid paralysis if waiting for a professional to move him. The damage to the victim and his family members is too high to bear.

If circumstances allow, immediately adjust the body part that hit the ground where bore the most force in order to avoid qi stagnation or blood stasis and causes other symptoms to appear.

The elderly usually have yang qi and/or blood deficiency. When they fall and disturb the oxygen supply to the head, it can cause brain damage in the head. Coma, memory loss, mental disorder, or a body part malfunction could be the result. You should be careful and take action to visit an acupuncturist to treat yang qi and blood deficiency in order to prevent that from happening.

Because you don't want to move the fallen person, when making an adjustment, you can stay in the front or the back of the person to adjust.

If someone falls suddenly, there will most likely be some qi stagnation. Unless in the center of a road where there is potential danger to be hit by car, do not change the person's position If not allowing the body to relieve the stagnated qi by itself, that will promote pain and other troubles later. The correct approach is to maintain the same posture and wait for the qi to straighten itself out. Then, slowly stand up and change the position. It is best to let the person slowly change posture and stand up again to minimize the damage.

There is an old saying: "Once fallen down, one has to stand up by oneself." The exception is if the person has no strength to stand up or received an injury that makes standing up impossible. Those who are unable to stand up by themselves need to be helped. If circumstances permit, it's better to use a wheelchair or a stretcher because bones, tendon, or muscles could be injured or damaged by walking or another fall.

Mental Stress

Please refer to the stress-induced problems chart at the end of this chapter. If you want to read the explanations, you can read the Stress Caused Problems[195]. You can adjust the liver first. Then, according to the symptoms, adjust the affected organ(s) that induced the symptom(s).

The method to adjust an organ is to put one hand on the top of the head Baihui 百會 (U3, GV 20 or DU 20) and one hand on the organ. It doesn't matter if it's in the front or back of the body. Alternatively, you can put both hands on the organ by putting one hand on the front of the body and one in the back of the body to let universal energy fully penetrate the body. By doing so, the organ will fully recover its functions and operate at its peak performance.

Remember that when there is a fire*, you can feel the heat. You can move your hand downward gently two to three times to guide the heat and the blockage downward.

> * Fire in Chinese medicine is extra heat that is generated from excess heat or yin deficiency heat. This fire has no flame.

When there is heat felt, it means that there is a blockage—usually caused by phlegm, blood stasis, tumor or cancer cells, or any kind of nodule—that reflected the yang qi back and generated heat. You can feel the extra heat on the hand that covers the area of blockage.

If the heat cannot be reduced and continues to accumulate after waving your hands, it's better to ask the client to consult professional medical services.

There are too many toxins that get into our livers by ingesting foods with toxic chemicals, taking drugs, or breathing in toxins from the air. Liver qi and blood flow get blocked by bad emotions or from toxins entering our body. No matter whether client is with or without mental stress, adjust the liver first. Patients usually feel emotionally lighter and often have a feeling of relief.

If the hand is behind the body on the back, it can cover both of an organ's back-shu points and its emotion control point located at the outer line of the Bladder Meridian. For example, to adjust the lungs, you can use one hand to cover the Feishu (BL13) and the Pohu 魄戶 (BL 42). To adjust the heart, you can cover the Xinshu 心俞(BL 15) and Shentang 神堂 (BL 44).

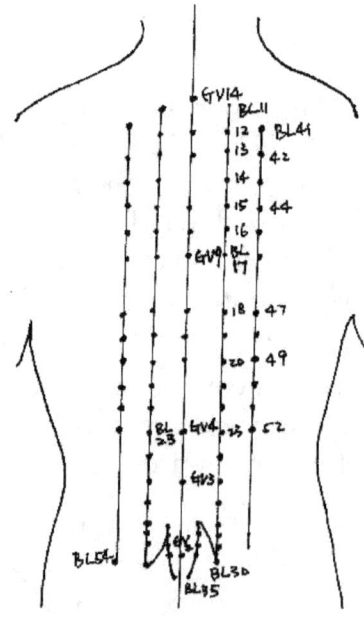

Fig 21 Points on the Bladder Meridian

This book is for the beginner and will not cover some of the more complicated diseases such as breast cancer, tremors, tumors, and infertility.

Insomnia

Insomnia Causes

Insomnia, according to the diagnostic and clinical experience of the Traditional Chinese Medicine, is diagnosed according to the following:

1. If by 11:00 p.m. to 1: 00 a.m., you cannot fall asleep, or you wake up during that time period, it's a problem of the gallbladder. Often, it also involves a liver problem.

2. If between 1:00 a.m. to 3: 00 a.m., you cannot fall asleep, or you wake up, it's a liver problem.

3. If between 3:00 a.m. to 5: 00 a.m., you cannot fall asleep, or you wake up, it's a lung problem.

4. If have a shallow sleep or wake up frequently, it's a heart problem.

A heart blood deficiency might accompany hair loss* on the head. Heart blood deficiency can be solved by an acupuncturist. In Chinese medicine, the spleen absorbs nutrition, the kidney controls bone marrow/original metabolism fuel of yang qi, and the lungs supply zhong qi to help produce blood. However, in Western medicine, only the bone marrow makes blood.

---

* In Chinese medicine, the liver controls head hair growth, and the kidney controls hair color.

Insomnia can also be caused by heart fire. The heart fire going upward and disturbing the heart doesn't host the shen to return to rest in the heart at night. You can confirm this by looking into the inner canthus of the eyes. If they have a red color, that causes heart and kidney disharmony.

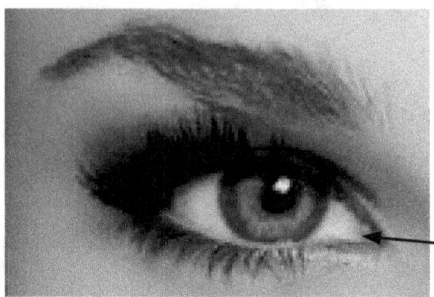

Inner Canthus

Pic 102 Inner Cantus

Heart fire can be caused by worrying or thinking too much or by any prolonged emotion. The other symptoms can be irritability, palpitation, little or no or yellow tongue coating, rapid pulse, hot in the hands, throat and mouth dryness, and red tongue tip.

Heart fire can also be caused by frequent intercourse. If this is the case, it can cause kidney yin (water) deficiency and cannot nourish the heart to lessen the heart fire. These two organs will be disharmonized.

Please refer to the Appendix Four Basic TCM Theory. In Traditional Chinese Medicine, the kidneys are water and the heart is fire. The kidney's water (yin) goes up to harmonize and nourish the heart to avoid the heart fire (yang) getting too hot. The heart fire goes down to warm up kidneys.

If the kidney is weak, accompanying symptoms could be a sore back, weak knees, nocturnal emission, dry mouth and throat, constipation, back pain, hot flashes, night sweats, dizziness, and tinnitus.

5. If waking up at night for urination, it is a kidney yang deficiency problem.

Kidney dialysis patients will take a longer time both in each session and in the whole period of the CHUEH adjustments. If under kidney dialysis treatment, it is difficult to get out of the treatment. The damage to the kidney is a tug of war with the other alternative treatments.

Especially when the patient does not want to change his diet to keep away from eating cold foods and/or drinks that put down kidney functions and kidney yang. A person with damaged kidneys should not increase their burden.

Kidney dialysis patients ought to follow the nutritionist-arranged diet and avoid eating high potassium foods to prevent potential irregular heartbeat, especially tachycardia* which could cause death[194].You may seek good quality TCM treatments.

*   Tachycardia is a heartbeat that is too fast.

As mentioned in the beginning of Insomnia Causes, we can know which organ has functional issues based on the time that one wakes up from sleep.

6. There is an old Chinese saying: "If the stomach is not in harmony, there is insomnia." It means that if the stomach is in discomfort, it affects sleep. Maybe you have experienced waking up after a big meal with stomach pain?

7. If you have a motor mind and your mind can't calm down and sleep, it's caused by a spleen problem. The root cause can also involve kidney or liver function issues. You sometimes have to wait until all of the organ functions are recovered to some extent, and then the insomnia will go away.

8. Sleep apnea is caused by the tongue falling backward and blocking the airway. It is caused by a cardiac problem. Sometimes the nose cannot breathe, and this is caused by lung problems or a Governor (Du) Meridian qi deficiency.

9. If have nightmares or weird dreams, they can be caused by liver fire and/or gallbladder fire, heart fire, and lung fire. You can follow the method mentioned in Chapter Seven, moving your hands downward gently to guide the fire down.

10. A lot dreams can be caused by a heart qi deficiency, a combination of heart and spleen deficiency, kidney and heart disharmony, a heart and gallbladder qi deficiency or a phlegm fire disturbance internally.

- If both the heart and spleen deficiency causes a lot of dreams, accompanying symptoms may be a pale face, palpitations, forgetfulness, loss of appetite, abdominal distention, loose stools, quietness, and tiredness.
- If kidney and heart disharmony causes a lot of dreams, additional symptoms may be irritability and insomnia, irritability and heart palpitations, waist and knee soreness and loss of strength, hot flashes, and night sweats, etc.
- Symptoms accompanying a heart and gallbladder qi deficiency are panic attacks, trances, emotional restlessness, and palpitations.
- Phlegm-generated fire (pyrophlegm) may cause extra phlegm, dizziness, irritability, palpitations, chest distention, and more.
- Ways to expel fire (heat) and phlegm are already mentioned in this chapter. If you forget, please find, read, and highlight this section. You will use it often.

11. If sleep-driving, it's due to accumulated toxins in the liver.
12. If sleep-speaking, it's caused by stress.
13. If sleepwalking or cooking or doing housework during sleep, it's due to mental stress or accumulated toxins in the liver from food additives or drugs or going to bed too late.
14. If waking up sweating during sleep, it's either a yin deficiency or cancer, It cannot be solved as a CHUEH beginner. Ask the client to get Chinese medicine and/or professional medical treatments.
15. Waking up from pain during sleep could be a simple muscle pain, trauma, or caused by surgery. If it is visceral pain, ask the client to get professional medical attention if the pain is severe or is not reduced by the CHUEH adjustment.
16. If waking up is due to a fear of the dark and being afraid to sleep, it's a kidney problem. Please read the Chapter Two—a case was mentioned there.

NOTE: For symptom and organ relationships, please refer to Appendix Four Basic TCM Theory.

Sleeping Adjustments

To adjust a person's insomnia should base on the insomnia symptoms and insomnia causes to make adjustments:

1. For the above items 1 to 11, put one hand to cover Shenting 神庭 (U2, GV 24 or DU 24) and Baihui 百會 (U3, GV 20 or DU 20) and put the other hand on the problem organ's position to adjust for twenty minutes or more. Or, put hands in front and behind the body on the problem organ's position to adjust until you can feel the energy penetrating between the front and back. It is the best adjustment.

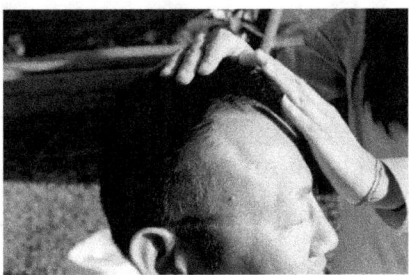

Pic 103 Hands cover covers U1, U2 and U3 in the same time

2. For the item 7 to 14 and 1, 2, 3, 16 items, please refer to the stress caused problems to adjust the organs.

3. Item 7 can focus two eyes on the nose tip or deep breathing until brain clam down or use the thumb and index finger nail to squeeze inside and outside of the pinno of an ear to let brain calm down without thinking too much.

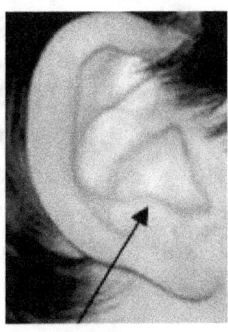

Pic 104 Pinno

It's a quick way to temporarily fix the issue. However, to treat the root problem, should adjust the organ as mentioned above. Until you can feel the energy can freely penetrate through the front and back as well as from the back to the front of the organ.

4. If be waked up from pain during sleep, it can be a simple muscle pain or caused by trauma or surgery, can put one hand at the head Baihui 百會 (U3, GV 20 or DU 20) and put one hand above the painful area with some distance to adjust.

    If it's a visceral pain, you can look for a good acupuncturist's treatments. If it's very sharp and or severe pain that is hardly tolerable, visit an emergency room.

    If it's the surgery pain, at the wound area, do routinely disinfection. Then, drop growth factor fluid or cover by a German poltice of Hirudoid or visit a MD to get a prescribed bandage or use the cheapest of the nature fresh and juicy meat of aloe vera to cover the scar and keep changing it to maintain freshness.

    For the old scar, use acupuncture and high concentrated growth factor with patience to reduce it.

    If there is a new thick and hard scar from injury or surgery, can do moxibustion on the scar to make it becomes thinner, narrower, smaller and softer. You can find an acupuncturist (in the US or a Chinese medicine physician in the other countries.) to use herbs or coat with high concentration growth factor to make it disappear. In case of a decades old scar, an acupuncturist can treat and make the scar be softer, no pain and/or disappear.

    If there is a nerve damage, within eighteen months of the damage, it is the golden time of nerve growth. It's better to grasp this period to get a good acupuncturist's treatment. Either the acupuncture treatments or CHUEH adjustments, all can speed up the nerve growth and along the normal nerve growth direction to grow. If you are unsure that your hands are hot enough and cannot conduct enough cosmic energy to conduct the nerve repairing work, you'd better to refer the patient to visit a medical professional.

If the client has a visceral pain, insomnia, night sweats, plus the painful area has a heat or burning sensation, let the client visit a medical professional immediately without delay.

If a cancer patient has pain and insomnia, a Chinese medicine physician (acupuncturist) will reduce the pain, treat the insomnia and change the cancer patient's internal environment to make it become an environment that does not fit the cancer cells to survive. Meanwhile, boost the cancer patient's immunity to let the body's macrophages to eat up the cancer cells. Please read How Does TCM Help Patients to Avoid Cancer?[193]

5. If your client takes sleeping pills, make sure besides to adjust the sleeping problem, you also need to do liver detoxification. The longer the time taking medication, the longer the time for each adjustment and the whole adjustment period are needed. Meanwhile, the time interval between the two adjustments should be shortened. If it is already for decades, it's better to make adjustments every day. It is also better to invite the client to do adjustment with you. As well as let your client do self-healing by himself as much as possible.

Investment Revenue Exercise

1. Gently close your eyes, take a deep breath for three to five times or until your brain can calm down.

    Imagine how happy you are, after you successfully adjusted yourself and your family members for their pain, stress and sleeping problem(s).

    Meanwhile, during your adjustments in your meditation, you have happily helped yourself and your family members feel the miraculous power of love, gratitude, sharing and collaboration. They also promised you to practice the four universal codes in their daily life.

    Then imagine, eventually, how a happy and harmonized environment that all of you created with your family members together! Remember this cheerful sensation always.

You can always do meditation and visualize this seen with your strong and vivid happy sensation.

2. Put down the names and your adjustment items for each person in your meditation.

3. Compare the item 2 and the table that you filled in the Chapter One Investment Revenue Exercise, cross out the repeated names. The final list are the targets for you to practice your adjustment.

4. For the people who are listed on your table, invite them one by one to make adjustment for them and fill in the Comprehensive Universal Energy Healing Adjustment Record to be your future reference. After accumulating for a while, you also can organize that data and do analyze. You will surprise the universe amazing love and grace as well as notice your progress. Meanwhile, you have more confidence in your learning ability. I will applause for your improvement.

5. Do you think that your adjustments can benefit the other people? If so, we expect that you can share your valuable adjustment experience(s). If you can use the Comprehensive Universal Energy Healing Adjustment Record to post all of the information, it can save a lot cost to do clinical trials. We can collect the data that you submitted to key into the computer to run the result. Therefore, your honest report is very important.

   Besides I give my sincere gratitude to you (can use a writer name to post), if share your adjustments experience, the universe will also accumulate the credit and give you reward someday. On behalf of all beneficiaries, I say: "Thanks!" to you.

6. At every step of medical progress and no matter how small it is, it is the great love heart person unlimited input even sacrificed personal leisure, time and money to generate the essence. That is not easily obtained.

7. Watch How to Make An Emergency Stretcher[185].

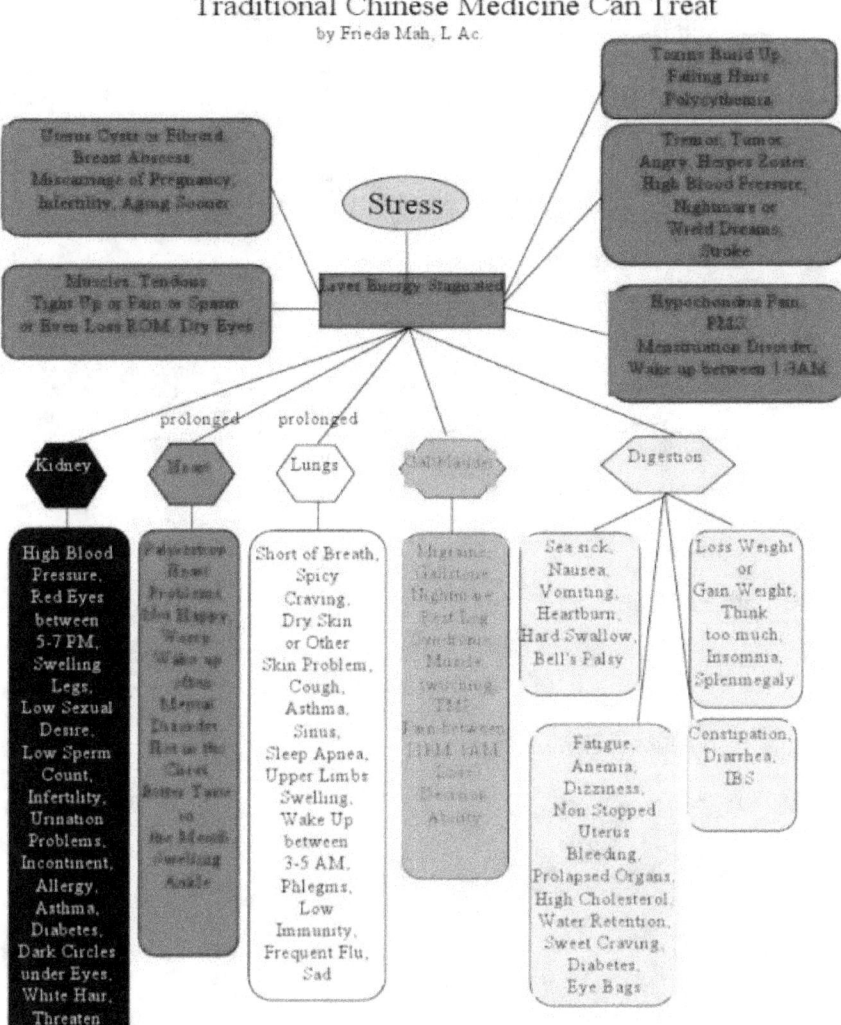

Fig 22 Stress Caused Problems

Back Pain
by Frieda Mah, L.Ac.

Causes	Results	Treatments
Arthritis	Emotional Stress	Bed Resting/Apply Cold
Diet	Pain	Pain Killer
Heavy Metal	Soreness	Muscle Relaxant
Dairy Products	Numbness	Cortisone Injection
Coffee, Soda, Processed foods, refine sugar, drugs	Insomnia	Narcotics Injection
Kidney Deficiency	Excessive Sleep	Stretch Machine
Legs not in Equal Length	Vertebra Bone Displacement	Surgery
Overuse (muscle/tendons tight up)	Vertebra Bone Fusion	Massage
Over Weight	Twisted Spine	Physical Therapy
Poor Posture	Compressed Lumbar Bones	Chiropractic Service
Cross Legs	Discs Degeneration	Tense Units
Not seat evenly	Narrow Disc	Acupuncture (quick & safe)
Not stand evenly	Crushed Disc	Herbs (solve root problems)
Not correct lifting	Sliding Disc	Herbal Bath
Pregnancy	Pinch Nerve (from bone pressed on nerve &/or muscle tapped the nerve)	Cupping
Scoliosis – birth defect		* Any one periodically needs chiropractic services, should have acupuncture treatments in order to balance the muscles pulling force from opposite directions i.e. to loosen the muscles
Sick		
Ankylosing Spondylosis		
Organ's Problems		
Lupus	Scoliosis (acquired)	
Fibromyalgia (It is not a life-long sickness.)	Sick	
	Bone Spur	
Stress	Lost ROM	* Acupuncture can relieve pain for narrow disks, bulging disks and herniated disks without surgery.
Tight Clothes	Numbness on Feet	
Improper Shoes/Bed	Chronic Fatigue	
Weight Lifting	Chronic Constipation	* Acquired scoliosis can be treated by acupuncture and chiropractic without surgery.
Injury		
Herniated Disk		
Outside Pathogens (wind, cold, dampness)		

Examples of Disc Problems

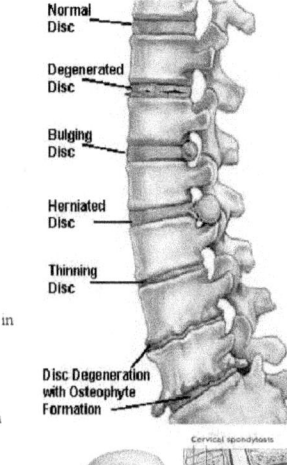

Normal Disc
Degenerated Disc
Bulging Disc
Herniated Disc
Thinning Disc
Disc Degeneration with Osteophyte Formation

Fig 23 Back Pain Problems

NOTES

CHAPTER TWELVE
Conclusion
•••••••••••••

Calm and let go, True Qi (great-self) resides.
Mental activities hold inner advices, illness has
nowhere to stay.

Huang Di Nei Jing • Chapter One Classic Natural Way Theory

Realize Our Healing Power

Since you've read the book, if you practice the Da Zhou Tian[152], until now, you should clearly feel its benefit for you. After practice loving, gratitude, sharing and collaboration, what are the changes in your life and your future life direction? When you need, there are people who have opened their hands to help you, how do you feel?

Please go to this book's website and write down what do you feel and share with the others.

At each chapter's investment return practice, you should fully realize the power of the Comprehensive Universal Energy Healing. When you feel proud of yourself that you are happy about that at any time you can heal yourself or help your family members, loved ones, friends and colleagues. You supposedly already have strong confidence i n y our h ealing a bility. D o y ou f eel s atisfaction a nd gratitude? Don't you?

Maintain Health is the Same Important as Eat Meals

Every day, you practice the Da Zhou Tian[152] or at least put one hand at U3 and the other hand put at U6 (use dorsal side) then put at the heart and the liver position to improve blood circulation and let yourself feel happier or speed up liver detoxification to reduce chances to get mad. Meanwhile, every night, before you sleep, you give gratitude to the person who gave you the most impression today.

This is an important homework that you clean out your emotional garbage and in charge your positive emotions. By doing so, your whole body's blood and qi have good circulation. Meanwhile, you keep good habit to keep your mood always feel happiness and gratitude. Then, you are hardly sick. Moreover, you pad foundation for your success.

To Experience the Magic Power of the Four Universal Codes Again

In Chapter Five, while you were first time to apply loving, gratitude, sharing and collaboration, I believe that the energy under your hands and your client's feedback can confirm the first three codes' magic powers. If you collaborate with the other person(s) to do healing, you should experience that reach the expected result is a lot quicker. Now, let review the magic power of these codes.

Love:

1. Rub your hands thirty times to make them have the same temperature. Put your two hands on your chest or on your upper legs. You can feel that they have the same temperature.
2. Try to blow to your left hand and tell your left palm by holding it nearby you: "I hate you, I hate you! "for three times.
3. Then blow to your right hand and tell your right palm by holding it nearby you: "I love you, I love you! "for three times.
4. Then, put your hands either back to your chest or upper legs, you can feel that your right palm is warmer than your left one. Even you can feel your left one is cold. There is nothing alive does not need love. Even a stone due to love and you put in your hands and play around with it, prolonged, it shines.

Gratitude:

1. For the person that you are always complaining about or dislike in the back of him. Think about any good characters or good deeds that he did. Even think that your complaint and/or bad manner could get into his ears. But he did not revenge to you, you should feel gratitude to this person.

2. Meditation

   After you fall into deeper meditation, you can imagine that you meet the person in step one mentioned, you think of all of his good stuffs and you talk to him to show your friendship and chat with him.

3. Write down both of your feeling and facial expressions.

4. You can share #3 with your closest one or go to online to share with the other readers at Chapter Twelve of this book.

5. When someone showed gratitude to you or said "Thanks" to you, or when you said "Thank You!" to the others, did you feel good? Your mood was excited. Right?

Sharing:

Sincerely to share good stuffs and expect to benefit the group.

1. When you hear A told B that: "Keep the good ones and bring the bad ones out to share with the others." How will you think?

2. When someone always shares good stuff with you, do you think he is a fool?

3. If you meet a stingy person, who only take in without give out, how will you feel about him?

4. If there is someone who only ask your favor but never think about your situation, how will you think?

5. If you share with someone who is worthy to share with, how do you feel?

6. When you are in a group, everyone is sincere to share out good stuff, happiness and sadness, how do you feel? Do you feel intimacy? Do you feel a sense of belonging in this group and would like to do more for the other members?

Collaboration:

Complimentary help each other, unite is the power.

1. In today's high technology era with open information, a person cannot own all talents or energy to handle all sorts of things. Will it be better if there is someone can share work or responsibilities with you?
2. Under the umbrella of collaboration, if there is someone lazy without doing his share, do you think is it right?

Many scientists finally acknowledged God's exist in the universe. Some religious respect He is the true God in order to differentiate with the other gods. He is sharp enough to know every tiny detail and His perspicacious reward is fair and unambiguous. If you see someone who steals, cheats or fraud takes away or robbery to gain illegal money, splurge and enjoy, please do not be blinded by short-term phenomenon, tribulations are waiting for him.

Let us return to our true self, back to nature, open our hands, help self, loved ones and countless the others! Make love, gratitude, sharing and collaboration to fulfill our society.

Build Up Self Confidence

Maybe you had never thought that you can help yourself or others to reduce pain, stress, make a loved one happier, sleep more soundly. Your efforts, not only not being wasted but have gratifying results. You have more confidence in yourself, there is a more self-satisfaction.

After you follow this and our later books (you can go to this book online page to recommend what kind health issues that you want to learn its healing method.) to remove yourself and your family member's discomfort, you might feel no more worries and would like to build up your dream, pursuing for wealth, talent, relationships or change job, or expect traveling during vacation, please visit NHUEH Training Programs[198] to find the appropriate course to register.

In some situations, you should look for professional(s)' help, do not rely solely on our book to do adjustment and delay client's needed treatment. Please re-read Chapter Nine for "time to refer" and How Does TCM (Traditional Chinese Medicine) view diseases?[139].

Conclusion

Use universal energy healing to do self-healing and preventive healthcare as well as practice universal codes can lead us enter into a better world, but also enhance the level of our life!

Please be aware about that the spiral universe is calling you to emerge into the spiral universe to raise up your frequency, expand the beauty inside you to enjoy the universal abundances.

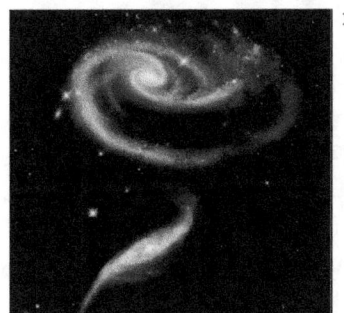 120

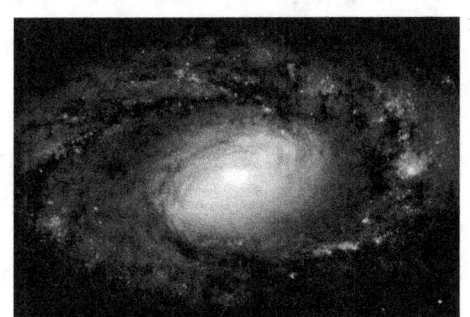 121

Pic 105   spiral universe   Pic 106   spiral universe

Therefore, be bold with love, joy, confidence, gratitude to toward to your divine life without doubt, fear, jealously and malicious competition cries kill, destroy and damage the interests of others to enrich sin illusory wealth.

By following this book series and put into actions, you can reach your dreamed life with healthy and wealthy step by step following book instructions to lead you transform from a self-constrained cocoon into a beautiful butterfly soars in the beautiful universe, enjoying the abundance of life it provides.

The power of reaching your expected dream and life is in YOU!

Investment Return Practice

1. Recall all kind benefits that you gain from this book including your health improvement. Write down on your diary or post at readers discussion[137].

2. Recall in the beginning, you did not know universal energy healing, until today, how many people got healed or improved from your service? What kind health issues have you ever helped? Please list them and write down how you feel. Give yourself a smile and post your achievement at reader's discussion[137].

3. Do you want to learn how to heal the other specific health issue(s)? Please go to new book content recommendation[166] to write down your suggestions. Thanks.

4. If you are a current medical staff, this book should touch your heart. If you would like to involve in health care reform, or to join or provide your feedback, please go to this book's website readers discussion[137] to express your great self-feeling. May our sacred mission to rescue the patient can be more satisfying. Thank you for your dedication input into the medical industry and precious sharing.

5. Please go to the book's website readers discussion[137] and to share what you gain from the Comprehensive Universal Energy Healing, self-healing and your experience to heal the others. Thank you!

Best Wishes for Your Health and Happiness!

APPENDIX ONE
Author's Medical Path
• •

I am a California licensed acupuncturist, NGH certified hypnotherapist, and global instructor. I am also an energy healer, Life Mastery Institute certified Dream Builder Coach, and Life Mastery Consultant.

The California licensed acupuncturist is equivalent to Taiwan and China's Chinese Medicine physician.

My Prior Experience

I have a bachelor's degree in industrial engineering from Chung Yang Christian Science and Engineering College (now Chung Yuan Christian University) in Chung Li, Taiwan. After graduation, I worked at a variety of electronics and watch USA factories in Taiwan in many different roles—industrial engineer, production engineer, system engineer, senior industrial engineer, and education and training supervisor. Their sizes were between three thousand to ten thousand employees.

Because of my unique thinking and observation, I often received assignments in solving the corporations' tough cases. My experience taught me to pay attention to innovation, cost reduction, quality and efficiency improvement.

Attached to the Chinese Medicine

In the beginning of 1993, at just over forty, an event caused me to become extremely disappointed, and the disappointment quickly evolved into an extraordinary anger. It severely disturbed my qi and blood circulation and transformed me from my usual energized self into a woman lacking in vitality. I had irregular menstruation, night sweats, hot flashes, half body numbness, and severe fatigue. Even with an overnight's sleep, I could not seem to generate more than fifteen minutes of energy. I couldn't barely do housework for more than five minutes. And when I did, I had to rest for two to three hours afterward. At that time, my kids were still young. I was hardly able to handle my life.

Because I had no healthcare insurance coverage, Western medical tests were not affordable. The only option I had was to visit an acupuncturist. I only visited a couple of times because the clinic was far away. Because the cost was high, I couldn't keep up with the treatments. Luckily for me, though, there were some Chinese book publishers holding a book show at Monterey Park around that time, and I found many inexpensive Chinese medicine books. I was thrilled and thought that I would buy the books and the herbs they recommended to treat myself.

In 1993, herbs were very inexpensive. The majority of them were no more than three dollars per pound. Within three months of self-treatments, not only had all of my symptoms of menopause, chronic fatigue, and body numbness disappeared, but my energy was approaching the level of my twenty-year-old self that only needed three to four hours of sleep a day to support a whole day of activities.

After recovery, I calculated that the cost for books and herbs was cheaper than any single Western test that an MD could have ordered for me. This experience excited me. My intuition told me that if Chinese medicine had such powerful treatment effectiveness and low cost, it was worth spreading the word. Immediately, I got the idea to go to school to learn Chinese medicine. So I found a weekend Chinese medicine school and planned to register.

But when I discussed my idea with an older friend who was born in a family with generations of Traditional Chinese Medicine (TCM) physicians, she stopped me from registering. She told me that in TCM, pulse diagnosis is very important. One should learn it at a young age while finger sensitivity is high. She led me to thinking about the importance of pulse diagnosis. I didn't want to mistreat my patients.

Though I gave up the idea of going to school to learn Chinese medicine, I continued to treat my own as well as my kids' health problems, and that included the asthma of my eleven-year-old, nocturne, headache due to neck pain from jumping and diving, flu, and abdominal pain. I started to use myself as a kind of lab rat. When I got a flu or cough, I would not treat myself immediately but would wait until my illness got severe enough to verify its prognosis with the Chinese medicine books. I continually challenged myself to see if I could treat more complicated situations and regain my health.

When I heard that a friend or relative was sick, I would run to the book store to buy a couple of related Chinese medicine books to study. I'd choose the pages that suited the illness best and mail copies to the sick person for reference.

Family Accident

In May or June, of 1998, my husband had a stroke. It was very surprising even considering his high work stress.

My husband's work compensation case only allowed reimbursement for Western medicine treatments. But for a stroke patient's hemiplegia, acupuncture is the most effective treatment. Because I had no stroke treatment experience, I used my own pocket money to hire an acupuncturist to treat my husband.

Because my husband's income was discontinued and insurance did not cover acupuncture treatments, medical cost after his stroke was a huge expense. The disability compensation was not even enough to cover our mortgage payment. After my husband recovered from hemiplegia, only Western medicine treatments were maintained. After six months of recuperation, my husband found a job with less pressure—and less income.

After this event, I studied numerous Western medicine books on stroke and stroke patients. I learned that stroke patients have no full recovery. Patients will continue to have strokes—whether insignificant or debilitating—until their lives end.

A Restart in Life

I realized that my husband could have strokes forever, and there may be a time when he would not be able to earn an income for our family. So in order plan for a time in the future when we would need money for our children's education, I decided I ought to have an income in place so that I could take over the economic burden if a tragedy hit our family again. However, in the greater Los Angeles area and Orange County, there were no factories' working environments compatible with my previously worked companies.

After much deliberation, I thought that since I had a strong logical thinking ability, it would be good to learn computer science because of the high job market demand. Even though I had no idea how to even use a mouse, I registered for computer classes at a community college. I earned my AA degree and planned to continue on to a master's degree and then find a job in preparation for my family's impending financial disaster.

Attracted to TCM Again

Just two semesters before my graduation from the community college, three weird events happened in three of my classes.

THE FIRST WEIRD EVENT: The computer graded my Scantron test sheet incorrectly, causing a shortage of fifty points in my computer class.

THE SECOND WEIRD EVENT: The IT Department Head was a very cautious person. He stopped us no fewer than five times during his class midterm to make sure every student had saved their answers to a floppy disk. I followed instructions each time, however, my floppy disk was totally blank!

THE THIRD WEIRD EVENT: The logic of my program for an HTML class assignment was perfectly correct. But I could not run out the expected answer. Both of my neighboring classmates and the instructor helped me to check my program and even helped me by retyping my program line by line on their own computers.

Still no answer. Eventually, the instructor allowed me to give him a blank floppy disk on which he copied and pasted his answer. The strange thing was that he tried five or six disks from the newly purchased pack of floppy disks, and not a single one of them could run out anything with the answer key on them!

All of these made me do some serious thinking. Before graduating with my master's degree in computer science, I would undoubtedly have to take out a student loan to finish my classes. After graduation, it was possible I'd find a job as a programming leader. Maybe the day before an important assignment was due, I would have everything on the computer, set and ready to go. But what would happen if—on the next day, in front of executives or a client—I turned on the computer and nothing worked? I would surely lose my job as a result. And then how would I feed my family? How would I repay my student loan?

While I was sinking into a deep feeling helplessness, I saw a new student recruiting booth from College of Acupuncture and Oriental Medicine of SCUHS (Southern California University of Health Sciences in Whittier, California). I gathered all of my courage—and borrowed some from the superpower—I approached the booth.

I said, "I am over fifty now. Is it still possible for me to learn Chinese Medicine? Will I still be able to do pulse diagnosis?" I received positive answers to my questions, and I thought to myself, why not give a try? So I changed all of my last semester's classes in the community college to prerequisite classes for SCUHS. It had been ten years since the moment when I first had the idea to learn Chinese medicine.

A thought came to my mind: *"It might be my mission to learn Chinese Medicine!"*

Suffering another Misfortune

Just when I felt fortunate and grateful that the first trimester had almost finished, my husband became permanently disabled.

Thereafter, I began to get student loans, and I did work study until graduation.

A Small Episode during School

One day in the fourth trimester's diagnosis class, we had a pulse diagnosis class. The instructor asked us to practice pulse diagnosis with the person in the neighboring seat.

When the instructor finished her instruction, I grasped my classmate's left hand to do a diagnosis. I thought to myself, *my goodness, I can't feel her pulse at all. My older friend was right after all. It's too late for me to learn Chinese Medicine.* I was feeling so upset about not listening to her advice, and my mind started running. *Now what can I do to earn a living? How am I going to repay my student loans? How can I feed my kids?* I cried out audibly and painfully. The instructor walked to my seat to ask what was wrong. I replied, "I can't feel her pulse."

My classmate began to laugh hysterically. She told me, "You'd have to be a magician to feel my left side pulse!" Then she told us she was a nurse. One day, she was escorting a two hundred pound patient through the garden, and the patient suddenly passed out. She was afraid that if he fell and hit the corner of a brick wall in the garden, his head would be injured. So, she used her left arm to hold him. As a result, some blood vessels and muscles in that arm were torn. Therefore, the pulse in her left side could not be felt.

The instructor had me take her right hand and give her my diagnosis. After the instructor double-checked the pulse, she told me I had done a good job. Next was the tongue diagnosis practice. The instructor double-checked my tongue diagnosis, and I had done well there, too. She told me I had been able to discover many detailed signs.

I Have My Acupuncturist License... Now What?

I started looking for a job. At that time, none of the job search sites like Monster, Indeed, Career Builder, and Salary had listings for acupuncturist jobs. I grasped the opportunity to promote Traditional Chinese Medicine and sent online suggestions to all of them to let them know the benefits of Chinese medicine. I told them it would be a high-demand job in the near future and recommended that they begin posting acupuncturist positions as soon as possible.

It was common practice for newly licensed acupuncturists to start in acupuncture clinics, spas, or chiropractic clinics pulling the needles out of patients' bodies, taking patient histories, doing tui-na (like massage but using more techniques), working at a front desk, or just being an intern. But I still couldn't get an offer even for this kind of job

So I went to school to ask advice from a clinical supervisor. He looked at me for quite a long time and then said, "At your age, employers may think that you already have decades of acupuncture experience. But you're just graduating. If they look at your resume first, potential employers may think that you're a young girl. But when they see you face by face, they see that you're old." Ah, that reply left me speechless.

By this point, I had honed my destiny for a couple of decades. How could I accept what the supervisor told me and give up looking for the job I dreamed of? Especially when my children had needs?

And then a thought came to my mind. I was born to do something meaningful with my life. There was a path God had prepared for me. If here wasn't the place I would find a better place!

With great hope and faith, I woke up at five every morning, prepared meals for the kids and let the older ones take care of their younger brothers. I searched Google every day for the entire day until near midnight. From the first page until the last page, I clicked every possible job that jumped out until I reached the very last one. Why?

Could I be an intern? Should I be blamed for everything by a picky employer according to his daily mood and whims? At my age, how could I put up with that treatment?

Should I remove needles from patients? How could I do that all day to earn only a tiny income not even enough to feed my kids?

Could I do tui-na service for patients? No way! At only halfway through the day, I would already be exhausted and would surely be fired.

Should I be willing to work at a front desk? My stilted English would probably lose my employer potential patients.

We need to know who we are and what we are capable of doing.

After two weeks of dedicated searching, I found an acupuncturist job at sea. I emailed my application, and almost within an hour, I got a phone call and passed the first interview. The second day, I passed my second interview. Later, I passed the training and accepted my assignment to work on a cruise ship! I carried out my dream to travel around the world and treat patients in need.

The Acupuncturist's Life at Sea

My life was filled with happiness after I got my license. Besides providing me with beautiful scenery all around the world, the broad sea helped me realize that we—and our lives—are such a small piece of the universe in which we live. There is nothing and no one in our lives that cannot be forgiven. Colleagues came to the ship from all over the world, and we had a good time working together.

The best thing about the patients on the ship is that most had a high level of education. They would ask, "What caused me to get sick? How can I avoid it?" Then they would follow my instructions. Sometimes the ship's restaurant manager would ask me, "Frieda, did you tell your patients to keep away from ice water and cold drinks? When we hear guests refusing to have ice in their drinks, we know they're your patients."

The patients' curious questions helped me to understand the theories of Chinese medicine more thoroughly, and this laid a strong foundation for my treatment skills. It stimulated my independent thinking ability. That's the biggest deficit in the training given in regular medical schools. The challenge of my patients' questions increased my knowledge, and for that I give to those patients my greatest gratitude and forever put them in my memory even though I cannot match their names and faces.

What touched me the most was when patients said, "Frieda, your treatment skills are so good. You sure work hard!" Another thing for which I am grateful is that many patients wrote testimonials so that they could share their treatment experience with others. That is tremendously powerful in spreading word of the benefits of Chinese medicine. And it helped my business.

One night at midnight, we were still in the spa for a last meeting of the cruise. One of my patients came in and whispered to our spa manager. I was called out to speak to the patient. She said, "After I put my kids in bed, I wrote this for you. Sorry that I interrupted your meeting." She handed to me a card filled with words that recorded most of the benefits she received from her nine treatments with me.

Every time I returned to the ship after my vacation, I was excited. I felt like I was going home. I hoped to stay on a cruise ship for the rest of my life.

For the cases and medical discoveries, please read Appendix Six Author's Cases Sharing and Medical Discoveries.

The Turning Point in Life and Healing Arts

On April 9, 2010, just before the ship that I worked on changed its itinerary to Europe, my boss forwarded a family emergency email to me, and I had to sign off immediately.

In summer of that same year, from July to September, I went to Merritt Island, Florida to accept Professor Ni, Hai-Sha's clinical training for severe and tough cases. This training tremendously raised my knowledge levels of medical theories, diagnosis, and treatment skills. It made me feel that no matter what kind diseases that I faced, I would have no more fear, and I would know how to treat without any doubt. This training will be forever memorable.

Later, I learned Longevitology. I combined it with the universe codes to do healing and gained amazing results. I also discovered that everyone was born with self-healing powers, and you do not have to rely on someone to open acupuncture points. I developed a number of ways to improve results and came up with Comprehensive Universal Energy Healing.

On another occasion, I earned my NGH hypnotherapist and instructor certificates. I used my hypnotherapy skills in my clinical treatments. When combining all methods, I can get three or four times more effective results. Adding hypnotherapy also solves the problem of the patient not following instructions to control diet, exercises, and change his lifestyle.

I also earned Dream Builder coach and Life Mastery consultant certificates from Ms. Mary Morrissey of the Life Mastery Institute. She teaches a proven formula by which you can create your ideal dream life if your desire is strong enough.

Since stepping into the world of Chinese medicine more than twenty years ago, I have learned that life, honor, and dignity are priceless. This is what I want to bring into the world as a gift to you. It is my life destiny. Health is a stepping stone. My desire is to integrate many different fields of medicines in order to create a healthy and happy global village. Because everyone has the right to be healthy.

My Future Goals

1. Integrate varying medical fields to develop better treatment results.

2. Develop a brand new concept of medical school based on prevention of illness and self-healing. Emphasize moral cultivation to guide people in avoiding disaster. Eventually, I would like to unleash people's great self to help each person to accomplish his life mission.

3. Invest in R & D to discover treatment methods for tough cases that have no side effects.

4. Educate people about the relationship between a person's energy frequency and sickness or health, severity of the disease, recovery speed and between his practical ability of self-actualization and completion of his life mission. I hope to continue writing my book series in order to teach Comprehensive Universal Energy Healing and universal codes to help self-cultivation, meditation, self-hypnosis, dream building, and to inspire even more awareness of the fate and destiny to fulfill one's mission in life.

APPENDIX TWO
Glossary
•••••••••••

The Chinese letter is following the English word(s) as a reference. With the trend of China's economic development, learning some Chinese is becoming a fad. As I discovered from the crews and guests on the ship, a lot people have tattoos of Chinese letter(s) on their bodies but don't know the letter's meaning. At least this book will give you pride in the meaning.

Some words or names might be repeated twice because the standard name and the commonly used name are different.

BIAO 表 means the superficial level of the body. It generally includes skin and body hair and the blood vessels that are nearby. It is also a relative location with the internal region of the body.

COLD 寒 means colder than normal and a temperature which is lower than the body's comfortable and normal functioning temperature.

COMPREHENSIVE UNIVERSAL ENERGY HEALING (CHUEH) uses the universe's positive energy to treat and prevent diseases. The cosmic energy contains radiated lights, electromagnetic waves, and many other kinds of waves and heat energy. There are some persons who feel it as a current flowing into their body. It has penetrating and distance transmission functions. But for the materials with condensed structure, its penetrating power is weak. The broad universal energy healing also includes promotion of virtue cultivation and spiritual lifting to link with everyone's great self and eventually finish the life mission if one's life and personal choice allow one to do so.

CONCEPTION (REN) MERIDIAN 任脉 runs from the lower abdomen of the uterus in the female and the seminal vesicle in the male to the Huiyin (between the lower two orifices). It goes up past the body hair and through the center of the abdomen to the Guanyuan (3 cun directly below the umbilicus), up to the throat, and then up the cheek along the face to the eyes. It travels the center of the front body.

Cun 寸 Cun is a unit of measurement in Chinese medicine. The below charts explain the measurement of the cun. It's a smart and easy way to measure everyone without mistake. From the pictures, you learn the wisdom of the ancient Chinese—it's surprising that everyone is born equal in this respect! Everyone has the same height of 75 cun, according to each one's natural constitution. You can learn more from the pictures below.

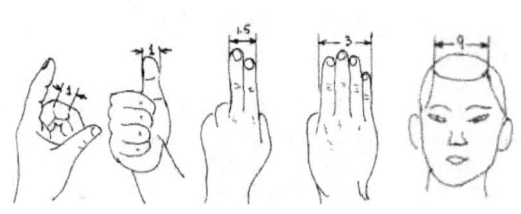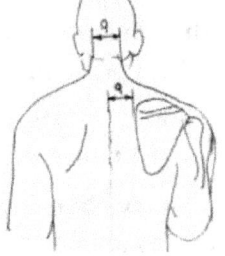

Fig 26 Cun Measurement

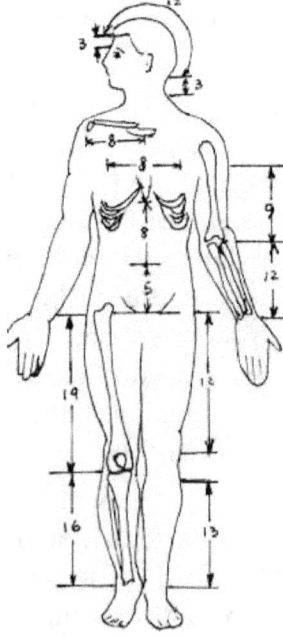

Fig 27 Body Part cun measurement

DEFICIENCY虚 means less than normal.

FENG SHUI風水is the concept of studying a place's environment and geographical characteristics to determine their impact on the health and life of a person.

A place's Feng Shui is its geographic environment and includes the form, quality, content of wind/space, water and ground/soil, as well as gathering the essence of the universe qi (both of energy and materials).

It was originally used to find a good place to bury a dead person but has gradually been applied to finding a living person's residence or business facility.

Many people believe being buried in a specific spot can affect later generations' fortunes in many ways—personality, wealth, happiness, ease of life, career, and social rank. However, a lot people dismiss it as superstition.

DU MERIDIAN督脈or the Governor Vessel as named by WHO (World Health Organization). It starts from the lower abdomen. It goes downward and exits at the Huiyin (It locates between the two lower orifices, is the meeting point for all of the yin qi). Later, it enters into the spine and travels upward to the neck. From the Fengfu, it enters the brain and travels to the top of the head. Then it goes downward from the forehead, along the bridge of the nose, and passes through Renzhong. It enters the mouth and stops at the middle point of the upper gums of the Yinjiao.

EXCESS實 **SHI** means more than normal.

GREAT SELF大我is relative to the small self (the self). In the spiritual field, the great self is the super self. It has super power and always protects the small self in the real world.

It also guides the small self to walk in the right way. Only when the small self is very calm can it hear the great self's reminding (a small voice inside). The great self can also direct our body to do self-repair. Our great self very clearly knows our inherent talents and our life mission—even we do not know.

Each person's great self also has the ability to help him accomplish his life mission or achieve his dreams.

Only when one lifts his frequency to a certain level can he communicate with his great self directly. Everyone's great self is from the same source, and all exist in harmony.

GU WEN GUAN ZI《古文觀止》was Wu, Chu-Cai and Wu, Tiao-Hou—uncle and nephew—collected and noted the book contents from Zhou to Ming Dynasties' classic literature articles to be used as their family's teaching material. It was done in the year of 1965 in Qing Dynasty. After its publication, it became a classic piece of literature and a popular teaching material in schools.108

HAN, YU 韓愈 was a famous poet in China's Tang dynasty.

HEART COUGHING 心咳[106] is a cough caused by heart problems. According to the *Huang Di Nei Jing • Su wen·Chapter Thirty-Eight—The Cough Theory*《黃帝內經•素問.咳論第三十八》: "The symptoms of a heart coughing, when coughing, the heart feels hurt, the throat feels something blocking in the throat, if even worse, can feel throat swollen and painful." Causes and SymptomsReview for All Diseases·Volume Fourteen- #1 Coughing Symptoms 《諸病源候論.卷之十四咳嗽病諸候一、咳嗽候》: "Cough and spitting blood that induces the Heart Meridian pulsing sensation…"

HOT 熱 means a higher temperature than the body is comfortable with and a higher than normal operating temperature.

LI 裡 means internal. It's relative to the superficial表. It refers to the deep tissues. Generally refers to the internal organs. TCM (Traditional Chinese medicine) used to use superficial or internal (Biao or Li表裡) to identify how deep the external pathogen had invaded the body. If it is more internal, it means the sickness is more severe.

MERIDIAN is our body's internal channel for qi circulation.

MOXIBUSTION[110] 灸 (Or called moxa that can be used as a noun or verb.) Uses Folium Artemisiae Argyi (also called mugwort leaf or Argy Wormwood Leaf) with or without other herbs to form a stick. The stick can be smoking or nonsmoking. The smoking one has better effectiveness. The stick can be burned for health maintenance, prolong life and avoid sickness, and to treat diseases when acupuncture alone failed. *Huang Di Nei Jing • Ling Shu • Guan*

Neng: "When acupuncture treatment does not work, it is pertinent to use moxibustion to treat."

Huang Di Neo Jing • Ling Shu • Chapter 73 Guan Neng 《黃帝內經 • 靈樞 • 官能第七十三》: "When acupuncture cannot treat, moxibustion is proper to treat…"

Bian Qie Xin Fa 《扁鵲心法》 [109] stated: "Even if people are healthy, often moxa Guanyuan (CV 4 or Ren 4), Qihai (CV 6 or Ren 6), Mingmen (L2), Zhongwan (CV 12 or Ren 12), although not giving longevity, can carry on life that lasts more than a hundred years…" In Chinese history, there were people who lived to be more than 200 years old[105].

If *Bian Qie Xin Fa* 《扁鵲心法》 can be translated, a lot of tough cases can become treatable. However, for those diseases, it takes long time to do moxa. Adding our external herbs can greatly shorten the moxa time.

If adding our external use herbal formula (refer to Appendix Eight for its applications), the treatment time saved and the effectiveness can be increased by two to six times. It can also treat severe cases such as patients with lost appetite or on kidney dialysis. For a detailed treatment method, please wait for our book for physicians or our clinical report.

I am used to moxa with our unique external herbal formula and acupuncture to treat tumors (all kinds), deficient organ functions, severe pain, qi stagnation, and blood stasis. It can shrink tumors and even make them disappear, boost organ function, raise immunity, activate blood and qi circulation, and warm up the body, all of which make the body healthier and form an internal environment in which the pathogenic bacteria, virus, tumor, and cancer cells cannot survive.

It also can turn white hair back to black, make dark circles around the eyes disappear, eliminate wrinkles, and rejuvenate the patient's body, both in function and outlook.

QI 氣 is comprised of two parts. The energy part lets the body function well, and the material part supports body activities, including growth (nutrients), defense (immunity cells, fluids), regulation (hormones, neurotransmitters), and moistening (fluids).

For the functions of the qi, please read the Basic Traditional Chinese Medicine Theory in Appendix Four.

Qi Bo 岐伯 had excellent Chinese medicine knowledge and skills. He was the subordinate of the Yellow Emperor. He had a lot conversations with the Yellow Emperor 黃帝 in the *Huang Di Nei Jing* and *Huang Di Wai Jing*.

Ren Meridian 任脈 is standardized by WHO (World Health Organization) as the Conception Vessel. It starts from the lower abdomen of the uterus for female and the seminal vesicle for male and moves down to the Huiyin (between the lower two orifices). Going up, it passes the body hair, goes through the center of the abdomen, up to the Guanyuan (3 cun directly below the umbilicus), up to the throat, and up the cheek along the face to the eyes. It travels the center of the front body.

Rong 榮 refers to the ying qi. It is the qi that contains nutrients. It is a relative to the wei qi and belongs to yin.

Shen 神 is the overall expression of one's health, alertness, conscience, intelligence, spirit, soul, and divine essence.

Superficial 表 Biao means skin and body hair—the superficial organisms that cover the body. It is also a relative concept versus the internal (Li 裡) without specific location.

Upper Jiao 上焦 refers to the body from the diaphragm to the throat—the heart, pericardium, lungs and all spaces between organs. It controls the respiratory and circulatory systems.

Wei Qi 衛(氣) is the defensive qi. It is an invisible shield outside the body that protects us from external pathogens invading our body. The defensive qi shields us from the wind, coldness, summer heat, dampness, dryness, and fire pathogens. Inside our body, the wei qi fights invading bacteria and viruses. The stronger the wei qi, the thicker the invisible shield and the stronger the immunity.

Doing meditation, practicing qi gong, or doing exercise can all strengthen the wei qi and increase its thickness.

Bad temperatures, stress, unhealthy body and mind settings, tightened muscles, not being able to close the pores of the skin (lung qi deficiency), or a deficiency in an organ's qi can harm the wei qi. Wei qi relative to the rong qi or ying qi belongs to yang.

Wei Shu 緯書[123] Wei 緯 is the Latitude. Shu 書 is the book. Wei Shu was completed mostly in the Han Dynasty and derived from interpretation of Confucian philosophy. There are three major fields included in the wei shu: philosophy, ancient scientific knowledge, and theological knowledge. The ancient scientific knowledge includes astronomy, the calendar, and weather. The wei shu is used mainly to interpret the seven Confucian classic books of Shi (Poetry) 「詩」— Shu 「書」,Yi (Easy) 「易」,Li (Ceremony) 「禮」,Yue (Music) 「樂」,Chuan Qiu (Spring and Fall—A war period in the Chinese history), 「春秋」 and Xiao Jing (Book of Filial Piety) 「孝經」.

Wen, Tian Xian 文天祥 is a late Song Dynasty poet (1236-1283). After he served in the military, his poems became very powerful and expressed his unyielding heroism[107].

Xia Jiao 下焦 **or Lower Triple Burner or Lower Jiao** is the area under the umbilicus. It includes the kidneys, urinary bladder, large intestine and small intestine, uterus, reproductive organs, and the space between the organs. It controls the excretory and reproductive systems.

Xiang Tian Yi 先天易 was the earliest tool to predict things happening in the universe and/or daily life.

Yang 陽 represents the male, light, brightness, heat, warmth, quickness, positivity, and function,

Yang Qi 陽氣 is the rightness qi. Without yang qi, there is no life. Yang qi has five functions. Please refer to Basic Traditional Chinese Medicine Theory in Appendix Four.

Yang Zai 陽宅 is part of feng shui, but it is specific to living persons. Please also refer to feng shui above.

Yin 陰 represents the female, darkness, slowness, coldness, negativity, and material.

Zhen Qi 真气 is the basic qi that maintains our daily activities. It is composed of the qi inherited from our parents and the qi we gain after birth.

Zheng Qi Ge 《正氣歌》 Its author was Wen, Tian Xiang 文天祥, born in Nan Song Dynasty. He wrote the poem when he was in his enemy Yuan Dynasty's jail. He never surrendered to the Yuan Dynasty and was killed by Yuan Shi Zu 元世祖—Hu Bi Lue 忽必略—the first emperor of the Yuan Dynasty.

Zou Li 腠理 refers to the space between the skin and muscles, among skin cells, and among muscle fibers. These are the channels for the wei qi, body fluids, and primary qi to flow. If the zou li is condensed with small spaces, then it is difficult for the pathogens to invade into the body, and the person will not likely get sick.

Zhu You Shu 祝由術 was one of the thirteen formal medical departments set up by the Huang Di (Yellow Emperor). Zhu You Shu is similar to today's hypnosis, but the therapist can use symbols to control the patient and prescribe herbs for treatment.

APPENDIX THREE

Testimonials

Cold and Flu

A fifty-year-old female client had the flu for a week. She had a productive cough and a runny nose:

I was coughing and had a runny noise. Frieda told me to put my hands over my middle body, and she put her hands over my chest and head. All of my symptoms were gone in about five minutes for my runny nose and less than five minutes for my cough.

By Zelena Coatagena in CA, USA on January 8, 2014

Note: After she stopped coughing, Zelena walked around because the qi was stuck in her throat. She coughed again, and I adjusted her throat for one minute more. She was no longer coughing.

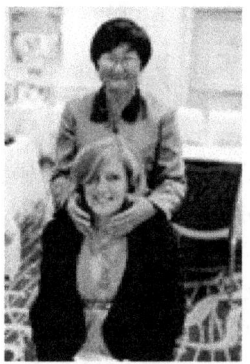

Pic 107 Adjust sore throat

Lisa had the flu and a sore throat. It was gone in a short time after my adjustment.

Shoulder Pain

I'd had periodic right shoulder pain for twenty years. When these episodes occurred, the pain level could reach as high as ten out of ten on a pain scale. The pain started after a childhood martial arts accident when I was eighteen.

When I showed Frieda where my painful area was, she asked me if it had been caused by a forceful hit. I confirmed that. I teach Arnis/FMA. She also noticed I had a thick nodule that was two inches in diameter.

Frieda put her hands on the top of my head and on my painful area. She also asked me to put my right hand on my left shoulder in order to reduce the pain quicker. My hand was colder than hers at the start, but pretty soon, my right hand had the same temperature as hers.

It took around forty or fifty minutes for my pain and the nodule to go away. Only a mild discomfort remained.

Frieda tested my hands for some heat. She told me to put my left hand on my torso where the heat was building up and wave off the pain. I felt totally fine the next day.

During the forty to fifty minutes, Frieda moved her hand from my head to the back of my shoulder to expel the coldness within the injured area. She also moved both hands away and then close to my painful right shoulder to help break the cold energy there. I did feel the energy. She also put hands on my neck, spine, liver, spleen, and heart areas to expel the coldness from my lungs. When she had me move my right hand to the area in front of my liver, I felt my emotions become lighter and happier.

During the process, Frieda demonstrated that the healing process can be made quicker by experiencing and channeling the powers of love, gratitude, and sharing.

This collaboration was an eye opener for me. I could feel the power increase with each experience of great loving feeling. It sped up the treatment.

I never thought that universal healing energy could be this powerful. I should have looked for this kind of help sooner.

By Ramses Sison in CA, USA on April 1, 2014

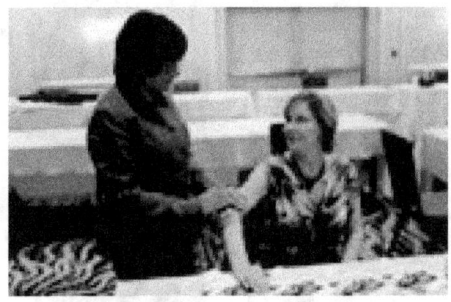

Pic 108 Adjust elbow pain

Kelly had elbow pain, and her pain was relieved after a five-minute adjustment.

Tiredness

- When I was tired, Frieda gave me energy by putting her hand on my head for about five minutes. I felt my head get warmer, and I started to wake up. I also had more energy throughout the day.

  By Hae-Song Hong in California, USA on April 4, 2014

- I was feeling very tired, and within two to three minutes of getting universal energy, I felt a lot of energy.

  By Zelena Coatagena

  CA, USA, on Jan 8, 2014

Pop-Up Veins

Pop-up veins can be effectively treated by universal energy healing. From the two cases posted, you can obviously that using cosmic energy only to do healing, as in Case 2, is a lot slower than using CHUEH with combined cosmic energy and TCM (traditional Chinese Medicine) knowledge, as in Case 1.

Case 1: Treated with CHUEH using cosmic energy plus TCM knowledge.

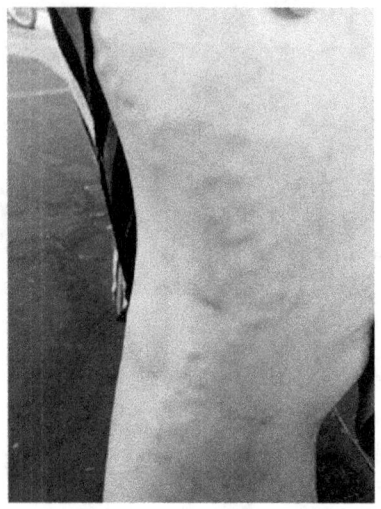

Pic 109 Before adjustment

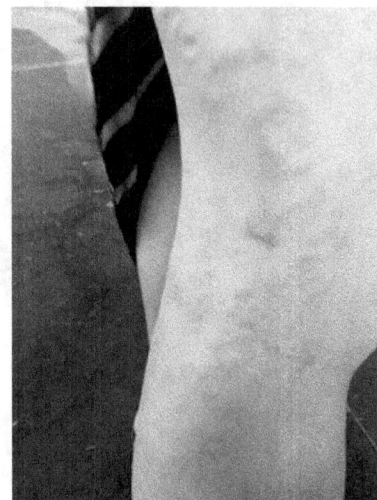

Pic 110 After 10 minutes of adjustment

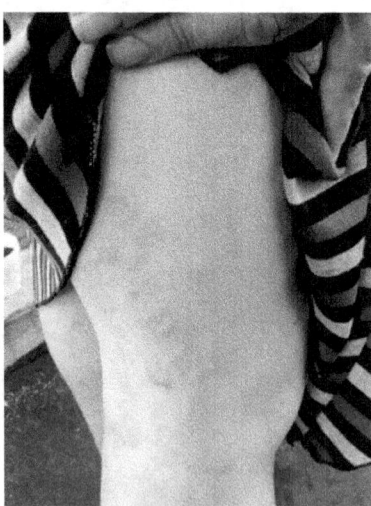

Pic 111 After additional 20 minute adjustment

The veins on the leg almost disappeared after the pain was gone. It's about two months on the leg.

Case 2: Treated by cosmic energy without any TCM knowledge.

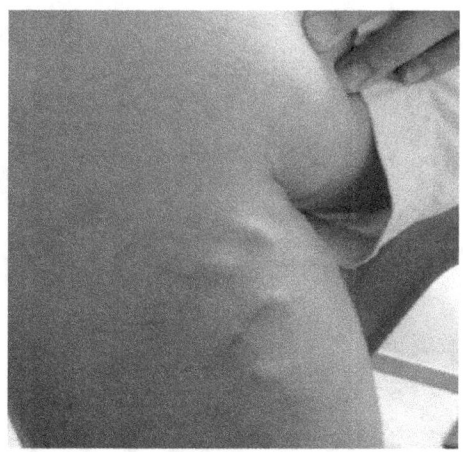 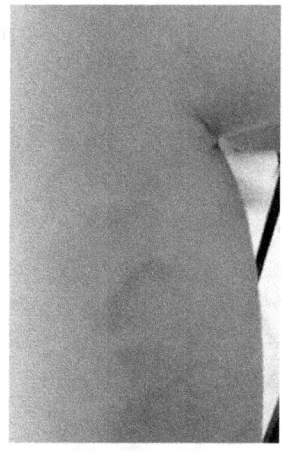

Pic 112 Before adjustment   Pic 113 After 1 hour and
                                   10 minutes adjustment

APPENDIX FOUR

Basic TCM Theory
•••••••••••••••••••••••••••

What is the Traditional Chinese Medicine (TCM)?

It is the humanity of medical science. It is rightness triumphing over evil!

Any natural way to prolong life is in the scope of TCM. It includes sickness prevention, health maintenance, disease treatments, and life nourishing.

- **SICKNESS PREVENTION:** Any approaches that prevent people from getting sick, including *food therapy, food tonifying, herbal tea, herbal foods, herbal bath, herbs, qi gong, exercises, moral cultivation*, massage, acupuncture, moxibustion*, tui-na, cupping*, hypnosis, and Comprehensive Universal Energy Healing and other kinds of energy healing.

  *   In Taiwan and China, people can do moxibustion and cupping by themselves without a professional treatment because they know Chinese folk medicine.

Sickness prevention is the cheapest medical intervention. As a car or a house must be maintained in order to avoid costly repairs, so with the body. Our body is the most valuable asset we have. Disease prevention is far more important and valuable than the maintenance for a car or a house.

The above listed includes both professional services and do it yourself (DIY) items. The DIY items are easy to practice and are designated with italics. Underlined items are things can do by yourself or seek professional service for.

You may not understand how to categorize exercises. Please read Chinese Exercises vs. Western Exercises[173] or The Differences between Chinese Exercises and Western Exercises chart[174].

Walking and jogging are the two most recommended exercises. However, it's also important for you to read Raise Your Legs 90 Degrees Up Against the Wall[175].

It is also valuable for you to read Cracking Sounds from Your Knee(s)[176] to avoid a Meniscus Tear[177] and an operation for certain delayed treatment cases. After you gain universal energy healing power on your hands, you can put your hands around your knees to relieve your discomfort and avoid them getting worse.

- **HEALTH MAINTENANCE:** In addition to disease prevention, early care for the sick is necessary to avoid a mild illness progressing into a severe illness.

- **DISEASE TREATMENT:** This includes sickness prevention and health maintenance methods. Disease treatment involves increased knowledge and skills. It is more challenging and involves more money and time to get better than does sickness prevention.

- **LIFE NOURISHING:** Life nourishing happens through a variety of methods which prolong life, enhance physical constitution, and prevent diseases in order to achieve good health and longevity.

Please refer to the TCM Health Concept Chart[178].

What is Qi

The universe is filled with enough qi to nourish all lives. Any living organism that loses the vital qi is dead. Period!

Qi contains energy and tiny material particles. The energy maintains a life's vitality. The material part is what provides the needed nutrients, fluids, neurotransmitters, hormones, and metabolic waste. We usually call the energy the yang part of the qi and the material part the yin part of the qi.

Because the material and energy are mutually exchangeable, the constant flowing of qi is one of the basic processes in the human body. It maintains life-sustaining activities and gives the energy to survive and maintain the body's functions. Qi is constantly flowing into the body and out to the universe. *Wei Qi* prevents toxic qi from entering our bodies.

The Varieties of Qi

There are more than sixty kinds of qi mentioned in Chinese medicine and literature books:

Primary qi元氣, true qi真氣, righteousness qi正氣, evil qi邪氣(negative qi that has pathogens and will hurt lives), *ying qi* 營氣, *wei qi* 衛氣, clean qi 清氣, turbid qi濁氣, grand qi谷氣, zong qi宗氣, pre-heaven (before birth) qi先天氣, after birth qi後天氣, *yang qi* 陽氣, yin qi 陰氣, spiritual qi靈氣, ghost qi鬼氣, violent qi戾氣, organ's qi臟腑之氣(each organ has its own qi to maintain function and emotion), meridian qi經絡之氣(every meridian has different characters and functions), joyful qi喜氣, anger qi怒氣, illness qi病氣, mood qi脾氣(it expresses personality, culture, environment, attitude, and other external manifestations. It is not the spleen qi.), etc.

There are many kinds of qi related to the Chinese medicine and diseases, and we will continue to introduce them in this series of books. In this book, we only explain a few and list them below:

- ## Yuan Qi or Primary Qi

  Yuan qi is from the heaven (before birth) where the great self resides to protect us.

- ## Righteousness Qi or Zheng Qi

  Righteousness Qi is related to our immunity. It can defend against outside pathogens such as bacteria and viruses. Inside, it will fight against allogeneic and abnormal cells. It also activates the self-healing function and stabilizes our immunity system to avoid hyper becoming auto-immune diseases or hypo becoming low immunity.

- **Evil Qi**

  Evil qi is the opposite of righteousness qi. It broadly refers to a variety of health risk factors such as wind, cold, summer heat, wetness, dryness, fire, phlegm, qi stagnation, and blood stasis. It also refers to negative thoughts, emotions, feelings, or behaviors such as laziness, a bad mindset, and unethical actions. Another concern is external injury from toxins in insects, birds, animal bites, and bacteria and/or virus from wounds, and so on.

- **Yang Qi**

  This is the qi that maintains body functions. It also maintains the body's best shape. It relaxes tightness and tightens looseness.

Functions of the Qi in Our Bodies

Qi is the driving force of life. It has the following five important functions:

1. **PROMOTING DELIVERY:** It delivers nutrients, detoxifies, and expels blockages (blood stasis/qi stagnation/phlegm accumulation). It controls qi, blood, lymph, and fluid circulation, sperm production, and endocrine secretion. It governs growth, reproductive functions, and all organs' normal functions as well as stabilizing nerve systems and emotions.

   Thus, the yang qi maintains the optimum performance of the body and promotes growth of the undeveloped body. The yang qi can even reverse the aging process.

2. **WARMING AND REGULATING FUNCTION:** The yang qi keeps a fixed body temperature range in order to provide energy for the body's physiological functions (i.e. heat provides the best

environment to execute the functions of material transport, metabolism, softness and elasticity of soft tissues. Once a person dies, the yang qi is gone, and the body gradually becomes hard.).

3. **DEFENSE FUNCTION:** The yang qi controls the opening and closing of the pores to resist wind, coldness, heat, wetness, dryness, fire and prevent other pathogens from invading the body. It also defends against invading bacteria, viruses, and parasites and expels from the body. It is responsible for repairing body organs, tissues, and cells to keep them healthy and functional.

4. **ASTRINGENT OR RETENTION OR CONSOLIDATING FUNCTION:** The yang qi keeps blood, body fluids, and essence (pure nutrients) from leaking and keeps the blood and body fluids flowing to the appropriate places.

    It regulates normal semen production, endocrine secretion, and menstruation. It maintains the nerves, blood vessels, and normal distribution of the meridian and ensures that various organs and tissues maintain their normal morphology and locations.

    We can use Comprehensive Universal Energy Healing and acupuncture to correct body distortion and prolapsed organs and to keep blood flowing in the blood vessels. It can also help to stop bleeding in mild cases.

5. **VAPORIZING FUNCTION:** It transforms the material and energy, connects body and spirit (i.e. controls and binds the soul and body relationship). It controls the state of water inside the body (such as absorbing water from the large intestine), vaporizes water and sends it to the lungs to distribute to the skin. It controls qi, blood, essence, and fluid mutual transforms and metaplasia i.e. control body metabolism.

When a person dies, his yang qi and soul leave the body. So by raising one's overall frequency, it increases spirituality and promotes one's health.

Yin and *Yang* that are the Fundamental Elements in Chinese Medicine

- ## What are the yin and yang?

  Yang represents male, bright, hot, heat, warm, quick, positive, movement, energy, light, hyper, and function, etc.

  Yin represents female, dark, cold, slow, negative, static, heavy, hypo, and substances, etc.

  Once you can clearly identify yin and yang, treating diseases and helping patients' recovery becomes very easy.

- ## The Relationship of Yin and Yang

  Yin and yang can represent anything in the universe. Please refer to the following picture of yin and yang:

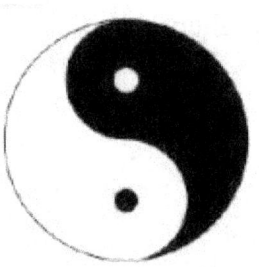

Fig 26 Yin and Yang

If the white part represents the yang, the black part represents the yin. You will see there is yin within yang and yang within yin. Yin and yang always coexist.

If you move a straight line passing through the center of the circle along the circumference, you will discover that yin and yang mutually grow and decline with each other. They change continuously. At the 12:00, 3:00, 6:00 and 9:00 o'clock positions, yin and yang are equal.

The relationships between yin and yang are interoperability and mutual interdependence[*1], mutually transforming[*2], dynamic balance and opposing constraints[*3], fix the yang first and the yin changes correspondingly[*4], forever changing[*5].

[*1] In the picture, yin and yang are forever coexisting. It represents vitality.
[*2] The ultimate hot becomes cold, and the ultimate cold generates heat is another characteristic of yin and yang.
[*3] Referring to the above picture, if there is more yang, then the yin will be less and vice versa.
[*4] Have the correct function first and then follow the healthy constitution.
[*5] Yin and yang are constantly changing, and that creates its eternal existence.

- ## What would happen if the yin and yang separate?

If the yin and yang begin to disengage, life moves towards death. When yin and yang completely separate, life ends.

- ## What is the relationship between yin and yang and health?

A person with balanced yin and yang is healthy. If the yin and yang are imbalanced, a person will get sick—or is already sick.

What is the Relationship of Age and a Balanced Yin and Yang?

A person with balanced yin and yang is healthy. In general, an eighty-year-old man's yin and yang balance at a lower level than a twenty-year-old man's. However, if an elderly person knows how to nourish his life properly, his balance level could be higher than a young person's.

What causes sickness?

- **EXTERNAL CAUSES:** Wind, cold, summer heat, wetness, dryness, fire, and climate or environment cause sicknesses. An improper diet also can cause sickness (please see Cold Foods Drinks Caused Problems Chart Rev 1[155]).

- **INTERNAL CAUSES:** Emotions can cause disease. Each organ associates with different emotions. Some degree of prolonged or intense emotions cause disease. Any prolonged mood affects the heart.

  The relationship between emotions and internal organs:

  - Lungs —sadness
  - Heart —happiness or joy
  - Liver —anger
  - Spleen —worry, contemplation
  - Kidney—fear

  Any organ if abnormal will show its emotions. Any emotion that is too strong will hurt its related organ.

  Causes before birth: congenital diseases, genetic diseases, alcohol consumption during pregnancy, medication, physical or emotional stress, disease.

- **NON-INTERNAL AND EXTERNAL CAUSES:** Unintentional injuries, insects, snakes, animal bites.

Five Elements Theory

Chinese medicine is an advanced science developed through long-term observation of the relationship and interaction between man's health and universal changes. It has passed the test of time for more than 250 million years.

It maps the five organs to the five elements: wood, fire, earth, metal, and water.

Five Elements Relationship Chart

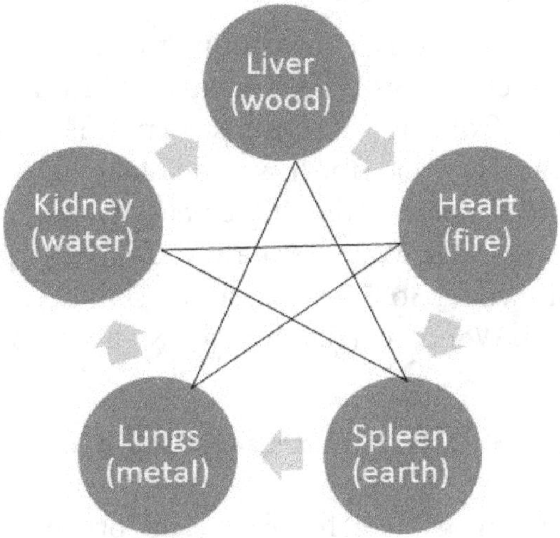

Fig 27 The five elements

In the above diagram, traveling clockwise depicts the mutually generating relationship: water irrigates wood, and wood grows well; burning wood produces fire; burning things with fire produces ashes, which return to the soil of the Earth; soil stores metal; metal melts into water. The diagonals show the mutually hurtful relationship. For example, wood hurts the earth (its roots break the soil), and it damages metal (burning wood melts metal).

We can use seasons to predict a disease. We also use seasons to treat diseases to get the best results.

You can refer to the five elements relationship and table 1. Heart and spleen problems will get worse in the winter. It's because winter benefits the kidney. Since the kidney is at the diagonal end of the heart and spleen, it causes heart and spleen diseases to become worse. One spleen disease is diabetes. It has been proven by Cambridge University's DNA research 217 that type-1 diabetes and heart disease peak in the winter. That is because DNA changes according to seasons.

According to Huang Di Nei Jing·*Su Wen·Chapter Twenty Theory for Organs' Qi Follows Seasons* 《黄帝内經•素向•脏气法时论

篇》, "Liver diseases can be relieved in summer. If not, they will get worse in the fall. If the fall does not kill them, it will be stable in the winter and will get better next spring."

The reason behind this is that summer is fire. Fire acts on metal. Therefore, the metal lungs cannot invade the liver. Liver disease is easier to recover from in the summer. If not, it goes to fall. Fall is metal. Metal invades wood (the liver) and makes liver diseases worse. It could cause the patient to die. If the patient is not dying, it goes to winter. Winter is water. Water is the wood's mother, and it does no harm to its son, wood. So liver disease can stabilize. And in the next spring, it's wood. Wood benefits the liver. So liver disease improves.

The Relationship between Zang and Fu Organs

In Traditional Chinese Medicine, each Zang organ corresponds with a Fu organ. They transmit qi to one another. For example, if the lungs are functioning poorly, that can cause the large intestine to function poorly (and vice versa).

- **SOLID ORGANS:** kidney, liver, heart, spleen, lungs.
- **HOLLOW ORGANS:** small intestine, large intestine, stomach, gallbladder, urinary bladder.
- **THE EXTRA FU ORGANS:** Brain, bone marrow, uterus, vessels, gallbladder.
- Chinese ancestors figured out a relationship between the five elements of nature and the universe. Based on this, they developed a lot of health theories. Please see Table 1—Five Elements.

Nature is the greatest instructor. It provides a billion years of evidence.

- **RELATIONSHIP BETWEEN SOLID ORGANS AND HOLLOW ORGANS:** They are internally and externally related and have a corresponding pairing as follows:

Heart - small intestine

Lung - large intestine

Spleen - stomach

Liver - gallbladder

Kidney - urinary bladder

Pericardium - triple energizer (san jiao) is an extra one to link the other organs.

This means that, using the internal - external relationship transfer can easily occur from one organ to its internally/externally-related organ. If there is disease in one organ, it will influence the other. Lung disease can make the colon not work properly. The patient may have constipation or diarrhea. Conversely, if you have constipation or blockage of the large intestine, it may cause coughing.

The Triple Energizer System

- The Triple Energizer System (San Jiao System) runs along the spaces between the zang and fu organs or between different tissues. The triple energizer system includes the uterus, the brain, the blood vessels, and the nervous and lymph systems. It is divided into upper, middle, and lower jiaos.

  o Upper Energizer (Upper Jiao): Above the diaphragm.

  o Middle Energizer (Middle Jiao): Between the diaphragm and the horizontal section of the umbilicus.

  o Lower Energizer (Lower Jiao): Below the horizontal section of the umbilicus.

Meridians—The transportation system in the human body.

The twelve main meridians:

There are six hand meridians and six foot meridians.

- **Six Hand Meridians:**

  o **THE LUNG MERIDIAN:** Passes through lungs and large intestine.

  o **THE LARGE INTESTINE MERIDIAN:** Passes through lungs and large intestine.

- o THE HEART MERIDIAN: Connects heart, lungs, and eyes.

- o THE SMALL INTESTINE MERIDIAN: Connects small intestines, stomach, heart, and eyes.

- o THE PERICARDIUM MERIDIAN: Connects pericardium with upper, middle, and lower jiaos.

- o THE TRIPLE ENERGIZER MERIDIAN (SAN JIAO MERIDIAN): Connects pericardium, upper, middle, and lower energizers (jiaos), ear, and eyes.

- **Six Foot Meridians:**

  - o THE STOMACH MERIDIAN: Connects forehead, cheeks, nose, upper gum, lips, stomach, and spleen.

  - o THE SPLEEN MERIDIAN: Connects spleen, stomach, and heart as well as the tongue's root and lower surface.

  - o THE BLADDER MERIDIAN: Connects eyes (inner cantus), forehead, brain, kidney, and urinary bladder.

  - o THE KIDNEY MERIDIAN: Connects heel, kidney, urinary bladder, liver, lungs, throat, and root of tongue as well as having branches linking lungs, heart, and pericardium.

  - o THE GALLBLADDER MERIDIAN: Connects ear, eyes (outer cantus), liver, and gallbladder.

  - o THE LIVER MERIDIAN: Connects genital area, liver, gallbladder, eyes, and top of the head.

- Every two hours, qi gathers to travel through a specific meridian to do renewal for that meridian.

- If the meridian is in excess: It happens in a blocked meridian. The meridian pathway has a smaller capacity. Then when there is plenty of qi flowing through, it will cause problems, and disease symptoms will appear.

- If the meridian is deficient: Under a deficiency, the meridian has insufficient capacity. When there is plenty qi flowing through it, it also brings problems and symptoms of disease.

- Judging by a disease's symptoms getting worse or better and their time of occurrence, we can figure out where the problem lies. It helps us in diagnosis and treatment.

- ## Qi's Flowing Time and Sequence Through the Twelve Main Meridians

  Qi flow sequence and times are depicted below for the twelve meridians.

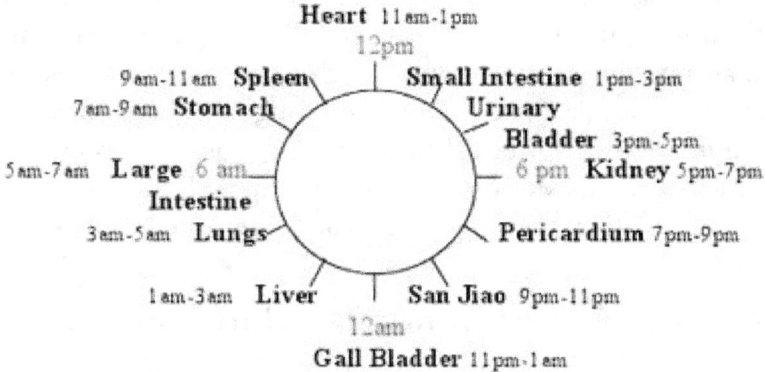

Fig 28 Qi flow in the twelve meridians

LIVER 1:00AM- 3:00AM

LUNGS 3:00AM- 5:00AM

LARGE INTESTINES 5:00AM- 7:00AM

STOMACH 7:00AM- 9:00AM

SPLEEN 9:00AM-11:00AM

HEART 11:00AM- 1:00PM

SMALL INTESTINE 1:00PM- 3:00PM

URINARY BLADDER 3:00PM- 5:00PM

KIDNEY 5:00PM- 7:00PM

PERICARDIUM 7:00PM- 9:00PM

TRIPLE ENERGIZER (SAN JIAO) 9:00PM-11:00PM

GALL BLADDER 11:00PM- 1:00AM

Branching Collaterals of the Twelve Meridians

The twelve main meridians have branching collaterals which start from the knee and the elbow and travel up or down. The branches enter the chest and the abdomen. They connect to their belonging meridians' luo connecting organs (internal-external related organs). For example, the Lung Meridian's luo connects to the large intestine. Therefore, the Lung Meridian branch connects both the lungs and large intestine.

In the neck area, the branch goes shallow to the surface. And here, the yang meridian's branching collateral merges with its original yang meridian, and the yin meridian's branching collateral merges with its original yin meridian's external related yang meridian. For example, the Large Intestine Meridian's branching collateral merges with the Large Intestine Meridian at the neck, and the Lung Meridian's branching collateral merge with the Large Intestine Meridian.

Twelve Meridian's Tendon Collaterals

They are the twelve meridian tendon collaterals, from the terminals of the extremities into the head and body muscles and joints, running parallel to the body's superficial surface. They do not enter the internal organs. Their qi knots at the joints in each meridian. Only the Liver Meridian's tendon collateral knots in the genital area, knotting all of the body tendons. It's because the liver controls the whole body's tendons. This control is achieved through the Liver Meridian's tendon collateral.

Twelve Divergent Meridians

Besides the twelve main meridians (often seen in regular acupuncture meridian pictures), there are also twelve divergent meridians that serve as extensions of the main meridians. They connect the internal-external meridians and the twelve cutaneous regions that split from collaterals and are distributed all over the body.

The Eight Extra Meridians

- **GOVERNOR VESSEL (DU MERIDIAN)**[117]: The Governor (Du) Vessel passes through the spine. All yang meridians get qi and blood supplies from the Governor (Du) meridian. The body's yang gathers here.

- **CONCEPTION VESSEL (REN MERIDIAN)**[117]: The Conception Vessel (Ren Meridian) passes through the spinal cord and the center of the front part of the body. It supplies qi and blood to the yin meridians and directly connects to the throat.

- **CHONG MERIDIAN:** The Chong meridian runs through the spinal cord, kidney, both sides of the abdomen, the throat, and the lips. In women, the "milk" in the lungs that makes the breasts distend before menstruation flows down along the Chong meridian to reach the uterus. According to TCM, on the way to the uterus, it turns the "milk" from white to red (due to the heat of the small intestine), leading to menstruation. This meridian runs inside the body.

- **DAI MERIDIAN:** The Dai meridian locates around the waist (like a belt). It transversely connects all twelve main meridians.

- **YANG QIAO MERIDIAN:** Pulls the foot outward and makes our steps move forward. Located between the Gallbladder meridian and the Bladder meridian on the legs, runs up the lateral side of the body to the back of the shoulder, passes through the neck, cheek, and eye and goes over the head to reach the back of the head.

- **YIN QIAO MERIDIAN:** Pulls the foot inward and makes our steps go backward. It runs along the medial side of the legs and passes through the abdomen, chest, and throat to the inner cantus of the eyes.

- **YANG WEI MERIDIAN:** It connects and coordinates all of the fu organs. It connects all of the yang meridians to hold them in position and looks like a cage.

- **YIN WEI MERIDIAN:** This meridian runs under the ribs to connect and coordinate all of the zang (solid) organs. It also connects all of the yin meridians to hold them in position and has the same function as the yang wei meridian.

The Meridian and the Collateral Meridians

- The fifteen collaterals are branches of the meridians. They run transversely and superficially across the whole body. There is one next to each main meridian, plus collaterals for the Governor Vessel (Du meridian) and Conception Vessel (Ren meridian), and the Major Collateral for the Spleen.
- Sub collaterals and superficial collaterals are small and crowded in order to distribute qi and blood to the terminals of the meridians and collaterals and nourish the body's organisms.

The Area the Meridians and Collaterals Cover

They cover our whole body—from skin to muscles, tendons, organs, and bone. They are mutually connected and overlapped. Depending on the blockage of the individual, stimulating any point of his body can induce stimulation to qi flow in meridians nearby.

If you look at the acupuncture chart and see places that have no meridians passing through, they are actually covered by several neighboring meridians and branches.

Acupuncture Points and Their Functions

Acupuncture points are the points that our body's innermost parts use to communicate with the external environment. External pathogens of wind, coldness, wetness, dryness, summer heat, and fire can invade the human being's body and cause sicknesses. Similarly, the energy and nutrients of the universe can also enter our body and produce positive effects.

Depending on whether the energy is good or bad, it can either strengthen or weaken a person's yang qi. For example, if there is the sunshine during the day, the sunshine is yang. So the sunshine can strengthen a person's yang qi.

At midnight, it is cold, and there is excess yin. The coldness will consume a person's yang qi. Thus, going to bed late at night can have a negative impact on health.

However, too much sunshine can cause extra heat inside the body and lead to sunstroke. In the Chinese culture and medicine, we talk about moderation and balance. Do not indulge too much in the good things. Too much can cause harm.

Typically, acupuncture points are located between bones, muscles, and tendons or between muscle and bone, tendon and bone, or muscle and tendon.

Each point is like a switch that can turn certain body functions on or off. It's also possible to do fine tuning of body functions. Needling at the "Xia Jin Jing" and "Xia Yu Ye" point can immediately produce more saliva. When doing an acupuncture treatment, if a patient feels thirsty, the acupuncturist does not need to pour water for him. Instead, putting needles on these two points can produce more saliva to relieve the thirst.

Each acupuncture point can be used as both a diagnostic and treatment point. When pressing on any acupuncture point, if there is tenderness (mild pain), it means that there is a local or remote congestion. It is the body's way of telling us, "Give me a needle here!" or apply the Comprehensive Universal Energy Healing here or at the remote area. When there is a kidney stone, there will most likely be pain around the KI 3 area. Needling on the specific area of pain near KI 3 can relieve some discomfort caused by the kidney stone.

If the sickness is more severe, the pain will also be more severe.

There are a total of 365 acupuncture points located in the twelve regular meridians (also called the main meridians) and the two extraordinary meridians - Governor Vessel (Du Meridian) and Conception Vessel (Ren Meridian).

There are more than one thousand extra points*, some of them located on the main meridians. The majority were found by ancient physicians who discovered that they could effectively treat specific symptoms at these areas of the body. As time passes, the discovery of extra points increases.

* Extra points are the effective points that were discovered after the 365 regular points were defined. Officially, they are called extra points or extra acupuncture points. Some of them are even located on the twelve meridians.

The Relationship of Organs and Emotions

In Western medicine, the brain controls the emotions. But in Chinese medicine, each organ controls a different part of the brain. Each organ has its own emotional expression, and each organ interacts with the brain.

Abnormal emotions can lead to illness in the related organ, and if an organ's function is not normal, it can affect your mood. An injured spleen can cause muscle pain, abdominal bloating, diarrhea, or motor mind. In addition, patients will be more likely to complain. They will feel they are being treated wrongly and that others should feel sorry for them.

When an organ is functioning properly or improperly, it will assert its unique mood. When an emotion is too strong, it will hurt the related organ's function. If prolonged, it will injure the organ. Any bad emotion kept for an extended period of time will hurt the heart. They are either live fire* or gallbladder fire.

* Meridians can be blocked due to emotional stress which can cause liver qi stagnation. When the regular flowing qi passes through the Liver Meridian blockage area, it generates heat due to friction. In Chinese medicine, too much heat is called fire, but it is fire without flame. However, like flamed fire, it can cause trouble in the form of more severe health problems. That can be insomnia, bleeding, anger or irritability, or high blood pressure.

If the five solid organs are not harmonized, it can lead to anxiety and endocrine secretion disorders.

If the heart function is normal, the person easily feels happiness and joy, is able to forgive others, and treats others fairly. If the heart qi is blocked or abnormal, the person will be unhappy or narrow-minded. Excessive happiness can cause death, and there have been real cases recorded.

Abnormal kidney function makes it easy to feel fear. If the kidney function is normal, the person feels ambitious and has a strong wills.

If there is sputum or fluid or sticky phlegm in the lungs, the person will feel grief or sadness or sensitivity to sad events. Excessive sadness will hurt the lungs and impair the large intestine's proper functioning.

If the spleen function is not good, the person will have a motor mind that causes extra thinking and worry. Excessive use of the brain or thinking too much hurts the spleen. It can cause ball-shaped stool or constipation.

When the liver accumulates excess toxins, it can cause fatigue, irritability, and an out-of-control temper. Similarly, the angrier a person gets, the more injuries to the liver he will experience. Please read Stress-Caused Health Issues in Chapter Eleven Some Commonly Seen Health Issues.

If the gallbladder is weak, it will be difficult to make a decision. In TCM, the gallbladder is in control of decision-making. For gallstones, if there is no sharp pain, you should visit a Chinese medicine physician to try to treat the stones. It requires either pushing the stone to a place that does not block the qi and blood flow, or it needs to be expelled from the body. If you visit an MD, he will most likely have the gallbladder removed. My patients have told me that after having their gallbladder removed, it's harder for them to make decisions than it was previously. One way to prevent gallstones is to not skip meals. If you skip a meal, the bile will have nowhere to go and will form stones.

If there is a sharp pain, it's a case for the emergency room.

The Relationship between Human Beings and the Universe

Human health and survival is inseparable from the universe. For example, a rapid change in the weather can make it easier for people to get sick. Volcanic eruptions, earthquakes, and tsunamis take away people's lives.

The universe is fulfilled with cold and hot flowing air, light, electricity, magnetic fields, and acoustic waves, etc. They have a great impact on a person's qi and blood circulation. Wind, coldness, wetness, dryness, summer heat, and fire invades the body and cause colds, flu, arthritis, sunstroke, diarrhea, pneumonia, meningitis, and a variety of other diseases.

On the other hand, universal water supports life on the entire Earth. The universe provides us with food, clothing, shelter, transportation, education, and music. The proper humidity, temperature, cosmic energy of light, heat, oxygen and nutrient particles are also aggregated to create our body's nutrition. They all supply the needs of our bodies. Please refer to Nutrition in Chinese Medicine[179].

The human body is a small universe unto itself. The space and the Earth belong to an even bigger universe. The human body map is connected with the universe. The body's health and genes are also affected by the universe. Human beings can receive information from the universe in order to develop special talents. In addition, the body can receive universal energy to help heal physical and mental problems. Something as small as a cell can carry universal information. Any part of the body can reflect the whole body's health and can be used to treat the whole body's diseases—ear acupuncture, foot massage, for example.

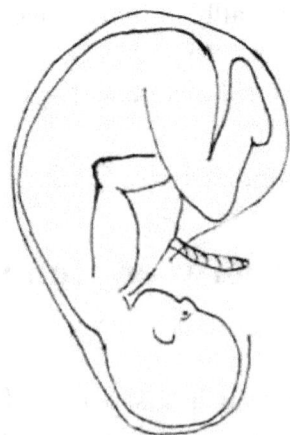

Fig 29 Ear looks like an upside down baby

One day, Dr. Ni visited his friend. His friend's mother answered the door. The entire family's four generations were all sick and in bed. But this old lady wasn't sick. Dr. Ni's friend told Dr. Ni that his mother has never been sick. So Dr. Ni asked his friend if she did any kind of exercise to keep her healthy. Dr. Ni's friend told Dr. Ni that she had never exercised.

Dr. Ni asked his friend to think further. What has his mother done to keep her healthy? His friend told him later that one day, he saw his mother leave the bathroom and both of her ears were very red.

He asked his mother why that was. She told him that in conservative Chinese culture, the girls from rich and higher ranking families were hardly seen outside because once an unmarried girl was seen by a man, she was supposed to marry that man no matter she likes or not.

So his grandmother had taught his mother to massage her ears all over for twenty minutes a day to keep her healthy instead of going outside to do exercises and be seen by a man. That was the only thing he could recall that his mother has done differently.

Thereafter, Dr. Ni taught his patients and students about this convenient health maintenance method. When stuck in traffic, don't complain—instead, do ear massage!

Health maintenance need not be expensive or complicated.

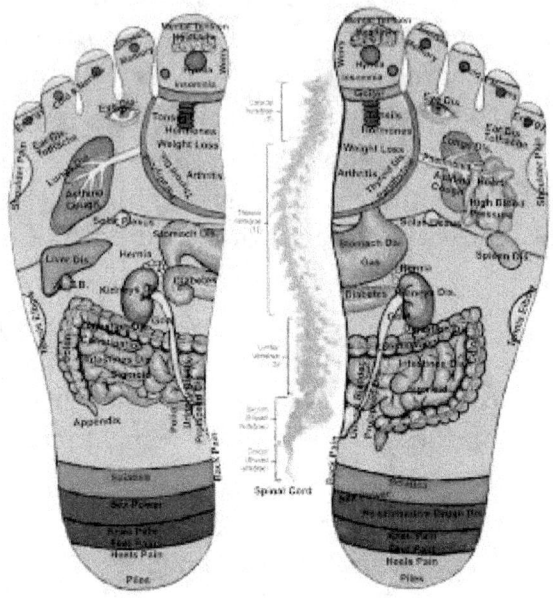

Fig 30 Foot reflexology200

Spine is in the inner edge of the feet

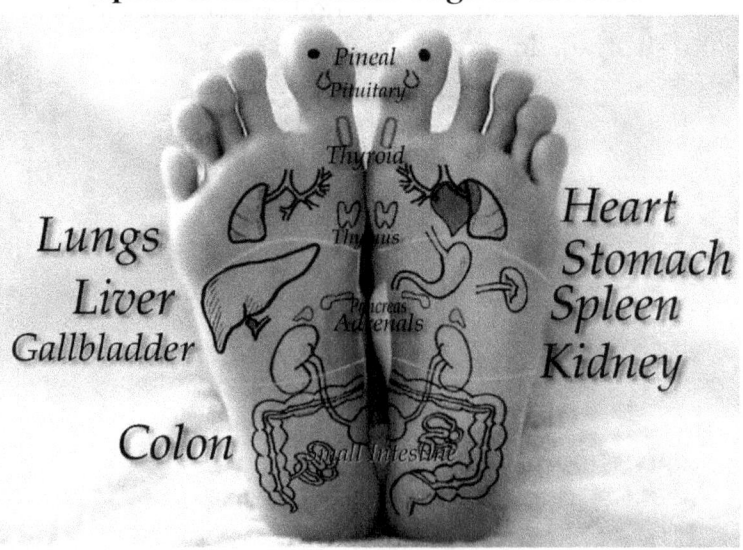

Fig 31 Foot reflexology can be used for foot massage201

Our body supplies signs that we can use to monitor our health situations. It is an earlier and more accurate notice than the medical machines and doctors can give us. That's why Chinese physician and acupuncturists do not usually order any tests but can treat patients well. It is 250 million years of development working well.

Methods of Diagnosis

TCM diagnosis is a product of 250 million of years[65] of observations and practices by many great physicians who had the kindness and desire to save people from sickness.

The diagnoses are quick and accurate if the practitioner is well-trained. There are four diagnostic methods—observation, auscultation and olfaction, inquiring, and palpation. There is a great sixty-episode video series of Huang Di Nei Jing from China[180]. If it could be translated into English, it would help people to learn the history and development of TCM.

There is another classic book called *Nan Jing*[111] 難經 which discusses about eighty-one difficult questions in the *Huang Di Nei Jing*. The sixty-first difficulty[112] is thus stated: "If a physician can diagnose diseases by observation, we can say his skill reaches a miraculous level. If he can diagnose diseases by auscultation and olfaction, we can say his skill has reached the holy level. If he can diagnose diseases by inquiring, we can say his skill has reached the professional level. If he can diagnose by palpation, we can say his skill has reached the craftsman's level."

Don't think an acupuncturist who doesn't do pulsing diagnosis can't treat diseases well. Taking the pulse can, however, be helpful to double check the diagnosis when false symptoms exist.

Sometimes in tough cases, symptoms and body signs conflict. If this is the case, a skilled diagnosis is critical. In these cases, a highly skilled acupuncturist is invaluable.

Observation means to observe vitality, color, appearance, the five sensory organs, the tongue, walking posture, body shape, the face, they eye, the palms, the nails, and the hair. There are so many things that can be used as diagnostic tools. Here are some of the most commonly used ones.

- **Auscultation and Olfaction are listening and smelling.**
- **Inquiring**

  Ask questions for internal medical problems: Are the body and limbs cold or warm or hot? How is the appetite? Thirsty? Sleepy? Is the patient sweating? Urination patterns? Regular or irregular bowel movements? How is the patient's energy? If the patient is female, is menstruation regular?

  Please refer to TCM Diagnosis for Internal Medicine – Ten Questions[181].

- **Palpation** means to palpate pulse and body for pain or organ problems such as enlarged organs, tumor, or body fluids.

  You must learn palpation from a professional, but the others you can learn them on your own from good TCM books.

TCM Eight Diagnostic Principals

They are *interior* and *exterior, cold* and *heat, deficiency* and *excess, yin* and *yang*. For their explanations, please see Appendix One.

Investment Revenue Exercise

This appendix covered a lot of things. They might be both strange and interesting to you. We don't want you to finish reading everything in one day. You're not reading a novel without using your brain to think. What is discussed here is the essence of the wisdom of Chinese ancestors that goes back 250 million years. It is a history and a guide for all of the Chinese medical in the whole world.

If you have time, come back to read this book over and over. Understand and imprint the TCM theory bit by bit in your brain. Try to apply the methods in your daily life. The more you understand, the more it will help your practice and your health.

If you need help, please go to Appendix Four of the book's website to post your question or search for answers.

When you do an adjustment, bring the book with you or study it beforehand.

The most important thing is to learn when you should refer your client out to avoid a delay in necessary professional services. Otherwise, you might take an extra-long time to do an adjustment and allow a treatable case to become untreatable.

CHUEH helps to increase the qi flowing inside body and therefore increase body functions. It does not cause any harm.

If you practice Da Zhou Tian[152] for yourself or teach other persons, you will improve your adjustment skills and effectiveness. It can make the universal energy on your hands grow stronger and can gradually shorten your adjustment time and make your adjustments more powerful. Moreover, your health will improve from practicing the Da Zhou Tian[152] and CHUEH. Binding with universal codes in daily life opens a bright future for you.

This book is an entry level book for TCM and CHUEH. You do not need to memorize each meridian's details. Having an idea of each meridian's route is enough. You should also be aware that the meridians are connected both internally and externally and they have a sequence of flow. All of the acupuncture points are directly or indirectly linked. If there is blockage in the body, apply energy to any point, and the energy can be transmitted to all of the other acupuncture points.

If you have time, we would like you take time here to remember each meridian's traveling route and the important acupuncture points listed in Appendix Five. If you can do so, it will bring you unlimited benefits and convenience for use in later adjustments.

1. Please write down the related emotion according to its organ.

Organ	Emotion
Kidney	
Liver	
Heart	
Spleen	
Lung	

2. In the right column, please write down the internal and external organ related to those in the left column.

Zang Organ (solid organ)	Fu Organ (Hollow Organ)
Kidney	
Liver	
Heart	
Spleen	
Lung	

3. Understand and write down the pathogens.

Classification	Pathogens
Internal causes	
External causes	
Non-internal and non-external causes	

Table 1 Five Elements Table

Five Elements	Four Seasons	Direction	Color	Plants	Environmental Factors	Zang Organs	Fu Organs	Sensory Organs	Tissues	Emotions	Tastes	Music Notes
wood	spring	east	green	germination	wind	liver	gallbladder	eyes	tendon	anger angry with someone injury liver	sour	jiao (Xu)
fire	summer	south	red	growth	heat	heart	small intestine	tongue	blood vessels	joy if hate, it injures heart	bitter	zheng, (He)
earth	2 weeks in between seasons	middle	yellow	transformation	dampness	spleen	stomach	lips	muscles	worry complain that injury spleen	sweet	gong, hu (Hu)
metal	fall	west	white	reaping, harvest	dryness	lungs	large intestine	nose	skin & hair	sadness, grief injuries of lungs	pungent	shang, si (Si)
water	winter	north	black	store	cold	kidney	urinary bladder	ear	bone	fear, injuries of kidneys	salty	yu, chui (Chui)

Table 1 Five Elements Practice

Five Elements	Four Seasons	Direction	Color	Plants	Environmental Factors	Zang Organs	Fu Organs	Sensory Organs	Tissues	Emotions	Tastes	Music Notes
wood												
fire												
earth												
metal												
water												

APPENDIX FIVE

Locations for Important Acupuncture Points and Organs

• •

We adopt the WHO (World Health Organization) names from the Meridian Alphabetic Code 117 (updated in 1989) in this book. Below is the table for your reference.

Number	Official Meridian Name	Other Common Name Used	WHO Code
1	Lung Meridian		LU
2	Large Intestine Meridian		LI
3	Stomach Meridian		ST
4	Spleen Meridian		SP
5	Heart Meridian		HT
6	Small Intestine Meridian		SI
7	Bladder Meridian	Urinary Bladder Meridian	BL
8	Kidney Meridian		KI
9	Pericardium Meridian		PC
10	Triple Energizer Meridian	San Jiao Meridian	TE
11	Gallbladder Meridian		GB
12	Liver Meridian		LR
13	Governor Vessel	Du Meridian	GV
14	Conception Vessel	Ren Meridian	CV

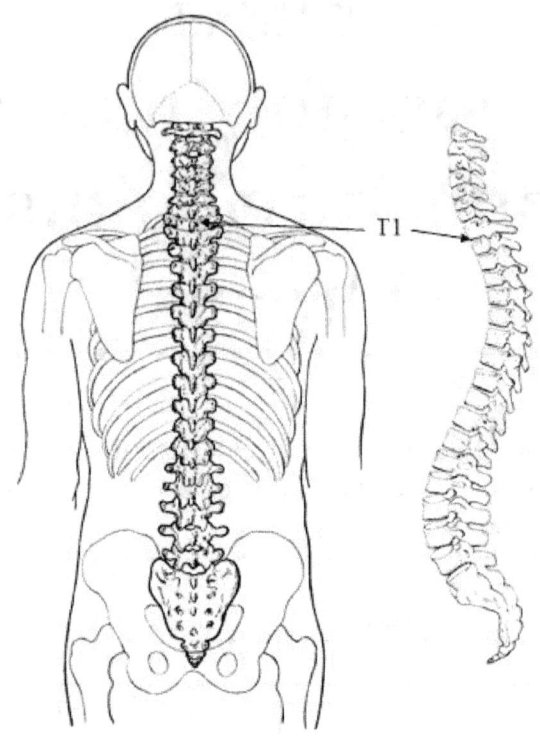

Fig 32 T1 protrudes below the neck and is easy to identify 209

The Important Acupuncture Points on the Governor Vessel

Symbols (This book code, Acupuncture Point Code)

Points & Code)	Location	Indications
Yingtang 印堂 (U1)	At the center of the two eyebrow heads.	Brain, consciousness and intelligence problems, insomnia, child convulsions, forehead headache, runny nose, nose bleeding.
Shenting 神庭 (U2, GV 24)	0.5 cun above hairline in the center of the front hairline.	Consciousness problems. With Baihui can adjust the pineal gland and the problems in the middle of the head. Strong tranquility, epilepsy, dizziness, sinus problems.

Baihui百會(U3, GV 20)	The crossing point of the two ear pix line and the nose line.	See Below.
Dazhui大椎 (U4, GV 14)	At the depression below the 7th cervical bone (C7).	An important point to control the body temperature. All of the yang meridians with heat start reducing heat from this point then enter the head.
Shendao神道 (U5, GV 11)	At the depression below the 5th spinal process (T5).	The qi passes through the heart and Xin Shu (BL 15), therefore, it can adjust for the heart, blood vessels, and blood problems. Heart coughing, poor memory, palpitations, spine and back pain.
Zhiyang至陽 (U6, GV 9)	At the depression below the 7th spinal process (T7).	Circulatory system, an important point to treat jaundice, cough and asthma, spinal stiffness, back pain.
Mingmen命門 (U7, GV 4)	At the depression of the 2nd spinal process (L2). At the same level of the navel.	Digestive, reproductive, and excretory systems, spinal stiffness and back pain.
Yaoshu腰俞 (U8, GV 2)	Below the tailbone, outside of the sacral hiatus.	Reproductive system, hemorrhoids, low back pain, lower limb paralysis, epilepsy.

BAIHUI百會 (U3, GV 20 OR DU 20) INDICATIONS

All of the yin meridians merge with the same named yang meridians in the neck. Then they go into the head. All of them gather at the Baihui. Therefore, the Baihui controls the all of the body's systems. The Triple Energizer System (many books used to call it the san jiao system—it includes nerves, the central nervous system, blood vessels, and the lymph, endocrine, skeletal and muscular systems) is an important acupuncture point for treating head problems, emergency cases, tumors, spinal problems, and pain syndrome,

DAZHUI 大椎 (U4, GV 14) INDICATIONS

It locates above the lungs and controls the respiratory system. Therefore, it also controls the respiratory organs—lungs, trachea, ears, throat, and esophagus. Because the lungs nourish the skin and body hair, it also can adjust the skin, body hair, and related issues. It is also the main point from which to cool down a high fever on the head.

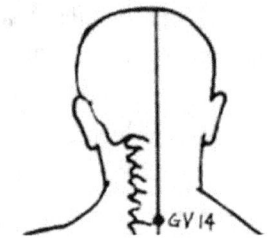

Fig 33 GV 14 (Dazhui) Location

Back-Shu Points—The Important Acupuncture Points on the Back

(Acupuncture Point Code)

Each Back-Shu point is a location where the qi of each organ converges at the back of the body. Each organ has a Back-Shu point. The Back-Shu point is used to treat its corresponding organ as well as the organ-related sensory organ and body limbs related diseases (please refer to Table 1). Often, it is used in conjunction with an organ's Front-Mu Point to treat its related organ.

Point & Code	Location	Indications
Feixhu 肺俞 (BL 13) The fei is the lungs.	1.5 cun lateral to the posterior midline (center of the back), under the lower border of the 3rd thoracic spinous process (T3).	Cough, asthma, chest pain, hot flashes, night sweats, vomiting blood.

Point & Code	Location	Indications
Xinshu心俞(BL 15) The xin is the heart.	1.5 cun lateral to the posterior midline (center of the back), under the lower border of the 5th thoracic spinous process (T5) i.e. 1.5 cun lateral to Shendao (U5, GV 11).	Heart problems, heart-caused coughing, vomiting blood, etc.
Geshu膈俞 (BL17) The ge is the diaphragm.	1.5 cun lateral to the posterior midline (center of the back), under the lower border of the 7th thoracic spinous process (T7) i.e. 1.5 cun lateral to Zhiyang (U6, GV 9).	Activate blood circulation, nourish (generate) blood, vomiting blood, shortness of breath, coughing, vomiting, hiccups, dysphagia, no appetite, hot flashes, etc.
Ganshu肝俞 (BL 18) The gan is liver.	1.5 cun lateral to the posterior midline (center of the back), under the lower border of the 9th thoracic spinous process (T9).	Liver problems: red eyes, blurry vision, jaundice, flank pain Manic, epilepsy; epistaxis, vomiting blood, etc.
Pishu脾俞 (BL 20) The pi is the spleen.	1.5 cun lateral to the posterior midline (center of the back), under the lower border of the 11th thoracic spinous process (T11).	Spleen and digestive problems: epigastric pain, bloating, vomiting, no appetite, diarrhea, dysentery, bloody stool, menstrual dripping, edema, jaundice, back pain, etc.
Sanjiaoshu三焦俞(BL 22) The san Jiao is the triple energizer.	1.5 cun lateral to the posterior midline (center of the back), under the first lumbar spinous process (L1).	Bloating, abdominal sounds, vomiting, diarrhea, dysentery, dyspepsia, edema, pain in the lower back, etc.

Point & Code	Location	Indications
Shenshu 腎俞 (BL23) The shen is the kidneys.	1.5 cun lateral to the posterior midline (center of the back), under the lower border of the 2nd lumbar spinous process (L2) i.e. 1.5 cun lateral to Mingmen (U7, GV 14).	Genital/urinary system problems: enuresis, nocturnal emission, impotence, lower back pain, weak waist, irregular menstruation, white vaginal discharge. etc.

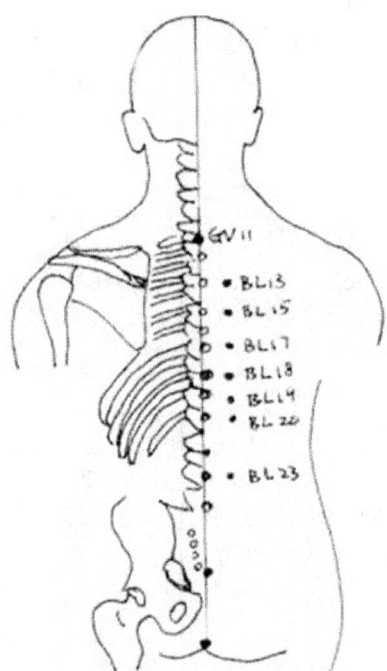

Fig 34 Back Shu Points

The Important Acupuncture Points on the Conception Vessel

Symbol (Acupuncture Point, Code)

Point & Code	Location	Indications
Zongji 中極 (CV 3)	On the center line of the abdomen, 4 cun below the umbilicus.	Reproductive system and urinary system diseases.
Guanyuan 關元 (CV 4)	On the center line of the abdomen, 3 cun below the umbilicus.	Reproductive system, digestive system, urinary system diseases, and the open type stroke.
Qihai 氣海 (CV 6)	On the center line of abdomen, 1.5 cun below the umbilicus.	Respiratory system, digestive system, reproductive system, urinary system diseases and open type stroke.
Shenque 神闕 (CV 8)	In the center of the umbilicus.	Digestive disorders, open type stroke. There is a deep channel linking the organs and thus it can treat each organ disease.
Zhongwan 中脘 (CV 12)	On the center line of abdomen, 4 cun above the umbilicus.	Insomnia caused by stomach diseases, jaundice and digestive system diseases, and so on.
Juque 巨闕 (CV 14)	On the center line of abdomen, 6 cun above the umbilicus.	If used together with Guan Yuan, it has better effectiveness with heart disease; also used in the treatment of digestive diseases with other points insanity, and epilepsy.
Tanzong 膻中 (CV 17)	At the level of the 4th intercostal space (between the 4th and 5th ribs), on the anterior median (front center) line of the chest (at the midpoint between the two nipples).	Qi problems in the upper body, asthma, shortness of breath, hiccups, dysphagia, chest pain, chest tightness, palpitations, lack of milk secretion.

Point & Code	Location	Indications
Tiantu 天突 (CV 22)	In the center of the suprasternal fossa.	Throat problems, cough, asthma, hiccups, dysphagia, sudden aphonia (loss of voice), goiter.

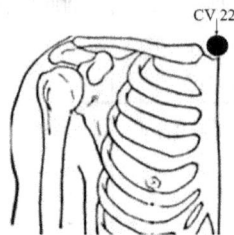

Fig 35 CV22 (Ren 22) Location

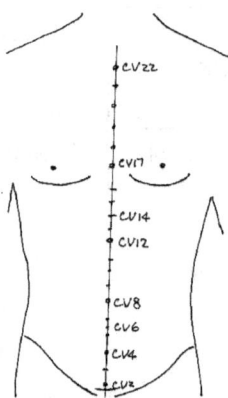

Fig 36 Important points on Conception Vessel

Front Mu—Important Points in the Front of the Body

Symbol (Acupuncture Point Code)

Each Front Mu point is the qi gathering place in the front of the chest and abdomen for its related organ. They are the important points from which to treat organs' diseases. Each organ has one Front Mu point. If an organ is sick, there is an abnormality in its respective Front Mu point. They are often combined with their related Back-Shu points in clinical practices.

Point & Code	Location	Indications
Zhongfu 中府 (LU 1)	6 cun from the center line of the chest. 1 cun below LU 2, at the level of the first intercostal space (between the st and 2nd ribs).	Coughing, wheezing, asthma, chest distention, shoulder and back pain.
Danzong 膻中 (CV 17)	At the level of the 4th intercostal space (between the 4th and 5th ribs), on the anterior (front) median (center) line of the chest—the midpoint between the two nipples.	Whole body systemic qi problems, asthma, shortness of breath, hiccups, dysphagia, chest pain, chest tightness, palpitations, lack of milk secretion.
Juque 巨闕 (CV 14)	On the center line of the abdomen, 6 cun above the umbilicus.	Heart disease, if used together with Guan Yuan has better effectiveness; also the treatment of digestive diseases with the other pints insanity, epilepsy.
Tianshu 天樞 (ST 25)	2 cun lateral to the umbilicus.	Bloating, abdominal pain, abdominal sounds, diarrhea, dysentery, constipation, pain around the navel, irregular menstruation, edema.
Shimen 石門 (CV 5)	On the center line of abdomen, 2 cun below the umbilicus.	Amenorrhea, vaginal discharge, bleeding, postpartum hemorrhage, hernia, abdominal pain, diarrhea, urinary incontinence, anuria (less than 50ml urine/ day), edema.
Guanyuan 關元 (CV 4)	On the center line of abdomen, 3 cun below the umbilicus.	Reproductive system, digestive system, urinary system diseases, and open type stroke.
Zhangmen 章門 (LR 13)	On the lateral side of abdomen at the free end of the 11th floating rib.	Vomiting, abdominal distention, abdominal sounds, diarrhea, indigestion, flank pain, etc.

Point & Code	Location	Indications
Qimen期門 (LR 14)	Below the nipple at the level of 6th intercostal space (between the 6th and 7th ribs).	Mastitis, hiccups, acid reflux, bloating, flank pain, diseases with fever, depression, mental stress.
Jingmen京門 (GB 25)	On the lateral side of the abdomen, on the lower border of the free end of the 12th floating rib.	Bloating, abdominal sounds, diarrhea, waist and flank pain.
Zhongwan中脘 (CV 12)	On the center line of abdomen, 4 cun above the umbilicus.	Insomnia caused by stomach diseases, jaundice, and digestive system diseases.
Riyue日月 (GB 24)	Below the nipple at the level of 7th intercostal space (between the 7th and 8th ribs).	Jaundice, nausea, vomiting, acid regurgitation (acid reflux), flank pain, mastitis.
Zongji中極 (CV 3)	On the center line of the abdomen, 4 cun below the umbilicus.	Reproductive system and urinary system diseases.

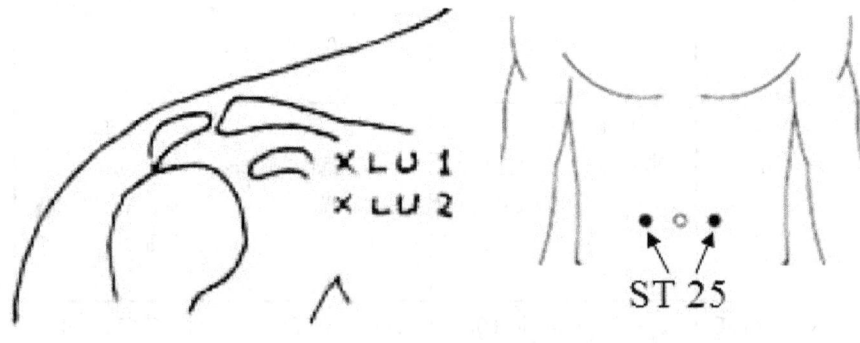

Fig 37 LU 1 & LU 2   Fig 38 ST 25

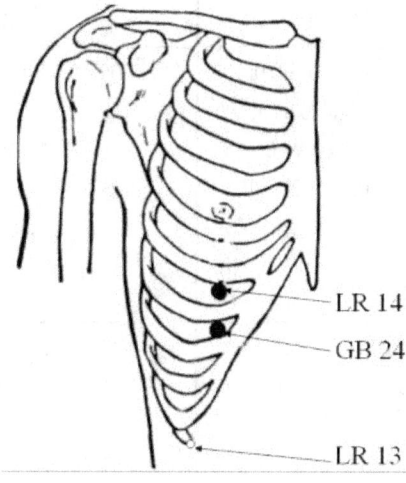

LR 14

GB 24

LR 13

Fig 39 LR 13, 14, GB 24

Eight Influential Points

There are eight points. The symbol is the acupuncture point code.

The eight influential points are the solid organs, hollow organs, tendons, blood vessels, qi, blood, bone, and bone marrow's eight essence qi (pure nutrition) confluence points.

Point & Code	Location	Indications
Zhangmen 章門(LR 13)	On the lateral side of abdomen, at the free end of the 11th floating rib.	All kinds of the solid organs' (kidneys, liver, heart, spleen, lungs) problems.
Guanyuan 關元 (CV 4)	On the center line of abdomen, 3 cun below the umbilicus.	All kinds of the hollow organs' (urinary bladder, gallbladder, small intestine, stomach, large intestine) problems.
Yanglingquan 陽陵泉 (GB 34)	On the external side of the lower leg, at the depression anterior (forward) and inferior (below) to the head of the fibula.	Whole body's tendon problems.

Point & Code	Location	Indications
Juegu or Xuanzhong 絕骨或稱 懸鐘 (GB 39)	3 cun above the tip of the external malleolus at the depression between the posterior border of the fibula and the tendons of peroneous longus and brevis.	Bone and bone marrow problems.
Geshu膈俞 (BL17) The ge 膈 is the diaphragm.	1.5 cun lateral to the posterior (back) center line, under the lower border of the 7th thoracic spinous process (T7) i.e. 1.5 cun lateral to Zhi Yang (U6, GV 9).	Activates the whole body's blood circulation and nourishes the blood.
Dazhou大柱 (BL 11)	On the back of the body, 1.5 cun lateral to the lower border of the first spinous process.	Bone diseases and its nearby organism problems such as fever, nasal congestion, headache, etc.
Taiyuan太淵 (LU 9)	At the radial (thumb) end of the transverse (horizontal) crease of the wrist, at the depression where the radial artery pulsates.	Blood vessel problems.
Danzong膻中 (CV 17)	At the level of the 4th intercostal space (between the 4th and 5th ribs), on the anterior median line of the chest at the midpoint between the two nipples.	Whole body qi circulation problems.

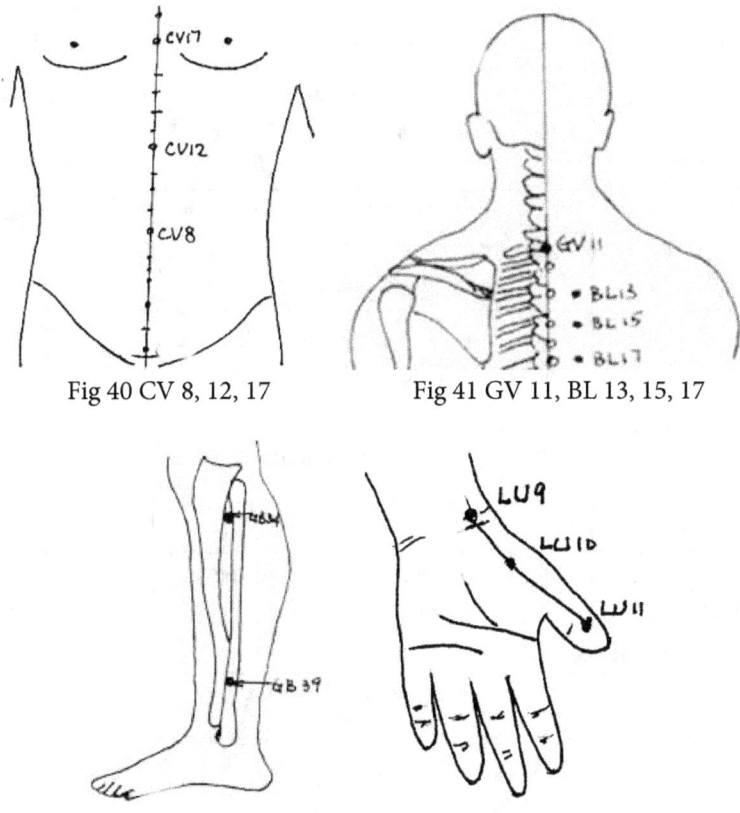

Fig 40 CV 8, 12, 17   Fig 41 GV 11, BL 13, 15, 17

Fig 42 GB 39 GB 34   Fig 43 LU9, LU10, LU 11

Eight Convergent Points

There are eight points. The symbol is the acupuncture point code.

The eight convergent points, also known as the eight intersection points of the eight extrameridians and the twelve regular meridians. The eight convergent points have every two points as a paired relationship.

Point & Code	Location	Indications
Gongsun 公孫 (SP 4) connects to the Chong Meridian	On the medial side (inside) of the foot, in the depression distal and inferior to the base of the first metatarsal bone.	Stomach, heart and chest
Neiguan 內關 (PC 6) connects to the Yang Wei Meridian	2 cun above the wrist crease between the two tendons of palmaris longus and flexor carpi radialis.	
Houxi 後溪 (SI 3) connects to the Governor Vessel	Keep a loose fist, it's under the pinky finger at the end of the Palmar crease and the junction of the white and red skin.	Inner canthus, neck, ears, shoulder blade
Shenmai 申脈 (BL 62) connects to the Yang Qiao Meridian	At the depression 1 cun below the tip of the external malleolus.	
Waiguan 外關 (TE 5) connects with the Yang Wei Meridian	On the dorsal (dark skin) side of the forearm, 2 cun above the transverse crease of the wrist between the ulna and radius.	Outer canthus, cheek, neck, back of the ear, shoulder
Zulinqi 足臨泣 (GB 41) connects Dai Meridian	On the lateral dorsal (outer of the back skin) side of the foot, at the depression 1.5 anterior (forward) to the 4th and 5th metatarsophalangeal joint.	
Lieque 列缺 (LU 7) connects to the Conception Vessel	1.5 cun above the wrist crease, superior to the styloid process of the radius.	Lung, throat, diaphragm
Zhaohai 照海 (KI 6) connects Yin Qiao Meridian	At the depression 1 cun below the tip of the medial malleolus.	

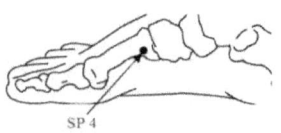
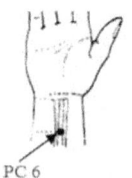
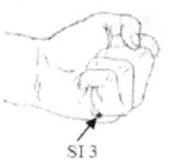

SP 4   PC 6   SI 3

Fig 44 SP 4, PC 6 and SI 3

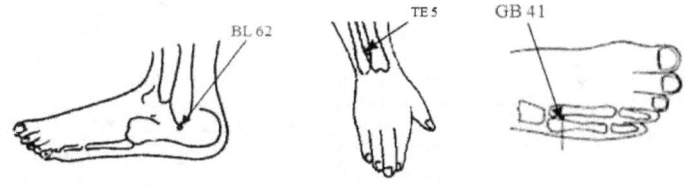

Fig 45 BL 62, TE 5, GB 41

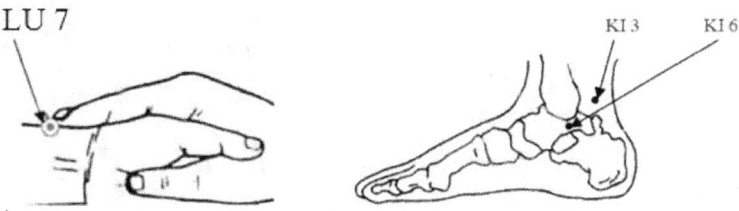

Fig 46 LU 7, KI 3 & KI 6

The Functions of the Eight Extra Meridians

In the *Huang Di Nei Jing • Ling Shu • Chapter Thirty-eight of the Rebellious, Smooth, Fat and Thin,* it is mentioned that the Chong Meridian is the sea of the organs' twelve regular meridians. In other words, all of the organs get the Chong Meridian's qi and blood nourishment. It is like the Chong Meridian serves as storage for the extra qi and blood and can supply both to the other twelve regular meridians and organs if needed.

The Dai Meridian is located at the abdomen. It binds the six vertically traveling foot meridians and the Yang Qiao and Yin Qiao Meridians horizontally and controls the waist and abdomen's curve.

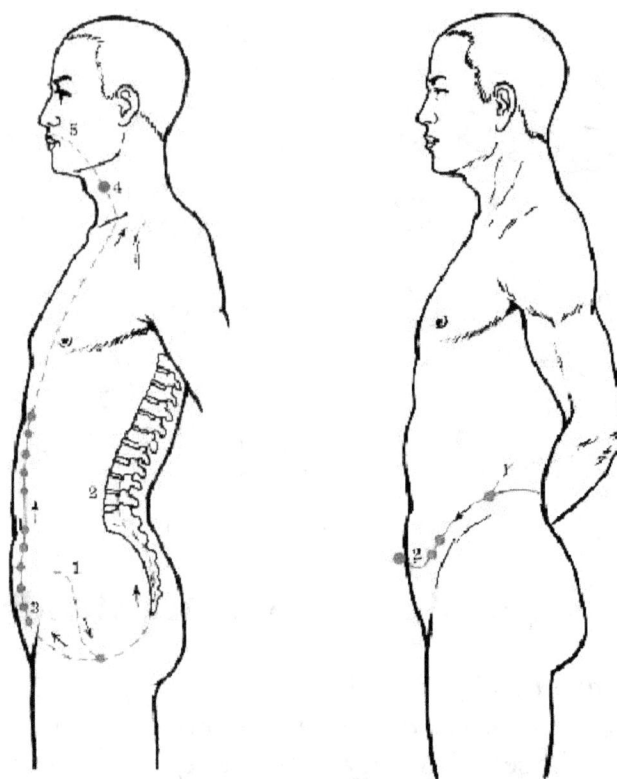

Fig 47 Chong Meridian[119]   Fig 48 Dai Meridian[199]

The Yang Wei Meridian connects with the hand's Small Intestine and and Triple Energizer as well as foot's Bladder and Gallbladder Meridians with the Governor Merdians. It maintains the yang meridians' connection.

The Yin Wei Meridian connects with the three foot yin meridians, the Pericardium Meridian and the Conception Vessel. It maintains the yin meridians' connection.

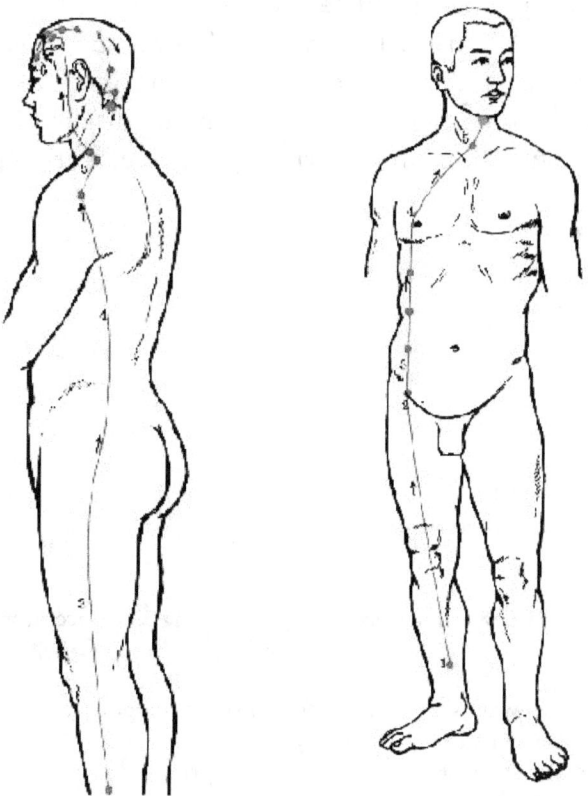

Fig 49 Yang Wei Meridian [216]   Fig 50 Yin Wei Meridian[138]

The Governor Vessel (Du Meridian)is found at the back of the body in the spine. It controls all of the yang meridians. Its pathway traces from the Yongquan (KI 1) up to the medial of the lower leg, to the back of the knee, and up to the abdomen. In the front, it goes through the Conception Vessel (Ren Meridian) and the Kidney Meridian. On the back of the body, it goes through the center of the spin and the Bladder Meridian.*

It's the main meridian of the eight extra meridians and the sea of all of the yang meridians. The Governor Vessel closely relates to the brain, bone marrow, and bone. The Governor Vessel and the Conception Vessel cross and meet lower around Huiyin** and at the lips.

The Conception Vessel (Ren Meridian) is located on the center line of the front body at the chest and abdomen. It controls all of the yin meridians. It's the sea of all of them and has the function of regulating menstruation and vaginal discharge, promoting reproductive function, and nourishing the fetus during pregnancy.

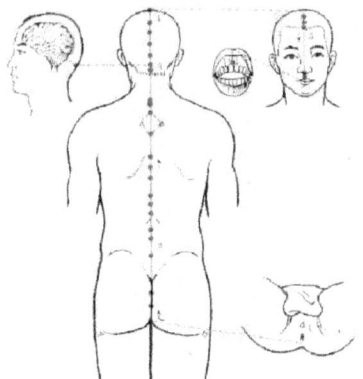 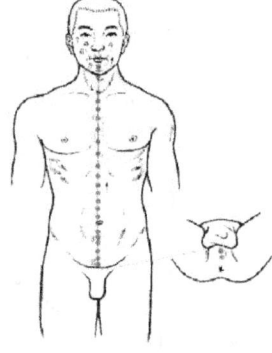

Fig 51 Governor Vessel[218]   Fig 52 Conception Vessel[219]

* This pathway is not mentioned in other acupuncture books, but I have discovered its existence in my clinical experience. To treat severely sick patients or boost a patient's yuan Qi (primary qi) or immunity, I use my external formula with wine and moxibustion and treat at the Yongquan (KI 1) to let the heat start at KI 1 and spread to the whole foot. It then travels the pathway mentioned above until the heat reaches the neck. At this point, I stop the treatment. I use what the acupuncture world calls the seven starts treatment. It can locate hidden blockages in the body that have been neglected or undiscovered by other therapists. It allows me to unearth and address the root problems that may have been seeded fifty or more years prior to the current symptoms.

For more detailed information about my external formula, please refer to Appendix Eight.

** Huiyin can be found between the body's two lowest orifices.
*** This book is not a textbook. Please Google the topic to find more information online.

The Yang Qiao Meridian is the branch from the Bladder Meridian and the Kidney Meridian. It starts from the foot heel at BL 62, travels along the yang (dark skin) side of the lower limbs, up and meets with the Small Intestine Meridian at the scapula. The Bladder Meridian, Stomach Meridian, and Yin Qiao Meridian meet at the eye and connect the main organs of the throat, eyes, and brain.

The Yang Qiao Meridian regulates muscle movement and communicates the yin and yang qi of the body. Its functions are making lower limb movements quick and light as well as moistening the eyes and controlling eyelid opening and closing.

The Yin Qiao Meridian is mainly distributed in the abdomen and neck. Its function is to communicate with the yin and yang qi that regulate a person's activities and sleep. Abnormalities in this meridian could cause the outside of the limb muscles to be loose and the inside muscles to be tight or sleeping too much.

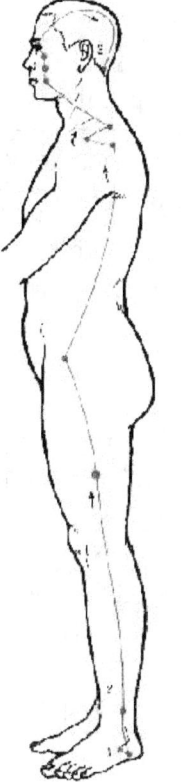
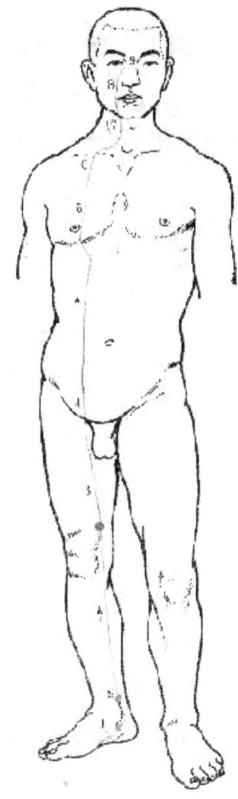

Fig 53 Yang Qiao Meridian[220]   Fig 54 Yin Qiao Meridian[221]

Lateral of the Body

Dabao (SP 21): Located at the center line of the lateral (side) of the body at the intercostal space between the 6th and 7th rib bones.

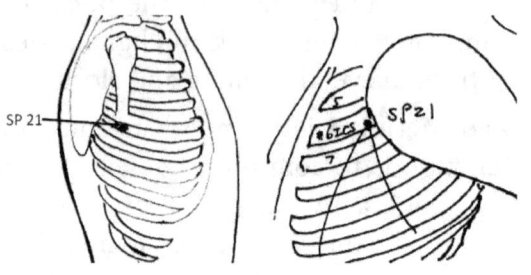

Fig 55 Dabao (SP 21)

The Important Points on the Arms

The symbol is the acupuncture point code.

Point & Code	Location	Indications
Hegu合谷 (LI 4)	On the dorsum (dark skin) of the hand, between the 1st and 2nd metacarpal bones, in the middle of the 2nd metacarpal bone on the radial (thumb) side.	Abdominal pain, diarrhea, constipation, pain/paralysis in the upper extremities. Craniofacial (head and face) problems such as headaches, red, swollen, and painful eyes, nosebleeds, nasal congestion or discharge, deafness, toothache in the teeth of the lower jaw, trismus (lockjaw), Bell's Palsy (facial paralysis), facial swelling, mumps, sore and swollen throat, neck/head pain. Lack of sweat or excessive sweating, fever, amenorrhea, prolonged labor, convulsions in young children, acupuncture anesthesia, etc.

Point & Code	Location	Indications
Quechi 曲池 (LI 11)	In the depression of the lateral end of the transverse cubital (horizontal elbow) crease. Or at midpoint between LU 5 and the lateral epicondyle of the humerus.	Abdominal pain with vomiting and diarrhea, paralysis of the upper limbs, sore throat, toothache of the teeth in the lower jaw, red eyes and pain, fever, skin diseases, high blood pressure.

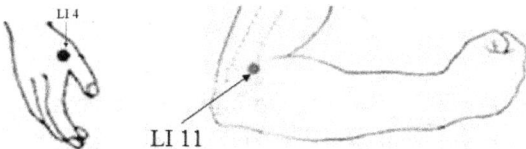

Fig 56 Hegu LI 4 and Quechi LI 11

The Important Points on the Legs

The symbol is the acupuncture point code.

Point & Code	Location	Indications
Zusanli (ST 36)	Locates 3 cun (four finger widths) down from the bottom of the knee cap, along the outer boundary of the shin bone and one index finger width outside of the highest line of the shin bone.	Gastrointestinal disorders: stomachache, vomiting, hiccups, acute/chronic gastritis, gastric or duodenal ulcer, acute/chronic enteritis, abdominal distension, abdominal sounds, appendicitis, constipation, diarrhea, dysentery, bacillary dysentery, appendicitis, undigested food, indigestion, acute/chronic pancreatitis, consumptive deficiency and emaciation, malnutrition, regulating gastric secretion. Other diseases: Tibia knee pain, athlete's foot, dizziness, cough, asthma, mastitis, insomnia, edema, mania, stroke, paralysis, mania, hepatitis, shock, nervous headache, hypertension, epilepsy, neurasthenia, schizophrenia, atherosclerosis, bronchial asthma, leukopenia, sciatica, lower limb paralysis, knee and surrounding soft tissue disorders, etc. It is an important point for longevity and immunity.

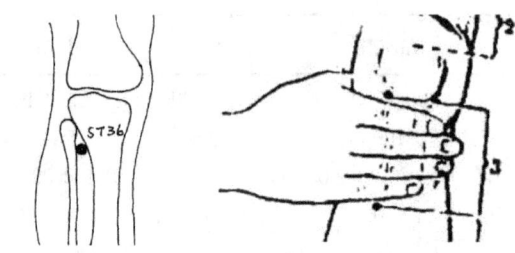

Fig 57 ST 36 Zusanli   Fig 58 Waixiyan

Organ Location Picture

Please note that looking at the image below is like looking into a mirror. As you can see from the picture, the location of the organs are on the *opposite* side of the body. For example, the liver is on the body's right side instead of on the left side as shown below.

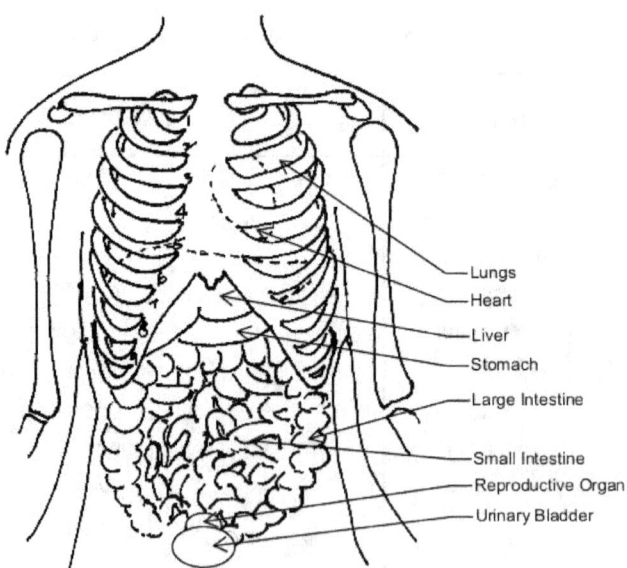

Fig 59 Organ Locations 214

Author's Cases Shared and her Medical Discoveries

● ●

Though the content of this appendix is not within the scope of Comprehensive Universal Energy Healing, you can learn here what diseases can be properly addressed by acupuncture treatments and could be converted to be CHUEH adjustments. You will also see how my skills can help people to be healthier, happier, be better more quickly.

My Medical Harvest on Cruise Ships

While I was at sea, food was prepared and readily available, and I had staff and crew to clean my room and wash my clothes. There was no need to drive, do shopping, or complete house chores. Basically, life was a lot simpler than it is on land. When stopping in a new port, I liked to go sightseeing and go on adventures either with my colleagues or by myself. Otherwise, I preferred to study in my cabin.

Maybe it's because of my mission, but I always seem to get extra help from the Super Power. Every time I would read a new case, soon after there would be real life patients asking for my treatment for that exact thing. The difficulty was how to gradually proceed without a huge jump.

Sometimes new cases would come in before I had studied that particular illness. Usually, I would insert some needles in the first treatment to gain general improvement for the patient. Then, during my evening studying, I would search for a more definitive answer. At times, I would crawl into bed and have a sudden inspiration which allowed me to figure out the pathology and etiology. That made the disease much easier to treat. Because of all of my studying and inspirations, my treatment skills and medical theories advanced quickly.

Below are some cases and the treatment results which came to my brain without even thinking about it:

1. Pain Syndrome

Pain syndrome is usually not hard for me to treat. From the patient's pain characters, I can tell how they were injured and from what kind activity—even if it happened decades ago injured and the pain symptoms didn't occur until they were sixty or seventy years old.

There were always the commonly seen problems—headaches, migraines, belt headaches caused by dampness, frozen shoulders, arm pain, hand pain, trigger fingers, inability to extend hand after stroke, lack of strength in hand, carpal tunnel syndrome, arthritis, swollen joints, rheumatoid arthritis, knee pain, leg pain, ankle pain, foot pain, heel pain, toe pain, abdominal pain, chest pain, back pain, neck pain, and edema. There were sports injuries from skiing, scuba diving (lower limb paraplegia), skating, dancing, ball games, and swimming and injuries from overuse from activities such as playing piano or typing. There was muscle strain, pain from surgery, fibromyalgia, sciatica, hip pain, lower back pain, and rare pain caused by things such as ankylosing spondylitis.

Acupuncture treatment can help many patients avoid surgeries for hip problems, spinal disc herniation, bulging or narrowing disks, partial spine scoliosis, frozen shoulder, big toe bone hyperplasia, meniscus tear, knee cartilage wear, carpal tunnel syndrome, and trigger finger, etc.

After reading even more medical cases and thinking about it more, it becomes easy to treat pain cases that other Chinese medicine physicians, doctors, and massage therapists can't.

A headache patient came to see me. She had already overdosed on the strongest painkiller her doctor had prescribed for her, and she still had no reduction in her headache pain. In only one treatment from me, her pain gradually faded, and she did not return later.

There was a special case where a patient had had back pain for more than ten years. One of the painkillers that he had taken had resulted in a heart surgery which left a one foot long, half inch wide scar on his chest. After heart surgery, he should have been taking medicine for his heart. But this medicine conflicted with his pain medicine. He was having three acupuncture treatments per week, but it wasn't reduce his back pain. Instead, the pain was worsening.

At my back pain seminar, he challenged me to see if I could treat his back pain better than his treatments. When I learned that the length of the needle his acupuncturist used was only one inch long, I promised him I could treat him. After only five treatments, I had loosened his neck, back muscles, the tendons besides his spine and had treated all kinds of painful disk problems which caused him to walk unevenly, tightening up his legs. Once all of the tendons and muscles that should be loose were taken care of, he was so happy that he no longer needed to take any drugs for pain.

Since a car accident forty years ago, a patient had continued acupuncture treatments once a week. But for those forty years, her pain had been getting worse. After four treatments with me, she felt no pain.

A Vietnam War soldier had a half foot by a foot area of flesh on his right upper leg sheared off by a bombshell. This area was bordered by a half inch wide scar that had lost elasticity. Each step he took caused pain. After one treatment, he recovered elasticity and could walk without pain.

My toughest pain case was a high pain tolerant male farmer. Both of his upper legs had a couple of string tendons that were as thick as a thumb and hardened like steel. They had lost their elasticity and could not extend without severe pain. On the cruise ship, we had only electrical needles—no moxibustion, no proper herbs.

Accompanying him to the spa was his pretty wife. She was a retired teacher. Both were eighty or ninety years old. It was their first cruise.

The wife was upset and said, "We've been on board for a week already, and besides our room, we haven't seen anything else on the ship. Today, we came here for an acupuncture treatment and at least can see what the spa looks like. Every day, we order meals to our room, plus tips, and money is flying out of our pockets like it has wings. It's terrible. We'd better just stay on our farm."

After getting the spa manager's permission, each three to four hour treatment was charged only as one hour for them. Gradually, after three treatments, the farmer could sit in a wheelchair by himself. The couples could dine at the restaurant, and there was no need to order meals to their room. Both were very happy.

The funniest memory I have is of a massage therapist who had back pain and could not straighten her back. I treated her once without results. The pain made her extra sensitive to needle insertion. It's used to be torture for me to treat this kind of patient.

The night after the first treatment, I turned to my *Huang Di Nei Jing • Su Wen • Needle the Back Pain Theories*. I saw a sentence that mentioned the same symptoms this massage therapist had—she could not straighten her back and had never stopped talking since entering my treating room! I found small nodules between her LR 2 and LR 3 and used a needle to dissolve them. Her back pain was gone, she could stand erect, and she stopped talking!

2. Insomnia

I was usually lucky in that my insomnia patients experienced improvement after only one treatment. Though there were patients who had taken sleeping pills for years, I hadn't met one who had taken them for decades. Otherwise, I might be able to share with you some very tough cases. I can, however, share some special ones:

A female patient who had high mental stress came to me for treatment. She was sleepwalking every night, waking up to do chores around the house. Her clients were VIPs spoiled by power and position. They all wanted to be her first priority.

After her first treatment, she told me that she was so lucky that all of the ship guests went to the shore on a port day. Even the security guards were busy at the gangways to serve guests and crews getting off or back to the ship. She yelled out very loudly and used her fist to hit the steel wall. There was no one to stop her. She only stopped when she lost her voice and her hands were too painful. Afterward, she felt much more comfortable. After the second treatment, she could sleep overnight without waking up.

A female police officer woke up every night to give a speech. After one treatment, her sleep-talking was gone, and she felt soothed and comfortable.

A seasick patient came to me for treatment. She had some pain and tough insomnia. She had visited Western physicians for two years and Chinese medicine physicians for more than two months, but it hadn't helped her insomnia. Within one hour of treatment, her body kept bringing out new symptoms. The needles I used for tranquility and sleeping aid wouldn't even help her to fall asleep on my treatment bed.

The second day was the end of my contract and sign off day. I woke up especially early to take some pictures of the sunrise and watch the ship entering the harbor. I met the seasick insomniac on deck, and she told me she had never slept so well as last night.

The most interesting case was a couple. Both of them had insomnia every night—they woke up and chatted. The wife came in for one treatment. That night, her husband could not wake her up. The second morning, she came in angry and told me that her husband gave her a hard time that morning because he could not wake her up. She was coming to see me that morning for her other health issues.

On the third day, her husband came in. He told me that he had never believed in Chinese medicine. However, for the past two nights, he could not wake his wife up and was bored awake alone in the night. He'd seen how happy his wife was at the improvement in her health, so he'd reluctantly come in to see me. After his treatment, I never saw the couple again.

3. Heart and Blood Pressure Problems

High blood pressure, palpitations, arrhythmia, somnolence (hypersomnia) and no energy after cardiac surgery, blood turbidity, high cholesterol, and angina are all treatable.

The most severe case I had was a woman whose husband had made her angry and induced angina. The day before visiting, she went to the ship's medical center and got a prescription. On the second day, her husband made her mad again, but the prescribed medication did not help. Her pulse was eight to nine beats per breath. My treatment battled for a while to reduce her pulse rate to a normal range—four to five beats per breath. I told her to avoid her husband, and I did not see her again.

Another case was a patient who'd previously had a stent. Because he's had a problem with it, his left side rib bones were cut in order to remove it. Afterward, he was always tired all day and slept the day away. On the ship, he used acupuncture treatments to boost his energy. At every port, he would have enough energy to get off the ship for fun, and then he would come back to the ship, take a shower, and come to the spa for his acupuncture treatment.

4. Breathing and Lung Problems

Some patients who carry oxygen tanks open the tank to its maximum flow volume but are still short of breath. After acupuncture treatment, their oxygen tanks can be used at a lower volume. Cold flu, asthma, phlegm in the lungs, pneumonia, yellow sputum, chronic cough (including cough caused by the lungs, the lungs and large intestine, the kidney, the kidney and urinary bladder, the heart and small intestine, the liver, the spleen and stomach, and other organs), chronic obstructive pulmonary disease, emphysema, smoking addiction, runny nose, watery nose discharge, sleep apnea, phlegm accumulation in the lungs, atopic dermatitis (AD or atopic eczema), dry skin, congenital systemic wrinkles, erythema, and eczema can all be treated.

5. Digestion Problems

Stomachache, morning sickness, vomiting, motion sickness, abdominal pain, diarrhea, constipation, food allergies, loss of appetite, overeating, pickiness in eating, poor digestion, cravings for sweets/fatty foods/salty foods/spicy foods, drinking (not too severe).

The most severe constipation:

A patient's severe constipation with a history of thirty years—along with his lower back pain—was fixed in three treatments. His constipation and back pain were caused by a lower back surgery. The surgery scar blocked his lower back qi and blood circulation.

The patient had been vomiting severely for twenty-four hours and could not ingest anything and keep it down, including water. After slightly more than an hour of treatment, he had no problem eating or drinking. This patient had severe mental stress which caused liver qi stagnation. In addition, South America's strong wind and big waves had induced seasickness. That prevented the stomach qi from descending, causing the severe vomiting.

There was a patient who came in with red rashes. Her doctor had told her that she had autoimmune disease and put her on medication. My examination discovered that her lungs had a lot phlegm, and she had a craving for spicy foods. Her symptoms were caused by mental stress. I soothed her stress and expelled the phlegm in her lungs. On the third treatment, she told me that she was not craving spicy food anymore. Her skin rashes had greatly subsided. After the third treatment, she did not come back. I met her on the ship later, and she was fine without a trace of rash.

6. Lower Limb Problems

General edema, sprains and swelling, poor circulation, pain, numbness—especially for diabetic patients' loss of sensation, rheumatism, arthritis, restless legs syndrome, and meniscus tears are treatable.

A male patient traveled to China and drank milk with toxins, and his lower extremities lost sensation. After one treatment, his sensation was recovered. The next day, he told me by telephone that his sensations had lasted only a half day, and then he felt numb again. I encouraged him to come back because continuing treatments would improve his chances of fully recovering. The efficacy time can be gradually extended until sensation is totally recovered. Unfortunately, he was extremely disappointed and gave up treatment.

One day, in the spa restroom and shower area, I met the above patient's wife. I approached her to explain to her that her husband must continue his acupuncture treatments in order to regain sensation in his lower limbs.

When I approached her, she began to shout at me in a high-pitched tone and her tears flowed. "You, the conscienceless Chinese people!" She did not give me a chance to speak. Her loud voice soon attracted a lot of stares.

I raised my voice and said, "Please calm down. I'm standing here listening to you instead of walking away, and that's completely for the benefit of your husband's health and the recovery of his sensation."

Seeing she had stopped blaming me, I continued, "China and Taiwan are two totally different political systems. I come from Taiwan. Unfortunately, China had a cultural revolution, and people lost their education and their sense of Chinese traditional morality. You should know that uncountable Chinese and Taiwanese were injured much more severely than your husband. If you want your husband to recover his health, please listen to me.

"Chinese medicine and treatment," I told her, "helps patients gradually restore their body's self-healing power in order to recover their functions. If we expel the toxins inside your husband's body, his sensation can come back. Once we achieve a period of time with improvement, no matter how short it is, it means his situation can continuously be improved. You should not give up."

The patient's wife had already stopped crying. However, there were still tears in her eyes. She talked in a nasally voice, "Yes. It reminds me of when I had a foot problem. I didn't stop the treatments, and it completely healed later. I understand what you're saying. But my husband has a bad temper after the toxic milk incident. We will get off the ship soon, and he might not have a chance to visit you again. But I will continue to try to explain to him. After we get back home, he can find an acupuncturist to continue his treatments. Thank you."

I treated a male and a female patient, both of whom had been in wheelchairs for a while. Acupuncture treatment brought them new hope in life.

After the first treatment, the female patient was excited and happy. She cried for a whole night because she felt that she would be able to stand up again and walk on her feet. Because acupuncture treatments in Los Angeles are cheaper than those at sea, she planned to go back home for further treatments. She made a special trip to the spa to show her gratitude to me.

7. Vision and Hearing Problems

Watery eyes, blurry vision, double vision (diplopia), painful and swollen red eyes, dry eyes, tinnitus, acquired deafness, machine noise-induced eardrum injury (can be improved).

An ophthalmologist told a patient that without surgery, there was no way to improve her vision. After two acupuncture treatments, the patient was able to see well without her glasses.

There was a patient who'd had three eye surgeries. His eyes were extremely dry. He needed to continuously use eye drops but still felt uncomfortable. After a couple of treatments, he did not need any eye drops for his eyes.

A female patient had blurry vision and intolerable pain in her eye. After five hours of treatment, her uncomfortable eye was fixed. Before the end of previous sessions, I had to pull needles quickly. Otherwise, I could not pull out any needle that was held very tightly by her eyes. Any slow needle withdrawal caused pain due to the muscles holding the needle tightly against the pulling force.

Our bodies are smart. When they need a needle to help in repairs, they don't allow the needle to be pulled out. Instead, they holds the needle tightly to avoid releasing it. During treatment, the body will gradually push the needle out of the body according to the speed of recovery.

8. Emotional Problems

Anxiety, easily feeling sadness, grief, mental stress, unhappiness, motor mind, panic attacks, anger, irritability, nightmares and dreams.

A patient came in for pain treatment. His body was extremely hot. Because he had a good sense of humor, teased him and said, "You'd better start living in a freezer. "The patient replied, "You're right. In the summer, I need to use five or six large ice packs on my body, otherwise it's as hot as an oven. Nobody can get close to me. Even my wife stands two to three feet away to talk to me." Three treatments got rid of his neck and shoulder pain. At the same time, I was able to restore his body temperature to normal. I told him that he could kiss and hug his wife now, and he left happy. This patient's body hotness was caused by tremendous stress.

Besides that, he' had the other two ailments for years—a mildly enlarged spleen, and every month he had to withdraw a half pint of blood because his blood was being over produced. Chinese medicine could have easily treated the case. However, his MD gave him chemotherapy. And eventually he got cancer.

His long-term high stress caused qi stagnation and blood stasis in the spleen, and that induced spleen enlargement. This kind of qi or phlegm stagnation or blood stasis case can happen anywhere and cause tumor or organ enlargement.

Stress caused blood stasis, and the red blood cells stacked together and carried less oxygen than normal. When blood circulated to the kidney and was filtered, the kidney didn't detect enough oxygen in the blood. Therefore, it released EPO protein in the blood. When EPO circulated to the spinal cord, the bone marrow detected the EPO and started to make blood. That's why he had to have blood drawn every month to get rid of the extra.

In TCM treatment, we soothe the liver, and the red blood cells will separate from each other. For mild spleen enlargement where there is mild blood stasis, we can use herbs or acupuncture or both to break the blood stasis.

Once the body organs' functions have been corrected, there are no stacked red blood cells, no qi or phlegm stagnation, and no blood stasis.

If the patient cooperates and does not continually make the situation worse, depending on the treatment method and the severity, the whole process takes one to six months or a little bit longer.

A Vietnam veteran who was an old Indian man could not walk well due to pain. Every night, he was awakened by nightmares of blood and bombs. Within the period of the seven-day cruise, he got my treatments, was able to sleep well without nightmares, and could walk well. The Vietnam War scenes that had bothered him in the past were out of his mind.

After that, his wife, young Korean lady, came in for treatment of her breathing problems and chest pain. This was a very affectionate and exotic couple with a huge age difference. They were very impressive, and it's hard to forget them.

9. Other Problems

Facial rejuvenation, weight loss, detoxification, Parkinson's disease, menopausal syndrome, detoxification, poor balance, nocturia, urinary incontinence, cloudy urine, poor energy, fatigue syndrome, prostate enlargement, dripping menstruation, no menstruation, menstrual syndrome, dysmenorrhea, internal medicines, carving the body curve. Too many to list!

A patient I treated who had the most severe case of poor balance I had seen had had many falls and a history of multiple fractures. After two treatments, she could even walk steadily without her walker on board the ship while South America's high waves tossed it about in the sea.

A two hundred and fifty pound patient came in for weight loss treatments. The second day he came to see me, he had already lost weight. He told me that after the acupuncture treatment, he had nonstop sweating and urination. His body began to feel more and more comfortable. Usually, his pants stayed on his abdomen without a belt, but that morning, his pants fell down to the floor.

Unforgettable Life Lessons on the Cruise Ship

This is the story of four couples who encountered family tragedy.

The first couple:

They were both busy with their own careers and were busy every day, not seeing each other much and hardly to talking to each other. After he was diagnosed with cancer, the husband quit his job. His wife slowed down and stopped working overtime. They seized every minute and every second that they could get to be together. They told me that their life became so very happy. In fact, they already had the world's most precious gift…their spouses. You don't have to work so hard without enjoying life!

The second couple:

The husband rode motorcycles. He had his first accident and had surgery for his fracture. He still had his mobility after the first surgery. After his second accident, he had to have a steel rod inserted in his upper leg. Thereafter, he had unbearable pain. He told me if I reduced his pain by even five percent, he would be grateful. After only the first treatment, the reduction in pain was already beyond what he had imagined.

He also told me that when he worked before, he always picked on his son and blamed him for everything. After his last injury, because he couldn't work and stayed at home, he discovered that his son had so many precious characteristics. His whole attitude toward his son changed. He was proud of his son. His family had more harmony than it did before the accident.

The third couple:

The husband was injured in a car accident. He had many spinal bones protruding externally. The couple discussed their options—having surgery and risking the high possibility of him being paralyzed for his rest of life or not having surgery and keeping his mobility but living with the pain forever. They chose the latter. They came to me to let the husband try an acupuncture treatment. The result was satisfying. They decided to continue the treatments.

The fourth couple:

After the husband's lower back surgery, he walked with a cane. He could not sit and could not maintain any position in bed more than three to five minutes due to unbearable pain. After the first treatment, he could sit. After the second treatment, he told me that he slept better because he didn't have to constantly shift his body.

After his second treatment, I was called to his room. He and his wife were stringing semi-precious stone necklaces and bracelets. They gave me a bracelet and told me that the number and type of stones represented different blessings to me. It was a gift designed by my patient especially for me.

I accepted the bracelet and thanked them.

These four couples have common characteristics—they deeply loved their spouses, and they had lost their family's major income. I asked them the impact of that and received the same feedback: They have a more harmonious family life.

Due to income reduction, their material desires were reduced. They connected with their family members through a sincere caring for each other rather than through expensive gifts. Shopping less, the family members had more time to staying together. All of these things combined to raise overall life happiness and satisfaction.

For friends' birthdays and other events that would normally be celebrated, instead of spending a great deal of money to buy fancy gifts, they spent a small amount to buy materials to make gifts. The gifts were always appreciated because they were created from the heart and couldn't be bought in a store.

Most memorable is their attitude in life. They do not complain, they always feel grateful, they keep life simple but meaningful, and they take a generous, sincere, and practical approach to their life.

Experienced Report from Years Working At Sea

1. When patients follow their healthcare provider's instructions, have an optimistic attitude, and hope to get better sooner, their sickness goes away sooner.

2. If patients maintain a good mood, it improves their qi and blood circulation, and almost any disease can be ridden off quickly.

3. For most patients, soothing their liver, removing their body stagnations, expelling phlegm, and activating blood flow can solve many health issues.

4. Within a certain scope of safety, acupuncturists can flexibly apply needle techniques that they think can help patients instead of following strictly what the book says. For example, at Fenglong ST 40, inserting a three-inch long needle and applying 200 to

300 Hz electrical stimulation can expel sticky phlegm. Jiexue has many magical applications, and I will share more in my later book about acupuncture treatments.

My Ideal Moves Me into the Marvelous Universal Medicine World

One day in September 2010, right after coming back from my clinical training with professor Ni, and during the break in a continuing education class, one of my friends who had decades of medical experience and was an MD in China and a licensed acupuncturist in the US invited me to work with her at her clinic which was located in a good area. She told me that wealthier people had more money to spend than financially comfortable people. People with more money didn't usually have severe ailments and were much easier to treat. They had the money to pay for her services. She said that those with less money saved more of their income for their life enjoyments, and they would bargain for better prices for their treatments. They also tended to have more severe ailments which were difficult to treat. She told me it was difficult to make money from them because of this.

At that time, we had only one car at home, and I needed to drive my youngest son between home and school. My friend's clinic was far away from my home, and Los Angeles' traffic is famously awful. If I worked in her clinic, I would not be able to take care of my youngest son. And taking care of him was my main reason for leaving the cruise ship.

And if I didn't treat the severe or tough cases and treated only the easy ones, then I had spent ten thousand dollars in medical materials for nothing. Since 2009, I'd bought Dr. Ni's book and DVD sets and had put all of my non-working hours into study. In addition, the two months of expenses for living in Florida, the plane tickets, and the car expenses from Merritt Island would all be wasted.

Since I'd left the ship to prepare myself for treating challenging cases, I'd had half a year with no income. In addition, a big curiosity for me was, why were the financially disadvantaged patients more difficult to treat?

The economy wasn't so good at that time. Los Angeles has the highest density of Chinese medical schools and acupuncturists in the whole world. And Southern California has the best weather and attracts new residents from all over. This meant a large influx of acupuncturists from Asian countries who had targeted to settle in Southern California. Many acupuncture clinics accepted subleases in order to relieve the financial pressure. I subleased a nearby clinic.

Because I had worked on a ship for years, I had spent a lot of time on the Internet studying Eastern and Western medical knowledge in order to communicate with my highly educated patients. My good friends lived far away, and I had no relatives living in Southern California.

That meant I had no patient base and no assistance to help me to pull in patients. When I started practicing, I charged my patients the local average, which was only one third of what I could have gotten if I had driven thirty miles north or south. The higher charge was what I deserved for the quality of my service.

The Difficulties of Providing Excellent Treatment to Financially Disadvantaged Patients While Still Making Money

The clinic had just opened when I immediately encountered difficulties. When patients came to visit, many of them tried to cut my price down or did not follow instructions and abused their health. Some always missed their appointments without notice, which makes treatment effectiveness drop and sometimes even causes new diseases or symptoms to crop up.

They had no concept of taking measures to prevent sickness and did not accept my advice. Many of them liked to complain—they saw what other people had and were not satisfied with what they had. They didn't appreciate or give gratitude to those who gave them favors and did not know how to cultivate morals or spirit to prevent sickness. Of course, they refused education on how to stay away from sickness and remain healthy.

The above stated things caused more severe blockage than that of my patients at sea. So although I could easily treat two patients in an hour at sea, in my own clinic, I had to focus all of my energy and work very hard for at least one and half to three hours per patient in order to attain my satisfied treatment result.

The most difficult part of that for me was that a lot of the severely sick patients had no money to pay my required fee. Moreover, they listened and trusted too much incorrect medical information. They had lost the ability and to apply attention to their body's warning signs and make their own decisions.

Treatment effectiveness is the summation of the sickness itself, the prognosis, acupuncture and herbs, the patient's effort and input, the patient's self-abuse, how well the patient follows the healthcare provider's instructions, the environment, and outside influences on health.

A patient's self-abuse includes going to bed late, keeping an irregular lifestyle, an unhealthy diet, lack of exercise, negative thinking and emotions, and overworking himself.

The patient needs to follow his health care provider's instructions, including visiting at the first sign of sickness or as instructed or as needed (in other words, be timely with medical treatment), taking medicines on time, maintaining a regular and healthy lifestyle, not overdoing activities, going to bed early, eating a healthy diet, exercising, pursuing the correct ethical/mental concepts, and maintaining positive thinking and a positive mood.

Timely medical treatment means getting the next treatment before the effects of the previous one start to diminish. By doing so, the sickness will continue to improve until you get rid of the root problem.

Both at sea and in the wealthier locales, I would ask patients to make their next appointment, and I could expect them to be very responsible about keeping it. But later when I practiced on land in the not-so-wealthy areas, unless requesting critically ill patients to return to the clinic on time, I learned to keep my mouth closed.

Those patients' health standards tended to be lower, and money was more important than their health. I was quickly educated by their uncomfortable glares when I would request them to schedule the next appointment.

Even some of the better educated patients would give me a list of excuses why they could not make the next appointment. As a proactive healthcare provider, I felt that I was not doing my job. It was a very helpless feeling.

So instead asking them to come back, I did my best to spend more time treating each patient in order to get the best results. That way, they could go a longer time without treatment.

Was there a solution to this? My previous solution was to ignore my meager savings and—no matter how much a patient paid me, and sometimes even without pay—treat the patient. It was because so many patients were their family's financial supporter, and I worried about them losing their jobs or spending money without getting the needed result.

For those patients who wanted to bargain the charge down, and whose illnesses were not severe, I let them find another acupuncturist.

I closed my clinic when I had no more room to spend money for patients. I am very grateful that I found Comprehensive Universal Energy Healing where it is so easy to uncover one's own self-healing power.

A satisfactory treatment result for a patient means totally unblocking the meridians I focus on in the treatment. For example, if I do moxibustion on Youngquan (KI1), the patient should feel the qi running in the Conception Vessel (Ren Meridian) and Governor Vessel (Du Meridian), to the front side kidney channels, to the back four urinary bladder channel lines, and then to the neck. Then I can stop the treatment.

The theory behind it is that a fully unblocked pipe is hard to get blocked. The total overall treatment effectiveness is higher. It can be maintain for a long time and avoid invasion from other diseases. The total treatment time and cost are lower than a regular treatment as well. The time needed depends on the individual. This approach is more beneficial for patients today. You can use Google Translate to read #109 item in Appendix Nine References. In Appendix Eight Reference also can benefit for your knowledge.

To deal with those difficulties, I found some solutions:

1. Often, the greatest way is the easiest way. I created a simple formula—raw herbs ground into powder and used with moxibustion treatments. It increased the treatment's effectiveness two to six times. It can be used to treat the following: harmonizing cancer patient's yin and yang, kidney dialysis, multiple sclerosis, pain syndromes, qi deficiency, qi stagnation and blood stasis, heart valvular insufficiency, myotonic myopathy, dizziness caused by Governor (Du) meridian qi deficiency, lack of energy in the morning, disc herniation or bulging disc, disc displacement, narrow disc, organ prolapse, and various yang deficiency cases. For pain, it does not apply to broken skin but can treat muscles, tendon tightness and hardening, common pain syndromes, abdominal pain due to a cold.

2. Because the general public needs to be educated in Chinese medicine, I set aside one hour a week to learn how to make a website. I started posting knowledge related to Chinese medicine. Most posts are original writing and reporting from my own learning and experience.

3. I teach patients to start practicing love and gratitude with their family members. Treatment effectiveness can be speeded up in this way, and it positively influences their interpersonal relationships, health, and good fortune. When living in a prolonged state of love and gratitude, many people are highly aware of their language and behavior, and they can think about what they should change in order to improve themselves to avoid making mistakes and hurting others.

4. I concluded that my patients' sicknesses were connected to their mindset. I posted Raise Up Your Energy Frequency to Avoid Sickness[160].

Learned Longevitology and Discovered Universal Codes

My classmate Catherine Lu, L.Ac. invited me to attend entry and intermediate level combined classes for Longevitology. I went with Catherine to learn about it. Later, I was assigned as a group leader to coordinate member's practice and do volunteer jobs.

At our first meeting, I was eager to spread love and gratitude. I thought that energy healing, love, gratitude, sharing and collaboration might be combined and spread out together. I found a member and did a demonstration for the members. Using the four universal codes combined with the cosmic energy healing, the healing power immediately increased. Afterward, I thought that might be my mission—to spread the ethical and cosmic energy together.

This discovery is a huge universal gift. People feel their power and benefit immediately.

Using universal energy and the codes to improve the general public's health depends entirely on people's input and efforts to make it a part of their daily activity and a social habit to change society's whole environment.

When using universal energy to do healing, if the person being healed can think about love and show gratitude to that source of love, the universal energy passing through his body immediately increases many times.

Two persons collaborating to do healing have far more power than a single person crossing his arms to do self-healing?

The universal codes are the key to opening yourself to cosmic help for your life.

Applications in Hypnosis

After I had earned my NGH hypnotherapist certificate, when I finishing needling in an acupuncture treatment, I would ask for the patient's consent to do hypnotherapy and obtained amazing results for a variety of illnesses. The speed for expelling phlegm, detoxifying liver toxins, and unblocking pain syndrome was often three or four times faster than regular acupuncture treatment alone.

The most amazing result was when I treated a patient who felt her yin and yang might be separated at any time. On her tongue was a black and gray coating. Her body was extremely cold, her pulse was very thin, and her shen (spirit) wasn't staying with her. She felt very blue. I used acupuncture and moxibustion, but it did not improve her mood.

With her permission, I tried hypnosis to solve her negative sensation.

I use hypnotherapy in many of my treatments. It's especially helpful in changing a patient's habits. Usually after only one session, the patient can make a change. After that, I don't have to act like a detective and try to figure out how a patient abused his body or which of my instructions he didn't follow. I also don't have to spend time trying to convince patients to adopt my advice to improve their health. What a relief for me!

Hypnosis can be used for longevity, rejuvenation, and self-healing.

In December 2013 at the monthly meeting of the LA Chapter of the NGH, I learned that only two percent of hypnosis certificate holders can use hypnosis to help clients solve their life or health issues.

In August 2014 at the NGH worldwide convention, I was one of the presenters to speak. My subject was "How to Combine Universal Energy and Hypnosis in Facial Rejuvenation: How to Treat Pop-Up Veins."

Some of My On-Land Cases

1. Pineal gland enlargement can cause an increase in intracranial pressure and pain. Two acupuncture treatments with moxibustion treatments made the pain go away.

2. Sjogren's syndrome, nearly fifteen years with Bell's Palsy, pain in multiple places, and chronic flu—overall improvement within eighteen hours of treatments.

3. Diabetes patient with hypertension, whole body edema which kept worsening, glucose level of 160. She'd had dialysis three times a week for more than a year. After one month of acupuncture and moxibustion treatments, the patient had clear urine, 1200 cc daily urine output, and a 110 in blood sugar level. Edema was gone and dialysis decreased to twice a week. The patient's husband told me the cost was $2,500 per dialysis.

4. A patient's lung capacity was only 1000 cc. I had her do qi gong by only and close arms and hands to expand her chest—every day for ten to fifteen minutes, once or twice per day. Two weeks later, her lung capacity had increased to 1500 cc.

5. A patient with urinary bladder cancer migrant to the lymph nodes had a loss of appetite. He refused to take herbs. In less than three months (and within that period always skipping treatments), there were two kidney function tests which showed an improvement in kidney function. This patient also gradually grew out black hair and a black beard. His cancer did not further spread, and his energy became better.

6. A female patient had pancreatic cancer which was migrating to her liver, spleen, stomach, duodenum, and small intestine. More than a month after surgery, she had no appetite, no energy, and an abdominal scar that was wide and thick. She could not fall asleep early and was awake until anywhere between one and three in the morning. Her hands and feet were icy cold.

   She had two moxibustion treatments. The first time was an hour and a half treatment. The second was a half hour treatment. Her appetite was restored after the first treatment. Her physical energy recovered, her hands and feet became warm, her whole body blood circulation improved, and her scar became thin and narrow. The first treatment was accompanied by hypnotherapy, and from that point on, she was able to fall asleep between ten and eleven at night and wake at 6:00 am the next morning to go a nearby park to exercise. Later, her MD checked her and told her that she had no more cancer cells.

7. A terminal stage nasal cancer migrant patient had no appetite, no energy, difficulty breathing, and discomfort in his nose because the nasal cancer cells were putting pressure on the brain. After one acupuncture and moxibustion treatment, his appetite recovered, his energy was good, his nose felt comfortable, and the pressure in his brain was gone.

8. After treatments, a myocardial infarction patient had no myocardial infarction, heartache, or chest pain.

9. A patient had severely watering eyes. After treatments, the eyes stopped watering.

10. Thirty years of chronic stomach pain was gone after treatments.

Other cases will be reported in future books.

Tribulations Revisited

My youngest son entered a regular university in the fall of 2013. I had intended to sell our house and move to a wealthier area to reopen my clinic. Unfortunately, reality set in, and I was unable to do so.

What could I do? Maybe I ought to change my job!

Mary Morrissey's Programs

Since 2013, I have participated in spiritual teacher Mary Morrissey's Brave Thinking Masters, DreamBuilder, Life Mastery Consultant, and Quantum Leap programs and training courses.

From Mary, I learned that our DNA has recorded on it our life missions for us to execute.

Unfortunately, that same DNA string can easily be covered in the dust of pursuing money, social rank, power, and sexuality. We must enrich our inner morals and culture to fortify ourselves against the dust, or our confidence to carry out our life mission will be constrained by improper concepts acquired from education or personal experience.

Everyone has the possibility of brilliant achievement in their lifetime.

The breadth and depth of my medical practice has covered almost everything. I've nourished couples before pregnancy so that the next generation will be robust. I've provided disease prevention to increase healing and minimize illnesses and have helped people to raise their body, mind, and spirit frequency to fight against diseases. I've guided people to follow their dreams and build a direction in life and have encouraged them to continuously generate even greater dreams.

Maybe it's my destiny, or maybe my mission has not yet been fulfilled. Every time I advance to the higher level courses, there are always patients referring others to me or potential patients who have read my website or patients who were attracted by my five-star reviews on Yelp or other acupuncturists or my friends or previous classmates who would come to me to ask about tough or severe diseases. Based on my humanity, I gave them free consultations, and it took away from my precious time to earn a living. These kinds of phone calls continued for four long months. My mind and heart were severely disturbed and hurt by hearing so many distressing stories of hardships and illnesses.

I started to ask myself why, instead of spending my precious time facing all these unseen challenges to save lives and answering all of these questions, why don't I write books that can guide people to the path of heaven or help them build ladders to reach heaven? It will be more meaningful—and a lot easier. It will take less effort on my part but give more productive results.

So at 6:00 am on January 1, 2014, I sat down to write my first book in Chinese. The interruptions for disease consultations were stopped. I concentrated on my book writing for a full six months without a single phone call. This peaceful time was unbelievably precious to me.

Concluding Report for my Experiences from 2010 - 2013

1. A person's health is his own business.

2. Bodies need exercises and movement, the mind needs cultivation, and spirit needs to be enhanced. They are indispensable to a person's health.

3. Rather than you looking for professional treatments, taking medicines by yourself, or using equipment to help improve your health, you should rely on your own effort to gain health and feel better.

   A Chinese Medicine physician is good for preventive health care, but there is no one cannot totally replace your own responsibility to activate your proper body functions, cultivate your mind, and promote your spirit.

4. Anyone who doesn't cultivate his mind and spirit can precipitate a lot of diseases.

5. Discontent or longing can cause health to be downgraded. Dream builder skills should be learned by everyone.

6. Anyone with severe sickness should use moxibustion or yang property herbs to treat it in order to improve the situation.

7. Every person has self-healing power. Self-healing power can be gained through universal energy or self-hypnosis. Moral cultivation, repenting for faults, and making up for mistakes can rid you of diseases. There are numerous real cases in China where diseases were cured in this way. There are featured videos of Philanthropist Liu[92] using talking to treat diseases.

   Philanthropist Liu is not a medical professional. He uses the traditional Chinese ethic of interpersonal relationship to educate people. Then, even cancer patients can sense their behaviors are wrong, corrected it, and recover. There are a lot cases posted on the YouTube.

8. Hypnosis has a unique effectiveness and can improve the body physically, mentally, and spiritually.

9. Psyche is also effective to treat patients.

10. Comprehensive Universal Energy Healing can help many health issues. But money and manpower is needed for medical research in this area.

11. Practicing universal codes has a positive impact on the body, mind, and spirit.

12. Moxibustion can help body functions recover, maintain a healthy longevity, and shrink cancer cells.

    It is a new direction to treat patients with cancers, deviated functions, and rare case diseases. It is worth doing more clinical research on moxibustion treatments even though Chinese medical records have recorded many successful cases reported. To be widely accepted by the Western world, extensive clinical research is necessary.

13. The herbal powder I created for external use in severe cases is worthy of clinical trials. It increases treatment effectiveness two to six times. It avoids the side effects of drugs, saves the time of practitioners, provides a simplified treatment, and reduces overall cost for both the patient and caregiver.

On the other hand, due to this herb's strong penetration ability, when a deep needle is needed to reach the tight/hard inner layer of the chest or abdominal cavities, it could cause damage to the organs. In this case, a shallower needle in a safer location of the outside muscle layer be used in order to avoid endangering the patient's life (pneumothorax or liver or any internal organ bleeding without notice).

Before I created this external herbal formula, in order to treat those patients well, I risk myself to needle patient with extra care and sometimes, I had cold sweating. Afterward, I kept praying until next time to see patient visiting me safely.

Usually, this kind patient does not have money to pay treatments. I do this way to avoid using intake herbs to add more treatment cost.

My next project is to produce it in bandage or another convenient form and perform clinical trials for a broader application.

14. I discovered an acupuncture point on the upper arm that can unblock many different body parts. If we can discover similar points on all four limbs, it would bring convenience to regular schools taught acupuncture points.* Patients could lie on the treatment bed in a comfortable position without having to remove clothing or change clothes. In addition, acupuncture treatments would require fewer needles.

> * Dong's acupuncture is not usually taught in acupuncture schools. It does not require taking off clothes or facing down to do needling, and it uses fewer needles.

15. Universe is great and amazing. It can be as big as no boundary or as small as the Planck **P length**, denoted ℓP, equal to $1.616199(97) \times 10^{-35}$ meters that contains ultimate mystery and fun. You may bounce between them as freely as you wish. They are "mutually linked and mutually influenced." How can we exclude them?

16. Hypnotic self-healing will be discussed in more detail in later books.

The above is an introduction to my medical path and medical discoveries in hopes that you will gain a preliminary understanding of my professional background, attitude, thoughts, and views on the medical field as well as its research challenges. It's my hope to have more people to join in self-healing, expand the universal codes and energy healing applications, and initiate clinical trials to open a new page for the medical field. For human health and for good fortune, let's paint together a beautiful picture for the future.

Life is priceless in its honor and dignity. This is the gift—and my mission—that I want to bring to people. Health is a stepping stone to achieving a rich life. My desire is to integrate the different fields of medicine to create one healthy and happy global village. Everyone has the right to be healthy.

Conclusion

1. Everyone has the right to be happy, healthy, and wealthy.

2. One cannot earn real happiness from selfishness. Treating other people well is fundamental to physical and mental good health.

3. To be happy and healthy is everyone's responsibility and obligation. Others can assist, but that cannot replace your job to achieve it.

4. Medical methodologies, policies, and systems should be simplified in order to avoid them being abused.

5. The highest level of medical field is the combination of medical ethics and art. It is the assertion of humanity!

6. A country's medical affairs and health concepts determine whether its foundation is strong or not.

APPENDIX SEVEN
Our Websites
•••••••••••••••••

1. This book's website: UniversalEnergyHealing.us

2. Our main site: universaltcmtc.com

Site Map

Home Welcome Our Value Knowledge Frieda Testimonials Services FAQ

Videos Qi Gong – Chinese Exercises Health Tips Privacy Policy Healthy Life

Life Wisdom to Healthcare Providers New Concepts Wrong Concepts

Research that We Support Thanks Blog Contact Us

傳統中文 tc.universal.com is the website for our traditional Chinese readers.

简体中文 sc.universaltcm.com is the website for the simplified Chinese readers.

Mobile mobile.universaltcm.com is a quick glance guide for TCM preventive healthcare.

Happy Pin happypinmasterhealer.com shares cases and clinical knowledge to let patients know their condition is treatable and let healthcare professionals know how to think and how to treat.

NBAARC nbaarc.com Natural Born Abundant Ability Recovery Center raises patients' energy frequency and fulfills their life missions in many ways. Currently, it is combined with the UniversalEnergyHealing.us training program.

1. Patients are involved in their own health and treatment.

2. We offer guidance, coaching, and consulting for your health and your dreams.

3. Patients staying here are givers and know how to give gratitude, respect, and rewards to others.

Self-Healing universalenergyhealing.us uses Comprehensive Universal Energy Healing as a tool to help you learn self-healing. The book(s) teaches people how to recover self-healing power and how to do self-healing.

This is intended to be a series of books. The first book teaches readers how to alleviate their pain, stress, and insomnia problems, under what circumstances they can do self-healing, and when to seek a professional's help.

APPENDIX EIGHT

Our Unique External-Use Herbal Formula

● ●

The basic concept is that after the Chinese medicine physician or acupuncturist has balanced a patient's body, the body's internal environment is not fit for diseases to exist. It changes the body's internal environment so that the virus, bacteria, and cancer cells die. Chinese medicine is a precious crystal of wisdom in the medical field with 250 million years of development.

My herbal formula is a pure, natural herbal product and totally green. For convenience of application, it would be best put into a bandage form or in environmentally friendly paper bags that can be cut to size for use with acupuncture.

The original product is in powder form and mixes with wine to form a paste. It is used with both acupuncture and moxibustion (if interested, you can Google to learn how).

It was originally created to treat a cancer migrant patient with no appetite and an extremely cold body. Then I gradually expanded its applications in my clinic and my acupuncturist friends began to use it as well. All of them received positive feedback from their patients.

The brother of a terminal stage nasal cancer patient with a bad mood, no appetite, and difficulty breathing called me to ask for help with his brother. He wanted his brother to feel more comfortable as he neared the end of his life. After one treatment with my formula, his mood and appetite recovered, and his breathing was much better. After using moving moxibustion without the herb, the pressure on his brain from his nasal cancer cells disappeared.

Benefits:

1. It can solve a lot tough cases, and it made many non- treatable diseases become treatable at a very low cost.
2. In general, the treatment effectiveness is two to six times higher than without using it.
3. It saves costs in herbal inventory, ordering, training herbalists, and preparation and treatment.

Application scope: External use.

1. Severe cases such as any kind of cancer, kidney dialysis, MS, chronic fatigue syndrome, low immunity, low organ functions, and any yang deficiency syndrome.
2. Pain caused by cold, tight muscles or tight tendons,

A friend in China did a clinical trial in China for a variety of pain, including cancer pain, and got positive results.

All tough cases are caused by a yang deficiency because yang qi controls the functions and has hot/warm properties.

All patients with cancer and tough-to-treat diseases have cold body and lower body functions.

This formula strongly promotes yang qi and its flowing. A professional must do the application.

If there is a pile of spoiled foods, it attracts flies, ants, and roaches. To expel these pests, it is necessary to keep a clean environment. Western medicine applies pesticide to kill the pests. TCM removes the spoiled foods and avoids the application of external poisons. That's the difference in their approach. TCM treatment does not require lab tests and does not use toxic poisons which cause side effects. That's why acupuncture is spreading so broadly in the Western world.

Please go to http://contest.techbriefs.com/2015/entries/medical/5310 to vote this formula for "Conquer Cancer and Hard to Treat Diseases."

APPENDIX NINE

References
• • • • • • • • • • • • • •

Appendix Nine References[231] lists all references used in the book. Though we do our best to cover all, we may be missing some due to reading a long time ago or forgetting the part of the content that was cited from somewhere. It's not our intention to do so. But it was used as a common sense and forgot to check its source. We'd appreciate if anyone can point mistakes out, and we will do our best to make it up. Thanks very much.

Meanwhile, due to academic research reports lagging behind what's available in the world, a lot of resources are from the internet. However, internet links change often. Therefore, we highly recommend you go to the book reference to check the most current ones. In case the material was deleted, we will find a similar or more advanced one to replace it. If we cannot find any substitute, we will let you know. Thanks for your understanding.

Citation is based on Journal citation http://www.easybib.com/reference/guide/mla/journal for journals.

1. Han, Yu. 古文觀止·韓愈〈進學解〉 *Advanced Study Solution of Gui Wen Guan Zhi.*

2. 黃帝內經 *Huang Di Nei Jing.*

3. Lao Zi. 春秋•老聃《道德经》 *Dao De Jing.*

4. 永不過時的50句名言#22, The #22 quote of 50 Timeless Quotes. <http://www.360doc.com/content/12/1011/15/535749_240858483.shtml>

5. 幾個小哲理故事 #6, #5, #4, #1 Several small philosophical stories: #6, #5, #4, #1. <http://www.360doc.com/14/0106/09/12338379_342965600.shtml>.

6. Sahng, Hui. 針灸穴位學速讀•商玉惠主篇 *A Quick Study of Acupuncture Locations.*

7. 長生學入門•國際版•長生學慈善基金會 *The Fundamentals of Longevitology.* International Edition, Chang Sen Xue Longevity Association.

8. 長生學進階•長生學慈善基金會 *The Advanced Longevitology*. Chang Sen Xue Longevity Association.

9. 再連結療癒法•艾力克•波爾著•黃愛淑譯•生命潛能出版社

10. 中華百科全書 傳記 黃帝 *Chinese Encyclopedia Biography of the Huang Di (Yellow Emperor)*. <http://ap6.pccu.edu.tw/Encyclopedia/data.asp?id=4884>.

11. Ritz, S. GRAVITATIONAL collapse, BLACK holes (Astronomy) GAMMA rays et al. *Overview of the GLAST Mission and Opportunities, AIP Conference Proceedings*. 92.1 (2007): 3-7.

12. Ulrich, H., Apel, W. D., ,Arteaga, J. C., et al. *The Knee of Cosmic Rays — News from KASCADE*. AIP Conference Proceedings. 928.1 (2007): 31-38.

13. Ciubotariu, Ciprian, Ciubotariu, Carmen-Iuliana, Ciubotariu, Corneliu. *Extracting Energy from Cosmic Electromagnetic Fields and Plasmas by a Chaotic Gun Effect for Relativistic Charged Particles*. AIP Conference Proceedings. 746.1 (2005): 1387-1394.

14. Quest, Penelope and Roberts, Kathy. *The Reiki Manual*.

15. Pearl, Eric. *The Origin of Reconnective Healing*. <http://connecttohealing.com/origin.html>.

16. *The Science of the Reconnection*. <http://connecttohealing.com/science.html>.

17. *Universal Human Body Energy* UDPHT, UHBE. <http://uhbe.org/?q=zh-hant/node/242>.

18. Schwartz, Gary E. and Simon, William L. *The Energy Healing Experiments (Science Reveals Our Natural Power to Heal)*. New York: Atria Books.

19. 瑜伽Yuga. *<http://zh.wikipedia.org/wiki/>*.

20. Noel, Mary *Network Spinal Analysis: A Review*. <http: //www.logan.edu/mm/files/LRC/Senior-Research /1999-Aug-51.pdf>.

21. Cross, John R. (2006). *Healing with the Chakra Energy System*. North Atlantic Books.

22. 旋轉查克拉中心-頂輪 *Lightweb*. <http://lightweb.uho.com.tw/articles3/96/381.html#.U35l9yitzXw>.

23. 七脈輪簡單介紹 *Brief Introduction to the Seven Chakras*. <http://airika.pixnet.net/blog/post/34429680-七脈輪簡單介紹>.

24. 清理脈輪 *Dying Consciously—The Greatest Journey*. <http://www.dyingconsciously.org/ceremony_cleansing_the_chakras-Chinese.htm>.

25. Gallob, R. "Reiki: A Supportive Therapy in Nursing Practice and Self-Care for Nurses." *Journal of the New York State Nurses Association*. 34.1 (2003): 9-13.

26. Catlin, Anita and Taylor-Ford, Rebecca L. "Investigation of Standard Care Versus Sham Reiki Placebo Versus Actual Reiki Therapy to Enhance Comfort and Well-Being in a Chemotherapy Infusion Center." *Oncology Nursing Forum*. (2011).

27. Baldwin, A.L. and Schwartz, G.E. "Personal Interaction with a Reiki Practitioner Decreases Noise-Induced Microvascular Damage in an Animal Model." *Journal of Alternative & Complementary Medicine.* Department of Physiology, College of Medicine, University of Arizona. 12.1 (2006): 15-22.

28. Baldwin, Ann Linda, Fullmer, Kirstin, and Schwartz, Gary E. "Comparison of Physical Therapy with Energy Healing for Improving Range of Motion in Subjects with Restricted Shoulder Mobility." *Evidence-Based Complementary & Alternative Medicine (eCAM).* 2013.

29. Bowden, Deborah, Goddard, Lorna, and Gruzelier, John. "A Randomised Controlled Single-Blind Trial of the Efficacy of Reiki at Benefitting Mood and Well-Being." *Evidence-Based Complementary & Alternative Medicine (eCAM).* 8.1 (2011): 1-8.

30. Morse, Melvin L. and Beem, Lance W. "Benefits of Reiki Therapy for a Severely Neutropenic Patient with Associated Influences on a True Random Number Generator." *Journal of Alternative & Complementary Medicine,* 17.12 (2011): 1181-1190.

31. Brooks, Audrey J., Schwartz, Gary E., Reece, Katie, et al. "The Effect of Johrei Healing on Substance Abuse Recovery: A Pilot Study." *Journal of Alternative & Complementary Medicine,* 12.7 (2006): 625-631.

32. Reece, Katie, Schwartz, Gary E., Brooks, Audrey J., et al. "Positive Well-Being Changes Associated with Giving and Receiving Johrei Healing." *Journal of Alternative & Complementary Medicine,* 11.3 (2005):455-457.

33. Johrei, *http://en.wikipedia.org/wik/iJohrei.*

34. Desy, Phylameana Lila. *What is Johrei Healing?* <http://healing.about.com/cs/holistictherapies/a/aa_johrei.htm>.

35. *Johrei - Divine Universal Energy.* <http://www.johrei-institute.org/>.

36. Allison, Nancy (ed.). *The Illustrated Encyclopedia of Body-mind Disciplines.*

37. *Dr. Michael Whelan on Network Spinal Analysis* <http://www.youtube.com/watch?v=1WVut4Ep0AI>.

38. *Advancing New Strategies for Living & Healing in our Rapidly Changing World,* NSA. <http://www.donaldepstein.com/nsa/network.shtml>.

39. "Spirituality, Healing, and Medicine." *The British Journal of General Practice.* 4.351 (1991): 425–427. <http://www.ncbi.nlm.nih.gov/pmc/articles/PMC1371827/>

40. 地球生物的DNA正在被改變 The DNA of Life on Earth is Being Changed. <http://www.ufotm.com/thread-1178-1-1.html>.

41. Ulrich, H., Apel, W. D., Arteaga, J. C., et al. "The Knee of Cosmic Rays — News." *KASCADE, AIP Conference Proceedings.* 928.1 (2007): 31-38.

42. Chertok, I. M., Grechnev, V. V., and Meshalkina, N. S. "On the Correlation between Spectra of Solar Microwave Bursts and Proton Fluxes near the Earth. *Astronomy Reports*. 53.11 (2009): 1059-1069.

43. Kirsanova, M. S. and Wiebe, D. S. "The Effect of the Ionization Rate on the Chemical Composition of Dense Cores of Dark Molecular Clouds." *Astronomy Reports*. 48.9 (2004): 705-715.

44. Launonen, T., Ashton, D., and, Keane, P. "Growth, Nutrient Acquisition, and Ectomycorrhizae of Eucalyptus Regnans Seedlings in Fertilized or Diluted Air-Dried and Undried Forest Soil. *Plant & Soil*. 268.12, (2005): 221-231.

45. Schwartz, Gary E. and Simon, William L. (2007). Unlocking the Mystery of Invisible Energy Fields. *The Energy Healing Experiments (Science Reveals Our Natural Power to Heal)*. Atria Books.

46. Stevenson, Richard J., Prescott, John, and Boakes, Robert A. "Confusing Tastes and Smells: How Odours can Influence the Perception of Sweet and Sour Tastes." *Oxford Journals*. 24.6 627-635.

47. *Alice in Wonderland Syndrome* <http://en.wikipedia.org/wiki/Alice_in_Wonderland_syndrome>.

48. 基本粒子*Basic Particles*. <http://zh.wikipedia.org/wiki/基本粒子>.

49. Earth shape picture from *NASA*. <*http://goo.gl/Sy4s1e*>.

50. 地球素顏照形狀醜陋網友稱毀三觀　*The Urgly Outlook of the Earth talked by Internet Viewers*. <http://www.youtube.com/watch?v=H7fTvD18SGc>.

51. *Probable Benefits and Risks – Gastric Electrical Stimulation*. <http://www.medtronic.com/patients/gastroparesis/device/probable -benefit-and-risks/>.

52. *Spinal Cord Stimulation for Chronic Pain*. <http://www.spine-health.com /treatmentback-surgery/spinal-cord-stimulation-chronic-pain>.

53. "Electrical Cardioversion (Defibrillation) for a Fast Heart Rate." *WebMD Home*. <http://goo.gl/Xi4sLO>.

54. *Electroconvulsive Therapy*. <http://en.wikipedia.org/wiki/Electroconvulsive_therapy>.

55. Massarweh, Nader N., Cosgriff, Ned, and Slakey, Douglas P. *Electrosurgery: History, Principles, and Current and Future Uses*. <http://www.albertahealthservices.ca/ps-1009154-electrocautery.pdf>.

56. "中醫史, A+醫學百科 >> 中醫史, *Chinese Medicine History*." *A + Medical Encyclopedia*. <http://cht.a-hospital.com/w/中醫史>.

57. 中醫刺灸水針療法, 醫學電子書 >> 《中醫刺灸》 >> 水針療法, *Chinese Medicine Acupuncture and Moxibution/Watery Injection Therapy*, Medical Ebooks >> "Chinese Acupuncture and Moxibustion" >> Watery Acupuncture <http://cht.a-hospital.com/w/中醫刺灸水針療法>.

58. 水疗法 Hydrotherapy,《理疗学》> 第九章　温热疗法 Physiotherapy > Chapter Nine Heat Therapy. <http://www.zysj.com.cn/lilunshuji/liliaoxue993-12-6.html>.

59. *Water Cure.* <http://en.wikipedia.org/wiki/Water_cure_%28therapy%29>.

60. 马王堆帛书，　开放分类：*书法设备历史文学秦汉考古编辑出版史,* Mawangdui Silk book, Open Category: Calligraphy Device Historical Literature, *Qin and Han Archeology Editing and Publishing History.* <http://www.baike.com/wiki/马王堆帛书>.

61. 拔罐療法的發展歷史 [原創 2007-9-20 10:52:43], *The History of The Cupping Therapy* [The Original 2007-9-20 10:52:43] <http://zhengtj.blog.hexun.com.tw/13048745_d.html>.

62. 王洪圖教授, 北京中醫藥大學, 黃帝內經 第二講 書名由來、作者、成書年代背景及流傳, *The Second Lecture of the Huang Di Nei Jing (Yellow Emperor) The Origin of the Book Title, Author, Book's background and Spread,* by Professor Wang, Hongtu, Beijing University of Chinese Medicine. <http://www.theqi.com/cmed/class/class7/nj_02.html>.

63. 《周易乾鑿度》 *Zhou Yi (Book of Changes), The Universe Forming Theory.* <http://baike.baidu.com/view/1383632.htm>.

64. Barlow, Fiona, Walker, Jan, and Lewith, George. "Effects of Spiritual Healing for Women Undergoing Long-Term Hormone Therapy for Breast Cancer: A Qualitative Investigation." *Journal of Alternative & Complementary Medicine.* 19.3 (2013): 211-6.

65. 伏羲 *Fu Xi.* < http://baike.baidu.com/view/13762.htm>.

66. 旧石器时代, *Paleolithic.* <http://zh.wikipedia.org/wiki/旧石器时代>.

67. Song, Mingjin, Lao Zi and Zhuang Zi Ethos. 宋明瑾, 老子思想與養生氣功, 臺灣大學老莊風貌, *Lao Zi Thoughts and Healthy Qigong.* National Taiwan University. <http://club.ntu.edu.tw/~davidhsu/New-Lao-Chuang -Lecture/LAO/lao-paperG001.ht>.

68. Peng, Shu Zhi. 彭述之, 老子的哲學及其社會思想, 中文馬克思主義文庫 -> 彭述之, 一九四六年四月, 原刊于一九四六年在上海出版的《求真杂志》第一卷第一期, *The Lao Zi's philosophy and His Social Thoughts.* <https://www.marxists.org/chinese/pengshuzhimarxist.org-chinese -peng-194604.htm>.

69. Huang, Chun-Lin 東方易經大學黃春霖校長之易經八卦命理風水名片姓名取名十大認識, 東方首頁 > 案例實證 > 易經(八卦)卜卦實證案例-易經風水大學, *The Ten Fundamentals of Understanding the Naming in The Eight Divinatory Trigrams, Numerology, Feng Shui and Name of The Yi Jing (The Book of Changes).* <http://www.oycu.org/Case/case-more.aspx?id=106&clsid=9>.

70. 郭璞, *Pu Guo,* The Feng Shui Originator in the Chinese History (276-324). <http://blog.sina.com.cn/sblog_5fa7641c0100cpwh.html>.

71. Indriolo, Nick and McCall, Benjamin J. "Investigating the Cosmic-Ray Ionization Rate in the Galactic Diffuse Interstellar Medium through Observation of H+3." *The Astrophysical Journal.* <http//:m.iopscience.iop.org /0004-637X/745/1/91>.

72. Ruini, Chiara and Vescovelli, Francesca. "The Role of Gratitude in Breast Cancer: Its Relationships with Post-Traumatic Growth, Psychological Well-Being, and Distress." *Journal of Happiness Studies.* 14.1 (2013): 263-274.

73. Stanley, Ruth. "Types of Prayer, Heart Rate Variability, and Innate Healing." *Journal of Religion & Science.* 44.4 (2009): 825-846.

74. Toussaint, Loren and Friedman, Philip. "Forgiveness, Gratitude, and Well-Being: The Mediating Role of Affect and Beliefs." *Journal of Happiness Studies.* 10.6. (2009): 635-654.

75. Puzeras, E., Tautvaišienė, G., and Cohen, J. G. "High-Resolution Spectroscopic Study of Red Clump Stars in the Galaxy: Iron-Group Elements." *Monthly Notices of the Royal Astronomical Society.* 408.2 (2010): 1225-1232.

76. 灵气疗法, *Reiki.* <http://zh.wikipedia.org/wiki/灵气疗法>.

77. Stein, Diana. (199-). *Essential Reiki—A Complete Guide to an Ancient Healing Art.* Freedom, CA: The Crossing Press, Inc.

78. *Interview with Scientific Hand Analysis Practitioner Jane Sanders.* <http://goo.gl/nDqMOY>.

79. 出手真靈光, *It Really Works by Press Your Hand On.* <http://www.simonchau.hk/Chinese_B5/cancer/letter28.htm>.

80. 拜見祖師爺~人電學第3關卡, *Meet the Original Master ~ Human Bio-Electrical Energy the 3rd Gate.* <http://blog.xuite.net/shy200415/twblog/116438678-拜見祖師爺~人電學第3關卡>.

81. *About Donald Epstein, D.C.* <http://www.donaldepstein.com/drepstein.shtml/>.

82. *SRI: 12 Stages of Healing.* <http://www.familynetworkchiropractic.com/sri-12-stages-of-healing/>.

83. 光子, *Photon.* <http://zh.wikipedia.org/光子>.

84. 2/24人體能量場的知識分享之後(小樹), *After Sharing the Human Energy Field Knowledge (Little Tree).* <http://blog.udn.com/scentiye/4930107>.

85. *Johrei.* <http:en.wikipedia.orgwikiJohrei>.

86. *Frequently Asked Questions.* <http://www.johrei-institute.org/faq.htm>.

87. Ahlers, Markus. "The Cosmic Triad: Cosmic Rays, Gamma-Rays and Neutrinos." *AIP Conference Proceedings.* 1535.1 (2013): 238-244.

88. Heydari-Fard, Jabar, Bagheri-Nesami, Masoumeh, and Shirvani, Marjan Ahmad. "Association between Quality of Life and Religious Coping in Older People. *Nursing Older People*, 26.3 (2014) 24-30.

89. 佛教历史, *The History of Buddhism*. <http//:zh.wikipedia.org/wiki/佛教历史>.

90. Testa, Gina and Manning, Maurie Jo. "Getting AAAs, not ZZZs, in the Classroom." *Children's Digest*. 47.6 (1997): 10.

91. Spencer, Kyle. "How Would You React in a Crisis?" *Cosmopolitan*. 238.6 (2005): 176-176.

92. Philanthropist Liu who uses the Chinese five cardinal relationship to educate patients in China to correct their concepts and behavior to treat others properly. The five cardinal relationships are parent-son, friends, boss-subordinate, husband-wife, and brothers. There is a proper attitude to treat each other. Patients learned how to correctly act on and execute what they learned. Their bodies expelled toxins through phlegm and diarrhea. Even cancer can be cured. Please refer to http:tc.universaltcm. com?page_id=17 if you understand Chinese.

93. 黃帝內經 *Huang Di Nei Jing*. <http://big5.wiki8.com/.A1.B6huangdineijing.A1.B7_6739/>.

94. 《静思書軒。心靈講座》看見自己的天才 (上), "Jing Si Book & Café– Mind Lecture." *Seeing Your Own Genius (Part 1)*. <https://www.youtube.com/watch?v=pEZUFT1BRyk>.

95. 意識的力量到底有多大？看看人家使用意識強大的人做的實驗吧, *How Powerful is the Awareness Strength?* <http://www.tudou.com/programs/view/YDcJ7hmQTEA/>.

96. *How Traditional Chinese Medicine (TCM) Can Balance the Body.* <http://universaltcm.com/how-traditional-chinese-medicine-tcm-can-balance-the-body/ or http://goo.gl/eZpzag>.

97. 脈輪圖, *Chakra Chart*. http://goo.gl/3dqpNi.

98. 人體器官圖, *Body Organ Chart*.< http://goo.gl/Z8btK8>.

99. 大包穴位圖, *Dabao*. <http://goo.gl/rbgdgI>.

100. 膀胱經背後穴位圖, *The Bladder Meridian Acupuncture Points*. <http://cht.a-hospital.com/w/足太阳膀胱经穴>.

101. *Gamma Wave*. <http://en.wikipedia.org/wiki/Gamma_wave>.

102. 鋸箭法, *Cut The Arrow Method*. <http://ihower.tw/blog/archives/1352>. **NOTE:** It means to eliminate only the "visible part" (i.e. only the symptoms).

103. Chu, Shu Zhang. 成树江, 从"赤脚医生"到世界医坛——记针刀医学创始人朱汉章 *From the "Barefoot Doctors" to the World Medical Forum*. Remember the Acupotomology Founder Mr. Hang Zhang Chu <http://www.cnki.com.cn/Article/CJFDTotal-KXZB200704190.htm>.

104. Xin, Hong Jun and Gao, Sheng Bing. 辛紅娟、高聖兵,追尋老子的踪跡一《道德經》英語譯本的歷史描述, *Follow Lao Zi's Foot Print*. <http://wenku.baidu.com/view/7cc3fd25ccbff121dd368363.html/>.

105. Wu, Yunqing. 吴云清中国长寿之星养生之道, *Chinese Longevity Stars' Good Health Methods*. <http://goo.gl/NsYXQo>.

106. 心咳, *Heart Caused Cough*. <http://cht.a-hospital.com/w/心咳>.

107. 文天祥, *Wen, Tian Xian*. <http://www.baike.com/wiki/文天祥&prd=so_1_pic>.

108. *Gu Wen Guan Zi* 《古文觀止》. <http://zh.wikipedia.org/wiki/古文觀止>.

109. *Bian Qie Xin Fa* 《扁鵲心書》. <http://jicheng.tw/jcw/book/扁鵲心法/index>.

110. 傳統中醫火灸療法, *Traditional Chinese Medicine Moxibustion Treatments*. <http://www.cn939.com/ft/zhongyihuoliao/huoliaochangshi/20071220 071226151043.htm>.

111. 《難經》 *Nan Jing* is a TCM theory book that explained eighty-one hard-to-understand questions in the *Huang Di Nei Jing*. Its original title was *Huang Di Eighty-One Difficulties*. There are three volumes. Its contents include pulse diagnosis, meridians, zang and fu organs, yin and yang, causes, etiologies, ying and wei, back shu points, and basic theories of acupuncture needling.
<http://cht.a-hospital.com/w/難經>.

112. 《難經》/論病 *Nan Jing Discuss Diseases*.< http://cht.a-hospital.com/w/難經/論病>.

113. *Huang Di Nei Jing* 《黃帝內經》 talks about disease etiologies and prognoses. It also includes some treatment methods. It's mainly for preventive health maintenance and for longevity. It was written by many authors over a period of time. It was completed in the Han Dynasty.

114. 《神農本草經》 *Shen Long Ben Cao Jing* was broadly used before the Ming Dynasty. Lee, Shi Zhen wrote the *Ben Cao Gamg Mu* 《本草綱目》. It has fewer herbs than the later one, but they are more powerful to treat diseases than the *Ben Cao Gamg Mu*. The latter was welcomed by Chinese physicians when the book was published in 1596 because the listed herbs are gentler and there are pictures to identify them. If prescribed incorrectly, the bad effects are mild. It gives people the wrong idea that treatment with Chinese herbs is slow. Actually, it's not. For TCM, herbs were used to treat acute and severe diseases with amazing results before the Ming Dynasty. However, it's been a long time since the Ming Dynasty, and there are many herbs that cannot be identified. Many of them are processed incorrectly today to make quick money instead of doing the right thing to save lives. <http://cht.a-hospital.com/w/神农本草经>.

115. *Shang Han Lun*《傷寒論》and *Jin Gui Yao Lue*《金匱要略》were written by Han Dynasty's Zhang, Zhong Jing 張仲景who treated cold-induced diseases and today's hard-to-treat diseases before the third century. His books are still being used by the best Chinese physicians as a reference bible when encountering diseases where treatments are not known.

116. *Huang Di Wai Jing*《黃帝外經》talks more about treatment principles for diseases. It talks about how to treat diseases' roots. <http://www.taiwantruth.com/waijingweiyan.pdf >.

117. *Standard Acupuncture Nomenclature Second Edition.* <http://www.centerfortraditionalmedicine.org/uploads/2/3/7/5/23750643 /standard_acupuncture _nomenclature.pdf>.

118. *How To Become Legendary - 23 Things Michael Jordan Taught Me About Entrepreneurship.* <http://onstartups.com/tabid/3339/bid/29878/How-To -Become-Legendary-23-Things-Michael-Jordan-Taught-Me-About-Entrepreneurship.aspx or http://goo.gl/WG6m Hz>.

119. *Chong Meridian.* <http://www.huangdineijing.com/thread-391-1-1.html>.

120. *Spiral Universe - Rose Galaxy* <http://www.nasa.gov/mission_pages/hubble/science/hubble-rose -gallery.html>.

121. *Spiral Universe.* <http://www.nasa.gov/sites/default/files/thumbnails/image/potw1448a.jpg>.

122. *Chapter 7 Deontological Theories: Natural Law Section 4.* In Ethics. <http://www.qcc.cuny.edu/SocialSciences/ppecorino/ETHICS_TEXT /Chapter _7_Deontological_Theories_Natural_LawNatural_Law_Theory.htm>.

123. *Wei Shu*《緯書》*includes seven of the Confucian classic books interpretations. Talk of the Han Dynasty Divination* 漫談漢代讖緯[124] (25AD-220AD) <http://zhuge.myweb.hinet.net/e-text/text004.html>.

124. 讖緯, *Qian Wei* is the "divination combined with mystical Confucian philosophy prevalent during the Eastern Han Dynasty (25AD-220AD). <https://chinese.yabla.com/chinese-english-pinyin-dictionary .php?define=讖緯 >.

125. *Electronvolt* <http:en.wikipedia.orgwikiElectronvolt>.

126. 漢典•中国历史朝代公元对照简表, *Han Allusion • Chinese History Dynasties and Their Western Calendar Years.* <http://www.zdic.net/appendix/f4.htm>.

127. 黃帝, 軒轅黃帝, *The Huang Di or Huan Yuan Huang Di.* <http://www.baike.com/wiki/軒轅黃帝>.

128. 移精變氣論, 南京中醫藥大學學報（社會科學版）2012 年3月第13卷第 1期 *Yi Jing Bian Qi Lun.* < http://www.cqvip.com/read/read.aspx?id=42115059>.

129. Tian, Gui-Min, Cao, Lina, Tian, Shu-Xiao. 移精变气论篇"琐谈, 田桂敏、曹麗娜、田淑霄, *A Talk on Yi Jing Bian Qi Lun*. http://www.cnki.com.cn/Article/CJFD_SIMINDEX_E-HZYX702.018.htm.

130. 道教符篆禁法祝由十三科, *Taoist's Zhu You Division of the Talisman and Prohibition Law.* <http://www.360doc.com/content/09/0824/15/9399_5212760.shtml>.

131. 中國武當山發現最早反映武當功夫的白話武俠小說. *China Wudang Mountain discovered the earliest martial arts novels that reflect the Wudang Gongfu.* <http://www.zwbk.org/MyLemmaShow.aspx?zh=zh-tw&lid=293695>.

132. 司馬遷 *Si Ma, Qian* (145 BC—90 BC) A great Chinese historian, writer, and thinker in the Western Han Dynasty. <http://www.zwbk.org/MyLemmaShow.aspx?zh=zh-tw&lid=87022>.

133. *Jnana Yoga - Brahman, Viveka, Advaita Vedanta and Jnana Mudra.* <http://www.himavanti.org/en/c/himavanti-1/jnana-yoga-brahman-viveka -advaita-vedanta-and-jnana-mudra>.

134. *Bhakti Yoga: The Nature of Devotion.* <http://www.ishafoundation.org/blog/yoga-meditation/demystifying -yoga/what -is-devotion/>.

135. *My Life is My Message.* <http://www.brainyquote.com/quotes/authors/m/mahatma_gandhi.html>.

136. Rand, William Lee. *What is the History of Reiki?* <http://www.reiki.org/faqhistoryofreiki.html>.

137. *Readers' Discussion.* <https://universalenergyhealing.us/reader-discussion>.

138. *Yin Wei Meridian.* <http://www.huangdineijing.com/thread-386-1-2.html>.

139. *How Does TCM (Traditional Chinese Medicine) View Diseases?* <http://happypinmasterhealer.com/?page_id=103>.

140. Videos. <https://nbaarc.com/?page_id=102>.

141. Lifting. <https://nbaarc.com/?page_id=100>.

142. Video 1. <https://nbaarc.com?page_id=103>.

143. Video 2. <https://nbaarc.com/?page_id=105>.

144. Video 3. <https://nbaarc.com/?page_id=108>.

145. Video 4. <https://nbaarc.com/?page_id=117>.

146. Video 5. <https://nbaarc.com/?page_id=125!>.

147. *The Power of CHUEH.* <https://universalenergyhealing.us/the-power-of -the-chueh>.

148. *Pain Relief.* <https://universalenergyhealing.us/pain-relief.>.

149. *Pop Up Veins.* <https://universalenergyhealing.us/pop-veins>.

150. *Cold Flu.* <https://universalenergyhealing.us/cold-flu>.

151. *Stop Bleeding.* <https://universalenergyhealing.us/stop-bleeding>.

152. *Da Zhou Tian.* <https://universaltcm.com/da-zhou-tian>.

153. *Q & A.* <https://universalenergyhealing.us/q>.

154. *Cold Foods & Cold Drinks Caused Health Problems.*
<https://universaltcm.com/cold-foods-and-cold-drinks-caused-health-problems >.

155. *Cold Foods Drinks Caused Problems Chart Rev 1..*
<https://universaltcm.com/cold-foods-drinks-caused-problems-chart-rev-1>.

156. *How Do I know that I Am Well Treated?*
<https://happypinmasterhealer.com/?page_id=105>.

157. *When can I stop my treatments?*
<https://happypinmasterhealer.com/?page_id=113>.

158. *How often should I get treated?*
<https://happypinmasterhealer.com/?page_id=136>.

159. *How long do you keep the happy pins (needles) in?*
<https://happypinmasterhealer.com/?page_id=142>.

160. *Raise Up Your Energy Frequency to Avoid Sick.*
<https://universaltcm.com/raise-up-your-frequency-to-avoid-sick-2>.

161. *Man invest machine to convert plastic into oil.*
<https://www.youtube.com/embed/qGGabrorRS8?rel=0>.

162. *Natural Born Abundant Ability Recovery Center.* <https://nbaarc.com>.

163. *Chapter One Introduction.* <https://universalenergyhealing.us/chapter-one>.

164. *Chapter Two.* <https://universalenergyhealing.us/chapter-two>.

165. 值得一读的20个经典励志小故事, *the seventh story of twenty classic inspirational stories worth reading.* <https://jiaren.org/2012/02/05/lizhi-9>.

166. *New Book Content Recommendation.* <https://universalenergyhealing.us/new-book-content-recommendation>.

167. *Chapter Three.* <http://universalenergyhealing.us/chapter-three>.

168. *How A Mother's Health Can Affect Kid's Health?* <http://universaltcm.com/how-a-mothers-health-can-affect-kids-health>.

169. *Emotional Disturbance During Pregnancy*
<http://universaltcm.com/emotional-disturbances-during-pregnancy>.

170. *Moral Cultivation.* <https://universaltcm.com/moral-cultivation-2>.

171. *The Dream Builder Coach Program.* <https://nbaarc.com/?page_id=150.>.

172. *New Book Announcement.*
<https://universalenergyhealing.us/new-book-announcement>.

173. *Chinese Exercises vs. Western Exercises.* <https://universaltcm.com/the-chinese-vs-Western-exercises>.

174. *The Differences Between Chinese Exercises and Western Exercises Chart.* <https://universaltcm.com/the-differences-between-chinese-exercises-and-Western-exercises-chart>.

175. *Raise Your Legs 90 Degrees Up Against the Wall.* <https//:universaltcm.com/raise-your-legs-90-degrees-up-against-the-wall/>.

176. *Crack Sound From Your Knee(s).* <https://universaltcm.com/crack-sound-from-your-knee>.

177. *Meniscus Tear.* <https://universaltcm.com/meniscus-tear>.

178. *TCM Health Concept Chart.* <https://universaltcm.com/tcm-concept-chart>.

179. *Nutrition in Chinese Medicine.* <https://universaltcm.com/nutrition-in-chinese-medicine/>.

180. Huang Di Nei Jing TV documentary. <https://tc.universaltcm.com/?page_id=504>.

181. *TCM Diagnosis for Internal Medicine – Ten Questions.* <https://happypinmasterhealer.com/?page_id=217>.

182. Dr Quantum - Double Slit Experiment. <https://universaltcm.com/to-healthcare-providers/>.

183. How do wolves change the river ecosystem? <https://m.youtube.com/watch?v=wwjjP77RZLk&hd=1 wolves>.

184. *You Can.* <http://nbaarc.com/?page_id=17>.

185. *How to Make An Emergency Stretcher.* <http://universalenergyhealing.us/make-emergency-stretcher/>.

186. *Cold Foods & Cold Drinks Caused Health Problems.* <http://universaltcm.com/cold-foods-and-cold-drinks-caused-health-problems/>.

187. *Cold Foods Drinks Caused Problems Chart Rev 1.* <http://universaltcm.com/cold-foods-drinks-caused-problems-chart-rev-1>.

188. "More Evidence That Milk Does Not Prevent Osteoporosis: A Harvard Nurses' Health Study." *Good Medicine. 12.3, (2003): 4.* This covers an eighteen-year follow-up on 72,000 postmenopausal women where a high-calcium diet did not reduce fracture rate.

189. Gerson, Charlotte. "Milk Ads and Osteoporosis: Complaint Filed with FTC (Federal Trade Commission)." *Gerson Healing Newsletter. 12.3* (1997): 5.

190. Robbins, John. *The Truth About Calcium and Osteoporosis.* (2009). <http://foodmatters.tv/articles-1/the-truth-about-calcium-and-osteoporosis>.

191. Kanigel, Rachele. "It raises diabetes risk and robs bone. It's wrecking our teeth. And it's making us fat. The culprit? SODA." *Prevention*. 58.10 (2006): 160-207.

192. Gelman, Lauren. "Which Food Boosts Your Bones?" *Prevention*. 61.9 (2009):18-32.

193. *How Does TCM Help Patients to Avoid Cancer?* <https://universaltcm.com /how-does-tcm-help-patients-to-avoid-cancer>.

194. Weisberg, Lawrence S. and Rachoin, Jean-Sebastien. "The Safety of Low-Potassium Dialysis." *Seminars in Dialysis*. 23.6 (2010): 556-560.

195. *Stress Caused Problems*. <https://universaltcm.com/stress-caused-problems/>.

196. *Poor Balance*. <https://happypinmasterhealer.com/?page_id=20>.

197. *Back Pain Chart*. <https://universaltcm.wordpress.com/back-pain-chart>.

198. *CHUEH Training Programs*. <https://universalenergyhealing.us/chueh -training-programs/>.

199. *Dai Meridian*. <http://www.huangdineijing.com/thread-387-1-2.html>.

200. *Foot Reflexology*. <http://www.sunshinekelly.com/2013/03/foot-reflexology -improves-my-health-and.html?>.

201. *Foot Reflexology*. <http://www.realbodywork.com/product/reflexology-for -the-feet-and-hands-dvd-video/>.

202. *Meridian Flowing Chart*. <http://www.ystjq.com/jlzs/jl-11.htm>.

203. *CHUEH Video 1* is the twelve strands of DNA for ascending. Video 1 explains DNA, especially the twelve strands' functions, and the relationship between human beings and the universe. <https://universalenergyhealing. us/video-1/>.

204. *CHUEH Video 2* discusses detoxifying your pineal gland (your third eye) and using meditation music to benefit you. Earphones are needed. Please find a comfortable and safe place to do meditation while you focus on your spiritual meditation. <https://universalenergyhealing.us/chueh-video-2/>.

205. *The Indigo Evolution Full Length Documentary Indigo Children*. <https://www.youtube.com/watch?v=fxvriVUk_5A>.

206. *Allegheny Candles' Blog*. <https://alleghenycandles.wordpress.com/2009/10/11/free-chakra -healing-meditation/>.

207. *Hypothalamus Florida Academic Cancer Alliance Body Map*. HealthLine Medical Team. 2015. <http://www.healthline.com/human-body-maps /hypothalamus>.

208. *DNA Can Be Influenced And Reprogrammed By Words And Frequencies.* <http://in5d.com/dna-can-be-influenced-and-reprogrammed-by-words-and-frequencies/>.

209. *Spine Chart.* <http://www.marysrosaries.com/collaboration/images/d/df/Spine_(PSF).png>

210. *Heart Pain Cases.* <http://happypinmasterhealer.com/?page_id=158>.

211. *Decades Stomach Problems.* <http://happypinmasterhealer.com/?page_id=154>.

212. *Bill Gates Quotes.* <http://www.brainyquote.com/quotes/quotes/b/billgates385136.html>.

213. Palm Reflexology. <https://www.pinterest.com/pin/420664421419965156/>.

214. *Emergency numbers around the world* <http://chartsbin.com/view/1983>

215. Governor (Du) Vessel. <https://www.pinterest.com/pin/425871708490974707/>.

216. *Yang Wei Meridian.* <http://www.huangdineijing.com/thread-389-1-1.html>.

217. Roberts, Michelle. "Seasons Affect How Genes and Immune System Work." *Health.* (2015). <http://www.bbc.com/news/health-32687313>.

218. *Governor Vessel.* <http://www.huangdineijing.com/thread-393-1-1.html>.

219. *Conception Vessel.* <http://www.huangdineijing.com/thread-392-1-1.html>.

220. *Yang Quo Meridian.* <http://www.huangdineijing.com/thread-390-1-1.html>

221. *Yin Qao Meridian.* <http://www.huangdineijing.com/thread-388-1-2.html>.

Author's Bio

• • • • • • • • • • • • • • • • •

My name is Frieda Mah, and I am a California licensed acupuncturist. I have a variety innovative clinical experiences and have treated some very tough and rare cases.

From treating the tough cases, I strongly felt that people do not need to suffer severe sicknesses. Therefore, I created Comprehensive Universal Energy Healing and have used it to help many patients improve their quality of life. So, they can be free of pain, stress, insomnia, and many other health issues. Therefore, people do not need to lose enjoyment to which they are entitled wealthy, healthy and happy life.

I deeply expect this book can help you. You can practice the Comprehensive Universal Energy Healing and let it be part of your daily meaningful life.

CONTACT INFORMATION:

Please post your adjustment experiences and questions at Readers' Discussion[137]. Your post is important so that we can know how to help you learn better.

Please contact us at support@universalenergyhealing.us or join Events.

Your Self-Healing Coach,

P.S. Please sign up at UniversalEnergyHealing.us Remember to check back often for more tips on self-healing at the Readers' Discussion[137]!!!

www.ingramcontent.com/pod-product-compliance
Lightning Source LLC
Chambersburg PA
CBHW072301200526
45168CB00014B/36